D1523468

Multiple Sclerosis

SOURCEBOOK

SECOND EDITION

Multiple Sclerosis
SOURCEBOOK

SECOND EDITION

Basic Consumer Health Information about Multiple Sclerosis (MS) and Its Effects on Mobility, Vision, Bladder Function, Speech, Swallowing, and Cognition, Including Facts about Risk Factors, Causes, Diagnostic Procedures, Pain Management, Drug Treatments, and Physical and Occupational Therapies

Along with Guidelines for Nutrition and Exercise, Tips on Choosing Assistive Equipment, Information about Disability, Work, Financial, and Legal Issues, a Glossary of Related Terms, and a Directory of Additional Resources

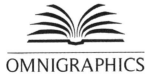

OMNIGRAPHICS

615 Griswold, Ste. 520, Detroit, MI 48226

LINDENHURST MEMORIAL LIBRARY
One Lee Avenue
Lindenhurst, New York 11757

Bibliographic Note
Because this page cannot legibly accommodate all the copyright notices, the Bibliographic Note portion of the Preface constitutes an extension of the copyright notice.

* * *

OMNIGRAPHICS
Angela L. Williams, *Managing Editor*
* * *

Copyright © 2019 Omnigraphics

ISBN 978-0-7808-1697-8
E-ISBN 978-0-7808-1698-5

Library of Congress Cataloging-in-Publication Data

Title: Multiple sclerosis sourcebook: basic consumer health information about multiple sclerosis (MS) and its effects on mobility, vision, bladder function, speech, swallowing, and cognition, including facts about risk factors, causes, diagnostic procedures, pain management, treatment, and physical and occupation therapies, along with guidelines for nutrition and exercise, tips on choosing assistive equipment, information about disability, work, financial, and legal issues, a glossary of related terms and a directory of additional resources / Lauren Parrott, managing editor.

Description: 2nd edition. | Detroit, MI: Omnigraphics, Inc., [2019]

Identifiers: LCCN 2019009454| ISBN 9780780816978 (hard cover: alk. paper) | ISBN 9780780816985 (ebook)

Subjects: LCSH: Multiple sclerosis--Popular works.

Classification: LCC RC377.M8638 2019 | DDC 616.8/34--dc23

LC record available at https://lccn.loc.gov/2019009454

Electronic or mechanical reproduction, including photography, recording, or any other information storage and retrieval system for the purpose of resale is strictly prohibited without permission in writing from the publisher.

The information in this publication was compiled from the sources cited and from other sources considered reliable. While every possible effort has been made to ensure reliability, the publisher will not assume liability for damages caused by inaccuracies in the data, and makes no warranty, express or implied, on the accuracy of the information contained herein.

This book is printed on acid-free paper meeting the ANSI Z39.48 Standard. The infinity symbol that appears above indicates that the paper in this book meets that standard.

Printed in the United States

Table of Contents

Part II: Symptoms of Multiple Sclerosis

Part III: Diagnostic Tests, Treatments, and Therapies for Multiple Sclerosis

Part IV: Living with Multiple Sclerosis

Part V: Multiple Sclerosis and Work, Financial, and Legal Issues

Part VI: Clinical Trials on Multiple Sclerosis

Part VII: Additional Help and Information

Preface

About This Book

Multiple sclerosis (MS) is the most common neurological disorder that strikes young adults. It is a difficult, unpredictable autoimmune disease that affects the central nervous system. It is estimated that about 400,000 Americans and 2.5 million people around the world are affected by the disease. It generally strikes people between the ages of 20 and 40 and more commonly affects women. Symptoms may include pain, sudden weakness, or difficulties with vision, speech, or mobility. Many people with multiple sclerosis experience problems such as fatigue, a limp, difficulties with bladder control, and need to use a wheelchair full-time. Currently, there is no cure, but several therapies can relieve the symptoms and, in some cases, delay disease progression.

Multiple Sclerosis Sourcebook, Second Edition provides information about risk factors, causes, and types of multiple sclerosis and its effects on mobility, vision, bladder function, speech, swallowing, and cognition. Treatments and rehabilitation therapies are described, guidelines for nutrition and exercise are discussed, and tips on choosing assistive equipment are provided. Information about issues related to disability resources, workplace concerns, financial planning, and clinical trials is also included, along with a glossary and directory of resources.

How to Use This Book

This book is divided into parts and chapters. Parts focus on broad areas of interest. Chapters are devoted to single topics within a part.

Part I: Multiple Sclerosis: Causes, Risk Factors, and Disease Course presents information about autoimmune disease and the cellular, genetic, and nerve processes involved with MS. It discusses the prevalence MS among women, children, and men. It includes facts about how toxic agents or infections may trigger MS and describes other demyelinating disorders and diseases that mimic MS.

Part II: Symptoms of Multiple Sclerosis describes the types of physical concerns that develop in people with MS, including movement problems, tremors, pain, fatigue, speech, swallowing, and vision problems. It deals with the complications that impact bladder control, cognition, and mental health.

Part III: Diagnostic Tests, Treatments, and Therapies for Multiple Sclerosis describes various ways MS is diagnosed, managed, and monitored, including drug treatments, pain management, and management of involuntary movement and tremor. Information is presented about rehabilitation methods, complementary and alternative medical treatments, and plasmapheresis. It also includes a separate chapter on how stem cell transplant induces multiple sclerosis remission.

Part IV: Living with Multiple Sclerosis includes information about nutrition and exercise and offers techniques for managing the symptoms of MS. Individual chapters provide tips for developing a support group, describe home accessibility guidelines, and discuss equipment that promotes self-care, mobility, and independence.

Part V: Multiple Sclerosis and Work, Financial, and Legal Issues describes how individuals with MS can navigate workplace challenges and prepare for the future. Financial planning needs, disability benefits, home care, assisted living, and skilled nursing healthcare options are described, and written advance directives are explained.

Part VI: Clinical Trials on Multiple Sclerosis discusses in detail about various researches that are performed to prevent, detect, and treat multiple sclerosis and its symptoms.

Part VII: Additional Help and Information includes a glossary of related terms and a directory of resources.

Bibliographic Note

This volume contains documents and excerpts from publications issued by the following U.S. government agencies: Bureau of Alcohol, Tobacco, Firearms and Explosives (ATF); Centers for Disease Control and Prevention (CDC); Centers for Medicare & Medicaid Services (CMS); *Eunice Kennedy Shriver* National Institute of Child Health and Human Development (NICHD); Genetic and Rare Diseases Information Center (GARD); Genetics Home Reference (GHR); National Center for Complementary and Integrative Health (NCCIH); National Council on Disability (NCD); National Eye Institute (NEI); National Heart, Lung, and Blood Institute (NHLBI); National Institute of Neurological Disorders and Stroke (NINDS); National Institute on Aging (NIA); National Institute on Deafness and Other Communication Disorders (NIDCD); National Institutes of Health (NIH); Office on Women's Health (OWH); Rehabilitation Research & Development Service (RR&D); U.S. Department of Justice (DOJ); U.S. Department of Veterans Affairs (VA); U.S. Equal Employment Opportunity Commission (EEOC); U.S. Food and Drug Administration (FDA); and U.S. Social Security Administration (SSA).

It may also contain original material produced by Omnigraphics and reviewed by medical consultants.

About the Health Reference Series

The *Health Reference Series* is designed to provide basic medical information for patients, families, caregivers, and the general public. Each volume takes a particular topic and provides comprehensive coverage. This is especially important for people who may be dealing with a newly diagnosed disease or a chronic disorder in themselves or in a family member. People looking for preventive guidance, information about disease warning signs, medical statistics, and risk factors for health problems will also find answers to their questions in the *Health Reference Series*. The *Series*, however, is not intended to serve as a tool for diagnosing illness, in prescribing treatments, or as a substitute for the physician/patient relationship. All people concerned about medical symptoms or the possibility of disease are encouraged to seek professional care from an appropriate healthcare provider.

A Note about Spelling and Style

Health Reference Series editors use *Stedman's Medical Dictionary* as an authority for questions related to the spelling of medical terms and the *Chicago Manual of Style* for questions related to grammatical structures, punctuation, and other editorial concerns. Consistent adherence is not always possible, however, because the individual volumes within the *Series* include many documents from a wide variety of different producers, and the editor's primary goal is to present material from each source as accurately as is possible. This sometimes means that information in different chapters or sections may follow other guidelines and alternate spelling authorities. For example, occasionally a copyright holder may require that eponymous terms be shown in possessive forms (Crohn's disease vs. Crohn disease) or that British spelling norms be retained (leukaemia vs. leukemia).

Medical Review

Omnigraphics contracts with a team of qualified, senior medical professionals who serve as medical consultants for the *Health Reference Series*. As necessary, medical consultants review reprinted and originally written material for currency and accuracy. Citations including the phrase "Reviewed (month, year)" indicate material reviewed by this team. Medical consultation services are provided to the *Health Reference Series* editors by:

Dr. Vijayalakshmi, MBBS, DGO, MD
Dr. Senthil Selvan, MBBS, DCH, MD
Dr. K. Sivanandham, MBBS, DCH, MS (Research), PhD

Our Advisory Board

We would like to thank the following board members for providing initial guidance on the development of this series:

- Dr. Lynda Baker, Associate Professor of Library and Information Science, Wayne State University, Detroit, MI

- Nancy Bulgarelli, William Beaumont Hospital Library, Royal Oak, MI

- Karen Imarisio, Bloomfield Township Public Library, Bloomfield Township, MI

- Karen Morgan, Mardigian Library, University of Michigan-Dearborn, Dearborn, MI

- Rosemary Orlando, St. Clair Shores Public Library, St. Clair Shores, MI

Health Reference Series *Update Policy*

The inaugural book in the *Health Reference Series* was the first edition of *Cancer Sourcebook* published in 1989. Since then, the *Series* has been enthusiastically received by librarians and in the medical community. In order to maintain the standard of providing high-quality health information for the layperson the editorial staff at Omnigraphics felt it was necessary to implement a policy of updating volumes when warranted.

Medical researchers have been making tremendous strides, and it is the purpose of the *Health Reference Series* to stay current with the most recent advances. Each decision to update a volume is made on an individual basis. Some of the considerations include how much new information is available and the feedback we receive from people who use the books. If there is a topic you would like to see added to the update list, or an area of medical concern you feel has not been adequately addressed, please write to:

Managing Editor
Health Reference Series
Omnigraphics
615 Griswold, Ste. 520
Detroit, MI 48226

Part One

Multiple Sclerosis: Causes, Risk Factors, and Disease Course

Chapter 1

Multiple Sclerosis Overview

Multiple sclerosis (MS) is a condition involving damage to nerve cells and is characterized by damage (lesions) on the brain and spinal cord. These lesions are associated with the destruction of the covering (the myelin sheath) that protects the body's nerves and promotes the efficient transmission of nerve impulses.

Multiple sclerosis is considered to be an autoimmune disorder; autoimmune disorders occur when the immune system malfunctions and attacks the body's own tissues and organs. In multiple sclerosis, the nervous system's tissues are affected.

Multiple sclerosis usually begins in early adulthood, between the ages of 20 and 40. The symptoms vary widely, and affected individuals can experience one or more effects of nervous system damage.

- Multiple sclerosis often causes sensory disturbances in the limbs, including a prickling or tingling sensation (paresthesia), numbness, pain, and itching.

- Some people experience a Lhermitte sign, which is an electrical shock-like sensation that runs down the back and into the limbs. This sensation usually occurs when the head is bent forward.

- Problems with muscle control are common in people with multiple sclerosis. Affected individuals may have tremors, muscle stiffness (spasticity), exaggerated reflexes

This chapter includes text excerpted from "Multiple Sclerosis," Genetics Home Reference (GHR), National Institutes of Health (NIH), March 12, 2019.

3

(hyperreflexia), weakness or partial paralysis of the muscles of the limbs, difficulty walking, or poor bladder control.

• Multiple sclerosis is also associated with vision problems, such as blurred or double vision or partial or complete vision loss. Infections that cause fever can make the symptoms worse.

There are several forms of multiple sclerosis:

• Relapsing-remitting MS

• Secondary progressive MS

• Primary progressive MS

• Progressive relapsing MS

The most common form of multiple sclerosis is relapsing-remitting MS, which affects approximately 80 percent of people with the disorder. Individuals with this form of the condition have periods in which they experience symptoms, called "clinical attacks," followed by periods without any symptoms (remission). The triggers of clinical attacks and remissions are unknown. After about 10 years, relapsing-remitting MS usually develops into another form of the disorder called "secondary progressive MS." In this form, there are no remissions, and symptoms of the condition continually worsen.

Primary-progressive MS is the next most common form, affecting approximately 10 to 20 percent of people with multiple sclerosis. This form is characterized by constant symptoms that worsen over time, with no clinical attacks or remissions. Primary progressive MS typically begins later than the other forms, around the age of 40.

Progressive relapsing MS is a rare form of multiple sclerosis that initially appears like primary progressive MS and has constant symptoms. However, people with progressive relapsing MS also experience clinical attacks of more severe symptoms.

An estimated 1.1 to 2.5 million people worldwide have multiple sclerosis. Although the reason is unclear, this condition is more common in regions that are farther away from the equator. In Canada, parts of the northern United States, western and northern Europe, Russia, and southeastern Australia, the condition affects approximately 1 in 2,000 to 2,400 people. It is less common closer to the equator; in Asia, Sub-Saharan Africa, and parts of South America, about 1 in 20,000 people are affected by MS. For unknown reasons, most forms of multiple sclerosis affect women twice as often as men; however, women and men are equally affected by primary progressive MS.

Chapter 2

Autoimmune Diseases: Is Multiple Sclerosis One of Them?

What Are Autoimmune Diseases?

The immune system is a complex network of special cells, organs, and tissues that defends the body from foreign invaders. One of the core responsibilities of the immune system is to protect the body from infection-causing microbes and organisms. When the immune system fails to effectively do this, the body makes autoantibodies that attack normal cells by mistake. Regulatory T cells are then unable to prevent opportunistic infections and diseases. This failed immune system response is called "autoimmune disease."

This chapter contains text excerpted from the following sources: Text beginning with the heading "What Are Autoimmune Diseases?" is excerpted from "Autoimmune Diseases," Office on Women's Health (OWH), U.S. Department of Health and Human Services (HHS), October 8, 2018; Text under the heading "Multiple Sclerosis and Autoimmunity" is excerpted from "Technique Selectively Represses Immune System," National Institutes of Health (NIH), December 3, 2012. Reviewed March 2019.

Who Gets Autoimmune Diseases

Autoimmune diseases can affect anyone. However, certain people are at a greater risk, including:

- **Women of childbearing age**—More women than men have autoimmune diseases, which often start during their childbearing years.

- **People with a family history of autoimmune disorders**—Some autoimmune diseases, such as lupus and multiple sclerosis, run in families. These families are susceptible to a range of autoimmune diseases. Inherited genes can make it more likely to have an autoimmune disease, but a combination of genes and other factors may trigger the start of the disease.

- **People who are exposed to specific environmental factors**—Certain events or environmental exposures may cause some autoimmune diseases, or make them worse. Sunlight, chemicals called "solvents," and viral and bacterial infections are linked to many autoimmune diseases.

- **People of certain races or ethnic backgrounds**—Some autoimmune diseases affect certain groups of people more severely. For instance, type 1 diabetes is more common in White people. Lupus is more common among African American and Latinx populations.

Types of Autoimmune Diseases

There are more than 100 autoimmune diseases. The following are some of the most commonly occurring autoimmune diseases:

- Alopecia areata
- Antiphospholipid antibody syndrome (APS)
- Autoimmune hepatitis
- Celiac disease
- Diabetes type 1
- Graves disease (overactive thyroid)
- Guillain-Barre syndrome

- Hashimoto disease (underactive thyroid)
- Hemolytic anemia
- Idiopathic thrombocytopenic purpura (ITP)
- Inflammatory bowel disease (IBD)
- Inflammatory myopathies
- Multiple sclerosis (MS)
- Myasthenia gravis (MG)
- Primary biliary cirrhosis (PBC)
- Psoriasis
- Rheumatoid arthritis (RA)
- Scleroderma
- Sjögren syndrome
- Systemic lupus erythematosus (SLE)
- Vitiligo

What Types of Doctors Treat Autoimmune Diseases

Juggling your healthcare needs among many doctors and specialists can be challenging. But specialists, along with your primary-care doctor, may help manage some symptoms of your autoimmune disease. Often, your family doctor may help you coordinate specialized care if you need to see one or more specialists. Here are some specialists who treat autoimmune diseases:

- **Nephrologist.** A doctor who treats kidney problems, such as inflamed kidneys caused by lupus. Kidneys are organs that clean the blood and produce urine.

- **Rheumatologist.** A doctor who treats arthritis and other rheumatic diseases, such as scleroderma and lupus.

- **Endocrinologist.** A doctor who treats gland and hormone problems, such as diabetes and thyroid disease.

- **Neurologist.** A doctor who treats nerve problems, such as multiple sclerosis and myasthenia gravis.

9

- **Hematologist.** A doctor who treats diseases that affect the blood, such as some forms of anemia.

- **Gastroenterologist.** A doctor who treats problems with the digestive system, such as inflammatory bowel disease (IBD).

- **Dermatologist.** A doctor who treats diseases that affect the skin, hair, and nails, such as psoriasis and lupus.

- **Physical therapist.** A healthcare professional who uses proper types of physical activity to help patients with stiffness, weakness, and restricted body movement.

- **Occupational therapist.** A healthcare professional who can find ways to make activities of daily living easier for you, despite your pain and other health problems. This could be teaching you new ways of doing things or how to use special devices. Or suggesting changes to make in your home or workplace.

- **Speech therapist.** A healthcare professional who can help people with speech problems from illness such as multiple sclerosis.

- **Audiologist.** A healthcare professional who can help people with hearing problems, including inner ear damage from autoimmune diseases.

- **Vocational therapist.** A healthcare professional who offers job training for people who cannot do their current jobs because of their illness or other health problems. You can find this type of person through both public and private agencies.

- **Counselor for emotional support.** A healthcare professional who is specially trained to help you to find ways to cope with your illness. You can work through your feelings of anger, fear, denial, and frustration.

Multiple Sclerosis and Autoimmunity

Multiple sclerosis (MS) is a neuroinflammatory disease that affects myelin, a substance that makes up the membrane (called the "myelin sheath") that wraps around nerve fibers (axons).

As with other autoimmune diseases, multiple sclerosis is a disease in which the immune system mistakenly attacks the body's own tissues. The resulting nerve damage in the brain and spinal cord can cause muscle weakness, loss of vision, numbness or tingling, and difficulty with coordination and balance. While MS sometimes causes severe disability, it is only rarely fatal, and most people with MS have a normal life expectancy.

Chapter 3

Multiple Sclerosis: Complex Disease of the Central Nervous System

Chapter Contents

Section 3.1

Nervous System: An Anatomical Overview

> This section includes text excerpted from "What Are the Parts of the Nervous System?" *Eunice Kennedy Shriver* National Institute of Child Health and Human Development (NICHD), October 1, 2018.

The nervous system has two main parts:

- The central nervous system (CNS) is made up of the brain and spinal cord.

- The peripheral nervous system is made up of nerves that branch off from the spinal cord and extend to all parts of the body.

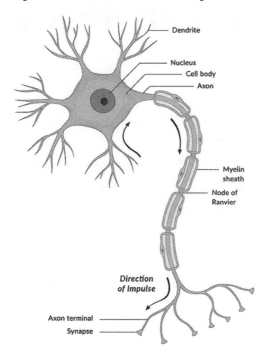

Figure 3.1. *Parts of the Nervous System*

The nervous system transmits signals between the brain and the rest of the body, including internal organs. In this way, the nervous system's activity controls the ability to move, breathe, see, think, and more.

The basic unit of the nervous system is a nerve cell or neuron. The human brain contains about 100 billion neurons. A neuron has a cell body, which includes the cell nucleus, and special extensions called "axons" and "dendrites." Bundles of axons, called "nerves," are found throughout the body. Axons and dendrites allow neurons to communicate, even across long distances.

Different types of neurons control or perform different activities. For instance, motor neurons transmit messages from the brain to the muscles to generate movement. Sensory neurons detect light, sound, odor, taste, pressure, and heat, and send messages about these elements to the brain. Other parts of the nervous system control involuntary processes, some of which include keeping a regular heartbeat, releasing hormones such as adrenaline, opening the pupil in response to light, and regulating the digestive system.

When a neuron sends a message to another neuron, it sends an electrical signal down the length of its axon. At the end of the axon, the electrical signal changes to a chemical signal. The axon then releases the chemical signal with chemical messengers called "neurotransmitters" into the synapse—the space between the end of an axon and the tip of a dendrite from another neuron. The neurotransmitters move the signal through the synapse to the neighboring dendrite, which converts the chemical signal back into an electrical signal. The electrical signal then travels through the neuron and goes through the same conversion processes as it moves to neighbor neurons.

The nervous system also includes nonneuron cells called "glia." Glia performs many important functions that help keep the nervous system working properly. For example, glia:

- Helps support and hold neurons in place

- Protects neurons

- Creates insulation called "myelin," which helps move nerve impulses

- Repairs neurons and helps restore neuron function

- Purges the body of dead neurons

- Regulates neurotransmitters

The brain is made up of many networks of communicating neurons and glia. These networks allow different parts of the brain to communicate with one another and work together to control body functions, emotions, thinking, behavior, and other activities.

What Does the Nervous System Do?

The nervous system plays a role in nearly every aspect of our health and well-being. It guides everyday activities such as waking up; automatic activities such as breathing; and complex processes such as thinking, reading, remembering, and feeling emotions.

The nervous system controls:

- Brain growth and development
- Sensations, such as touch or hearing
- Perception (the mental process of interpreting sensory information)
- Thought and emotions
- Learning and memory
- Movement, balance, and coordination
- Sleep
- Healing and rehabilitation
- Stress and the body's responses to stress
- Aging
- Breathing and heartbeat
- Body temperature
- Hunger, thirst, and digestion
- Puberty, reproductive health, and fertility

Neuroscientists study these and other nervous system functions in both healthy and diseased states. Studying and understanding the nervous system is important because it affects so many areas of human health and well-being.

Section 3.2

How Multiple Sclerosis Targets Myelin

This section includes text excerpted from "Multiple Sclerosis: Hope through Research," National Institute of Neurological Disorders and Stroke (NINDS), July 6, 2018.

Multiple sclerosis (MS) is a neuroinflammatory disease that affects myelin, a substance that makes up the membrane (called "the myelin sheath") that wraps around nerve fibers (axons). Myelinated axons are commonly called "white matter." Researchers have learned that MS also damages the nerve cell bodies, which are found in the brain's gray matter, as well as the axons in the brain, spinal cord, and optic nerve (the nerve that transmits visual information from the eye to the brain). As the disease progresses, the brain's cortex shrinks (cortical atrophy).

The term multiple sclerosis refers to the distinctive areas of scar tissue (sclerosis or plaques) that are visible in the white matter of people who have MS. Plaques can be as small as a pinhead or as large as a golf ball. Doctors can see these areas by examining the brain and spinal cord using a type of brain scan called "magnetic resonance imaging (MRI)."

While MS sometimes causes severe disability, it is rarely fatal, and most people with MS have a normal life expectancy.

What Are Plaques Made Of and Why Do They Develop?

Plaques, or lesions, are the result of an inflammatory process in the brain that causes immune-system cells to attack myelin. The myelin sheath helps speed up nerve impulses traveling within the nervous system. Axons are also damaged in MS, although not as extensively, or as early in the disease, as myelin.

Under normal circumstances, cells of the immune system travel in and out of the brain, patrolling for infectious agents (viruses, for example) or unhealthy cells. This is called the "surveillance" function of the immune system.

Surveillance cells usually won't spring into action unless they recognize an infectious agent or an unhealthy cell. When surveillance cells notice an infectious agent, they produce substances to stop the agent. If they encounter unhealthy cells, they either kill them directly or clean out the dying area and produce substances that promote healing and repair among the remaining cells.

Researchers have observed that immune cells behave differently in the brains of people with MS; they become active and attack what appears to be healthy myelin. It is unclear what triggers this attack. MS is one of many autoimmune disorders, such as rheumatoid arthritis (RA) and lupus, in which the immune system mistakenly attacks a person's healthy tissue as opposed to attacking foreign invaders, such as viruses and bacteria. Whatever the reason, during these periods of immune system activity, most of the myelin within the affected area is damaged or destroyed. The axons also may be damaged. The symptoms of MS depend on the severity of the immune reaction as well as the location and extent of the plaques, which primarily appear in the brain stem, cerebellum, spinal cord, optic nerves, and the white matter of the brain around the brain ventricles (fluid-filled spaces inside of the brain).

Chapter 4

Understanding the Genetics of Multiple Sclerosis

Although the cause of multiple sclerosis (MS) is unknown, variations in dozens of genes are thought of as being involved in multiple sclerosis risk. Changes in the *HLA-DRB1* gene are the strongest genetic risk factors for developing multiple sclerosis. Other factors associated with an increased risk of developing multiple sclerosis include changes in the *IL7R* gene and environmental factors, such as exposure to the Epstein-Barr virus (EBV), low levels of vitamin D, and smoking.

The *HLA-DRB1* gene belongs to a family of genes called the "human leukocyte antigen (HLA) complex." The HLA complex helps the immune system distinguish the body's own proteins from proteins made by foreign invaders, such as viruses and bacteria. Each *HLA* gene has many different normal variations, allowing each person's immune system to react to a wide range of foreign proteins. Variations in several *HLA* genes have been associated with an increased risk of multiple sclerosis, but one particular variant of the *HLA-DRB1* gene, called "*HLA-DRB1**15:01," is the most strongly linked genetic factor.

The *IL7R* gene provides instructions for making one piece of two different receptor proteins: the interleukin 7 (IL-7) receptor and the thymic stromal lymphopoietin (TSLP) receptor. Both receptors are

This chapter includes text excerpted from "Multiple Sclerosis," Genetics Home Reference (GHR), National Institutes of Health (NIH), March 12, 2019.

embedded in the cell membrane of immune cells. These receptors stimulate signaling pathways that induce the growth and division (proliferation) and survival of immune cells. The genetic variation involved in multiple sclerosis leads to the production of an IL-7 receptor that is not embedded in the cell membrane but is instead found inside the cell. It is unknown if this variation affects the TSLP receptor.

Because the *HLA-DRB1* and *IL7R* genes are involved in the immune system, changes in either might be related to the autoimmune response that damages the myelin sheath and nerve cells, leading to the signs and symptoms of multiple sclerosis. However, it is unclear as to what role variations in either gene plays in the development of the condition.

CYP27B1 *Gene—Normal Function*

The *CYP27B1* gene provides instructions for making an enzyme called "1-alpha-hydroxylase (1α-hydroxylase)." This enzyme carries out the second of two reactions that converts vitamin D to its active form, 1,25-dihydroxyvitamin D3, also known as "calcitriol." Vitamin D can be acquired from foods or can be made in the body with the help of sunlight exposure. When active, this vitamin is involved in maintaining the proper balance of several minerals in the body, including calcium and phosphate, which are essential for the normal formation of bones and teeth. One of vitamin D's major roles is to control the absorption of calcium and phosphate from the intestines into the bloodstream. Vitamin D is also involved in several processes unrelated to bone and tooth formation.

HLA-DRB1 *Gene—Normal Function*

The *HLA-DRB1* gene provides instructions for making a protein that plays a critical role in the immune system. The *HLA-DRB1* gene is part of a family of genes called "the human leukocyte antigen (HLA) complex." The HLA complex helps the immune system distinguish the body's own proteins from proteins made by foreign invaders such as viruses and bacteria.

The HLA complex is the human version of the major histocompatibility complex (MHC), a gene family that occurs in many species. The *HLA-DRB1* gene belongs to a group of MHC genes called "MHC class II." MHC class II genes provide instructions for making proteins that are present on the surface of certain immune-system cells. These proteins attach to protein fragments (peptides) outside the cell, and MHC class II proteins display these peptides to the immune system.

If the immune system recognizes the peptides as foreign (such as viral or bacterial peptides), it triggers a response to attack the invading viruses or bacteria.

The protein produced from the *HLA-DRB1* gene, called "the beta chain," attaches (binds) to another protein called "the alpha chain," which is produced from the *HLA-DRA* gene. Together, they form a functional protein complex called the "HLA-DR antigen-binding heterodimer." This complex displays foreign peptides to the immune system to trigger the body's immune response.

Each MHC class II gene has many possible variations, allowing the immune system to react to a wide range of foreign invaders. Researchers have identified hundreds of different versions (alleles) of the *HLA-DRB1* gene, each of which is given a particular number (such as "*HLA-DRB1*04:01").

IL2RA *Gene—Normal Function*

The interleukin 2 (IL2) receptor alpha (IL2RA) and beta (IL2RB) chains, together with the common gamma chain (IL2RG), constitute the high-affinity IL2 receptor. Homodimeric alpha chains (IL2RA) result with a low-affinity receptor, while homodimeric beta (IL2RB) chains produce a medium-affinity receptor. Mutations in this gene are associated with interleukin 2 receptor alpha deficiency.

IL7R *Gene—Normal Function*

The *IL7R* gene provides instructions for making a protein called "interleukin 7 (IL-7) receptor alpha chain." This protein is one piece of both the IL-7 receptor and the thymic stromal lymphopoietin (TSLP) receptor. These receptors are embedded in the cell membrane of immune-system cells. The IL-7 receptor is found in B cells and T cells, as well as the early blood-forming cells that give rise to them. The TSLP receptor is found in several types of immune cells, including B cells, T cells, monocytes, and dendritic cells. These cells identify foreign substances and defend the body against infection and disease.

At the cell surface, the IL-7 receptor interacts with a protein called "IL-7." IL-7 is a cytokine, which is a protein that regulates the activity of immune-system cells. The receptor and cytokine fit together like a lock and its key, triggering a series of chemical signals inside the cell. In early blood-forming cells, signaling through the IL-7 receptor ensures the development of mature B cells and T cells. IL-7 receptor signaling also stimulates the later growth and division (proliferation) and survival of these cells.

Similarly, the TSLP receptor interacts with the cytokine TSLP. Attachment of TSLP to its receptor triggers a set of signals that support proliferation and maturation of a variety of immune system cells.

TNFRSF1A *Gene—Normal Function*

The *TNFRSF1A* gene provides instructions for making a protein called "tumor necrosis factor receptor 1 (TNFR1)." This protein is found spanning the membrane of cells, with part of the TNFR1 protein outside the cell and part of the protein inside the cell. Outside the cell, the TNFR1 protein attaches (binds) to another protein called "tumor necrosis factor (TNF)." The interaction of the TNF protein with the TNFR1 protein causes the TNFR1 protein to bind to two other TNFR1 proteins, forming a three-protein complex called a "trimer." This trimer formation is necessary for the TNFR1 protein to be functional.

The binding of the TNF and TNFR1 proteins causes the TNFR1 protein to send signals inside the cell. Signaling from the TNFR1 protein can trigger either inflammation or self-destruction of the cell (apoptosis). Signaling within the cell initiates a pathway that turns on a protein called "nuclear factor kappa B," which triggers inflammation and leads to the production of immune system proteins called "cytokines." Apoptosis is initiated when the TNFR1 protein, bound to the TNF protein, is brought into the cell and starts a process known as the "caspase cascade."

How Variation in These Genes Causes Multiple Sclerosis

Variations in the *HLA-DRB1* gene have been associated with an increased risk of developing multiple sclerosis. This condition affects the brain and spinal cord (central nervous system), causing muscle weakness, poor coordination, numbness, and a variety of other health problems. One variant of this gene, called "*HLA-DRB1**15:01," is the most strongly linked genetic factor for the risk of multiple sclerosis.

Because the *HLA-DRB1* gene is involved in the immune system, changes in it might be related to the autoimmune response and inflammation that damage nerves and the protective coating surrounding them (the myelin sheath), leading to the signs and symptoms of multiple sclerosis. However, it is unclear exactly what role *HLA-DRB1* gene variants play in the development of multiple sclerosis.

A combination of genetic and environmental factors is likely involved in this condition.

A common variation of the *IL-7R* gene increases the risk of developing multiple sclerosis. This condition affects the brain and spinal cord (central nervous system), causing muscle weakness, poor coordination, numbness, and a variety of other health problems. The genetic variation involved in multiple sclerosis affects a single protein building block (amino acid) in the IL-7 receptor alpha chain, specifying the amino acid isoleucine at position 244 instead of the amino acid threonine. The IL-7 receptor that contains this version of the alpha chain is not embedded in the cell surface, but is instead found inside the cell. It is not clear if this alpha-chain variant affects the TSLP receptor.

Because the *IL7R* gene is involved in regulation of the immune system, changes in it might be involved in the autoimmune response and inflammation that damage nerves and the protective coating surrounding them (the myelin sheath), leading to the signs and symptoms of multiple sclerosis. (Autoimmunity occurs when the immune system malfunctions and attacks the body's own tissues and organs, in multiple sclerosis it attacks tissues of the nervous system.) However, it is unclear exactly what role the *IL-7R* gene variant plays in the development of multiple sclerosis. It is likely that a combination of genetic and environmental factors is involved.

Chapter 5

Multiple Sclerosis in Women, Children, and Men

Multiple sclerosis (MS) is an autoimmune condition that affects the brain and spinal cord of the central nervous system (CNS). According to the National Multiple Sclerosis Society (NMSS), epidemiology estimates that:

- MS has been prevalent since 1975.

- About 2.3 million people are living with MS globally.

- Nearly 200 patients are diagnosed with MS each week in the United States.

- MS is more commonly seen in Caucasians that are far above or far below the equator.

- The incidence of MS is higher in colder climates (i.e., Native Americans, Africans, and Asians who lie on the equator are at low risk of developing MS, whilst people of Northern European descent, Canada, and Scotland are at increased risk of developing MS).

The exact cause of MS is yet to be discovered, but age, environmental and genetic factors, and sex all play their respective roles in making people susceptible to this disease.

"Multiple Sclerosis in Women, Children, and Men," © 2019 Omnigraphics. Reviewed March 2019.

- **Age**—The average onset of MS is approximately at 30 years of age or older. It mostly affects people in between 20 and 50 years of age. Some children and teens younger than the age of 18 are affected by MS, which is called "pediatric multiple sclerosis."

- **Environmental factors**
  - Exposure to Epstein-Barr virus (EBV)—A virus that causes infectious-glandular fever, otherwise called "kissing disease"
  - Minimal exposure to sunlight (causes vitamin D deficiency—a known causative agent of MS)
  - Smoking, alcohol, or drug usage
  - Obesity and feeling emotionally stressed

- **Genetic component**—Having a parent with MS increases the risk of having MS to three to five percent.

- **Gender bias**—Most people receive a diagnosis between their twenties and fifties.
  - The risk of a female developing MS is three times greater than a male's chance of developing the disorder, and it is even higher for children.
  - It is believed that sex hormones and other intense alterations that occur during menstrual cycles, pregnancy, and childbirth play an active role in the onset of MS.
  - Girls with MS tend to have greater initial sensory symptoms, such as numbness and tingling, when compared to boys; similarly, symptoms tend to retreat more quickly for females than they do for males.

Symptoms in the General Population

Symptoms vary from person to person, so there is no standard set of symptoms that everyone will definitely experience. However, the most common symptoms are:

- Weakness in all parts of the body
- Feeling dizzy
- Feeling extremely tired and lethargic (fatigue)
- Vision problems, such as blurry or double vision and, sometimes, loss of sight

- Balance issues due to walking difficulties, poor coordination, stiffness, and tremor (shaking)
- Urinary urgency along with hesitation
- Lhermitte phenomenon—tingling and electrical shock-like sensations on the arms, legs, and back, especially if the neck is bent forward
- Sensitivity to heat
- Emotional and cognitive changes
- Sexual dysfunction

Usually, however, no physical trauma or surgical needs have risen due to MS. Furthermore, people living with MS do not develop severe disabilities, and most of them have a normal to near-normal lifespan.

Women-Specific Multiple Sclerosis

Due to hormonal fluctuations and low testosterone (sex hormone) levels, women are more prone to having MS than men, but it does not hinder a woman's ability to get pregnant and have children.

During puberty, the incidence of MS increases due to hormonal changes, so puberty is considered as a key risk period in developing MS, particularly for females.

During pregnancy, women may find it easier to handle MS, as the pregnancy hormones control/improves symptoms, especially during the second and third trimesters. However, relapse is common after delivery.

During menopause, MS symptoms may worsen due to a drop in the estrogen (steroid hormone) levels.

Women-specific symptoms of MS include:

- Increased bouts of symptoms, such as imbalance, depression, fatigue, and weakness during the menstrual cycle

- **Sex-specific dysfunctions.** Sex is a process in which the nervous system provokes the feelings of sexual desire, and the endocrine system drives the hormones for which the body of an individual responds and reacts. MS damages those nerve pathways, which destroy both the desire and the bodily response of an individual.

  - Hypoactive sexual-desire syndrome (a low sex drive and trouble reaching the climax of sexual excitement)

- Decreased sexual interest and ability due to fatigue, muscle spasms, and pain

- Numbness and impaired clitoris (sensitive erectile part of the female genitals) stimulation

- Decreased vaginal lubrication (dry vagina), causing difficulty during intercourse

Pediatric Multiple Sclerosis

MS can occur at any age for children and adolescents. According to data collected, in the United States, 8,000 to 10,000 adolescents (18 years of age or older) have MS, and 2 to 5 percent of young children (18 years of age or younger) experience symptom onset.

- MS is mostly diagnosed in children following the nerve disorder called "acute disseminated encephalomyelitis (ADEM)," which causes headache, confusion, stiff neck, seizures, coma, fever, and a lack of energy.

- Young children are more likely to have seizures when compared to adults, but once diagnosed, all children are considered to have relapsing-remitting MS, as children often experience frequent relapses (worsening of symptoms).

- Although the disease progresses notably slower in children than in adults, it affects children emotionally, as they feel that their school work, social image, and relationship with peers are getting affected with symptoms of MS.

In 2006, the NMSS established a nationwide network that consists of 6 pediatric multiple sclerosis centers of excellence that provide evaluation and care to children and teens (up to the age of 18) with MS and other related disorders.

Men-Specific Multiple Sclerosis

As established, MS is more prevalent in women than men due to the fact that men are protected by high levels of testosterone. When MS occurs in men, it produces similar symptoms to that of females, but the experience may differ, especially because of the gender norms that typically establish a male as the "protector." When men become ill with this kind of debilitating disease, it becomes challenging, and sometimes impossible, to upkeep societal expectations. Other symptoms that men may experience include:

- Changes in vision, such as blurry eyes or loss of sight

- Extreme tiredness and lethargy (fatigue) due to pain

- Balance issues and falls, due to stiffness and difficulty with walking

- Numbness and tingling sensation (like electric shocks)

- Constipation and urinary problems, such as false urgency and hesitation

- Sexual dysfunction

References

1. Kim, Steve MD. "Multiple Sclerosis: Facts, Statistics, and You," healthline, June 20, 2018.

2. Calabresi, Peter Arthur MD; Mowry, Ellen MD. "Healthy Woman," Johns Hopkins Medicine, August 13, 2017.

3. Matt Allen G. "Living as a Male with Multiple Sclerosis," multiplesclerosis.net, July 1, 2014.

4. "Pediatric Multiple Sclerosis," Cleveland Clinic, March 25, 2006.

Chapter 6

Causative Agents of Multiple Sclerosis

The ultimate cause of multiple sclerosis (MS) is damage to myelin, nerve fibers, and neurons in the brain and spinal cord, which together make up the central nervous system (CNS). But how that happens, and why, are questions that challenge researchers. Evidence appears to show that MS is a disease caused by genetic vulnerabilities combined with environmental factors.

Although there is little doubt that the immune system contributes to the brain and spinal cord tissue destruction of MS, the exact target of the immune system attacks and which immune system cells cause the destruction is not fully understood.

Researchers have several possible explanations for what might be going on. The immune system could be:

- Fighting some kind of infectious agent (for example, a virus) that has components which mimic components of the brain (molecular mimicry)

- Destroying brain cells because they are unhealthy

- Mistakenly identifying normal brain cells as foreign

This chapter includes text excerpted from "Multiple Sclerosis: Hope through Research," National Institute of Neurological Disorders and Stroke (NINDS), July 6, 2018.

The last possibility has been the favored explanation for many years. Research now suggests that the first two activities might also play a role in the development of MS. There is a special barrier, called "the blood-brain barrier," which separates the brain and spinal cord from the immune system. If there is a break in the barrier, it exposes the brain to the immune system for the first time. When this happens, the immune system may misinterpret the brain as foreign.

Genetic Susceptibility

Susceptibility to MS may be inherited. Studies of families indicate that relatives of an individual with MS have an increased risk for developing the disease. Experts estimate that about 15 percent of individuals with MS have 1 or more family members or relatives who also have MS. But even identical twins, whose deoxyribonucleic acid (DNA) is exactly the same, have only a one in three chance of both having the disease. This suggests that MS is not entirely controlled by genes. Other factors must come into play.

Current research suggests that dozens of genes and possibly hundreds of variations in the genetic code (called "gene variants") combine to create vulnerability to MS. Some of these genes have been identified. Most of the genes identified so far are associated with functions of the immune system. Additionally, many of the known genes are similar to those that have been identified in people with other autoimmune diseases, such as type 1 diabetes, rheumatoid arthritis (RA), or lupus. Researchers continue to look for additional genes and study how they interact with each other to make an individual vulnerable to developing MS.

Sunlight and Vitamin D

A number of studies have suggested that people who spend more time in the sun and those with relatively high levels of vitamin D are less likely to develop MS. Bright sunlight helps human skin produce vitamin D. Researchers believe that vitamin D may help regulate the immune system in ways that reduce the risk of MS. People from regions near the equator, where there is a great deal of bright sunlight, generally have a much lower risk of MS than people from temperate areas, such as the United States and Canada. Other studies suggest that people with higher levels of vitamin D generally have less severe MS and fewer relapses.

Smoking

A number of studies have found that people who smoke are more likely to develop MS. People who smoke also tend to have more brain lesions and brain shrinkage than nonsmokers. The reasons for this are currently unclear.

Infectious Factors and Viruses

A number of viruses have been found in people with MS, but the virus most consistently linked to the development of MS is Epstein-Barr virus (EBV), the virus that causes mononucleosis.

Only about five percent of the population has not been infected by EBV. These individuals are at lower risk for developing MS than those who have been infected. People who were infected with EBV in adolescence or adulthood, and who, therefore, develop an exaggerated immune response to EBV, are at a significantly higher risk for developing MS than those who were infected in early childhood. This suggests that it may be the type of immune response to EBV that predisposes to MS, rather than EBV infection itself. However, there is still no proof that EBV causes MS.

Autoimmune and Inflammatory Processes

Tissue inflammation and antibodies in the blood that fight normal components of the body and tissue in people with MS are similar to those found in other autoimmune diseases. Along with overlapping evidence from genetic studies, these findings suggest that MS results from some kind of disturbed regulation of the immune system.

Chapter 7

Multiple Sclerosis: Disease Course and Exacerbation

Multiple sclerosis (MS) is a complex neurologic disease that affects the central nervous system (CNS), which includes the brain, spinal cord, and vision pathways. In MS, the immune system attacks the myelin sheath, the fatty tissue that surrounds and protects nerve fibers, as well as the nerve fibers themselves. This damage is called "demyelination," and the scar tissues that develop when myelin is damaged are called "sclerosis," also known as "lesions" or "plaques."

When any part of the myelin sheath or nerve fiber is damaged or destroyed, nerve impulses traveling to and from the brain and spinal cord are distorted or interrupted, causing a wide variety of symptoms. Sometimes the myelin can repair itself, and the MS symptoms go away after the immune attack or relapse. However, over time, the myelin and underlying nerve fibers cannot recover and suffer permanent damage. This may lead to a decline in function, depending on the disease course. Several MS disease courses have been identified.

This chapter contains text excerpted from the following sources: Text in this chapter begins with excerpts from "About Multiple Sclerosis," U.S. Department of Veterans Affairs (VA), August 20, 2018; Text under the heading "What Is an Exacerbation or Attack of Multiple Sclerosis?" is excerpted from "Multiple Sclerosis: Hope through Research," National Institute of Neurological Disorders and Stroke (NINDS), July 6, 2018.

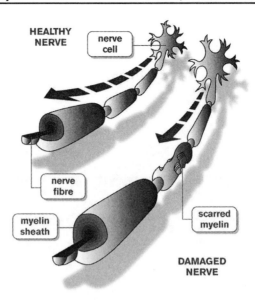

Figure 7.1. *Healthy Nerve vs MS Nerve*

Relapsing-Remitting Multiple Sclerosis

Relapsing-remitting multiple sclerosis (RRMS) is the most common MS disease course. About 85 percent of people with MS are first

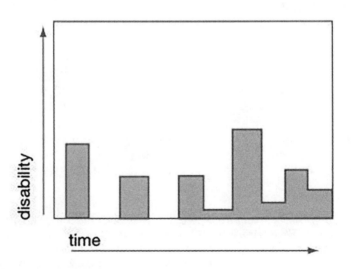

Figure 7.2. *Relapsing-Remitting MS Graph*

diagnosed with this course. It is characterized by clearly defined relapses. These relapses are followed by periods of partial or complete recovery with no apparent progression of the MS disability between relapses.

MS relapses, also called "attacks," "exacerbations," or "flares," are rapid, significant worsening of existing symptoms or development of new symptoms, last at least 24 hours, and are not caused by infection, fever, or other stress. A relapse is different from the daily fluctuations in symptoms, which are caused by the variable function of the nervous system due to already existing MS plaques. In contrast to fluctuations, relapses are caused by new areas of inflammation and demyelination in the brain, spinal cord, or visual pathways. Most symptoms of relapses clear up with time, rest, and, if needed, therapy. There are treatments that can speed up the rate of recovery from a relapse. However, if there is partial recovery, those remaining symptoms can become permanent. MS relapses typically last a few days to weeks. If not participating in a disease-modifying therapy, people with RRMS typically experience 1 to 3 relapses a year; however, some can go decades between relapses.

Infection, fever, and stress can all lead to significant worsening of neurological function, which can look like an MS relapse. This is called a "pseudo-relapse" because, like fluctuations, there is no new inflammation and demyelination occurring. A magnetic resonance image (MRI) can be helpful in distinguishing between MS relapses and pseudo-relapses. A pseudo-relapse is managed by treating the underlying infection or source of stress.

Primary and Secondary Progressive Multiple Sclerosis

Primary progressive multiple sclerosis (PPMS) is characterized by progressive worsening of the disease from onset without clear relapses. There may be changes in the rate of progression or periods of stability during the course of the disease. About 15 percent of people with MS are first diagnosed with this course.

People with secondary progressive multiple sclerosis (SPMS) are initially diagnosed with RRMS and then transition to this progressive form of the disease. This course is characterized by progression of disability over the years, with fewer or no further relapses. In addition, there are fewer or no further new or enhancing plaques seen on the MRIs. Not everyone with RRMS will transition to SPMS.

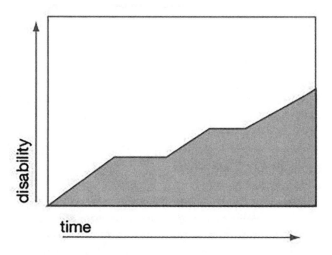

Figure 7.3. *Primary Progressive MS Graph*

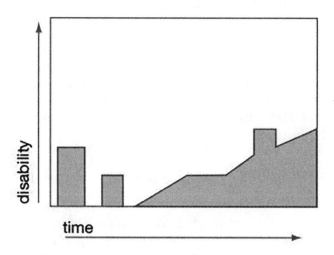

Figure 7.4. *Secondary Progressive MS Graph*

Clinically Isolated Syndrome

Clinically isolated syndrome (CIS) is a term that describes an event similar to a typical MS relapse in a person not previously diagnosed with MS. People who experience a CIS are at higher risk of developing MS, but not all go on to have MS.

What Is an Exacerbation or Attack of Multiple Sclerosis?

An exacerbation is a sudden worsening of MS symptoms or the appearance of new symptoms that lasts for at least 24 hours. MS relapses are thought to be associated with the development of new areas of damage in the brain. Exacerbations are characteristic of relapsing-remitting MS, in which attacks are followed by periods of complete or partial recovery with no apparent worsening of symptoms.

An attack may be mild or its symptoms may be severe enough to significantly interfere with life's daily activities. Most exacerbations last from several days to several weeks, although some have been known to last for months.

When the symptoms of the attack subside, an individual with MS is said to be in remission. However, MRI data have shown that this is somewhat misleading because MS lesions continue to appear during these remission periods. Patients do not experience symptoms during remission because the inflammation may not be severe or it may occur in areas of the brain that do not produce obvious symptoms. Research suggests that only about 1 out of every 10 MS lesions is perceived by a person with MS. Therefore, MRI examination plays a very important role in establishing an MS diagnosis, deciding when the disease should be treated and determining whether treatments work effectively or not. It also has been a valuable tool to test whether an experimental new therapy is effective at reducing exacerbations.

Chapter 8

Rare and Unusual Variants of Multiple Sclerosis

Chapter Contents

Section 8.1

Schilder Disease—Tumefactive Multiple Sclerosis

This section includes text excerpted from "Schilder's Disease
Information Page," National Institute of Neurological
Disorders and Stroke (NINDS), June 21, 2018.

Schilder disease is a rare progressive demyelinating disorder
which usually begins in childhood. Schilder disease is not the same
as Addison-Schilder disease (adrenoleukodystrophy).

Symptoms

Symptoms may include dementia, aphasia, seizures, personality
changes, poor attention, tremors, balance instability, incontinence,
muscle weakness, headaches, vomiting, and vision and speech impairment. The disorder is a variant of multiple sclerosis (MS).

Treatment

Treatment for the disorder follows the established standards for
MS and includes corticosteroids, beta interferon or immunosuppressive
therapy, and symptomatic treatment.

Prognosis

As with multiple sclerosis, the course and prognosis of Schilder
disease are unpredictable. For some individuals, the disorder is progressive with a steady, unremitting course. Others may experience
significant improvement and even remission. In some cases, Schilder
disease is fatal.

Section 8.2

Marburg Variant Multiple Sclerosis—Malignant

This section includes text excerpted from "Malignant Multiple Sclerosis," U.S. Social Security Administration (SSA), March 28, 2018.

Malignant multiple sclerosis (malignant MS) is an aggressive and rare form of multiple sclerosis (MS). It is characterized by rapidly progressive inflammation and destruction of myelin (protective covering surrounding the nerves) and increased formation of lesions and plaque in the brain and spine. The loss of myelin affects the brain's ability to transmit electrochemical impulses between nerve cells of the brain and the spinal cord, resulting in diminished or loss of neurological functioning. People with this form of MS experience weakness in their extremities, difficulties with coordination and balance, spasticity, and paresthesias (abnormal sensory feelings of numbness and prickling sensations). Speech impediments, tremors, dizziness, hearing loss, changes in vision, bowel and bladder difficulties, falls, and cognitive impairments are other frequent complaints. As the disease progresses, lesions develop in the areas of the brain responsible for information processing; this results in cognitive impairments, such as difficulties with concentration, attention, memory, language, and judgment. People with malignant MS can have damage to regions of the brain responsible for behavior and emotions, resulting in psychotic disorders, such as manic depression and paranoia.

Onset and Progression

People with malignant MS experience a rapid decline in functioning. They require assistance with ambulation within five years from symptom onset due to the loss of the ability of the nerve cell (neurons) to transmit impulses to muscles that control motor functioning. Assistance with activities of daily living (ADL) is required.

Treatment

There is currently no cure for malignant MS. Treatment generally consists of immunomodulatory therapy and the management of symptoms. Physical and occupational therapies can help the person perform daily activities, such as handwriting, buttoning, and using eating utensils. Ambulatory aids, such as canes, walkers, and wheelchairs, are prescribed for gait and ataxia.

Chapter 9

Other Demyelinating Diseases

Chapter Contents

Section 9.1

Chronic Inflammatory Demyelinating Polyneuropathy

This section includes text excerpted from "Chronic Inflammatory Demyelinating Polyneuropathy (CIDP) Information Page," National Institute of Neurological Disorders and Stroke (NINDS), June 15, 2018.

Chronic inflammatory demyelinating polyneuropathy (CIDP) is a neurological disorder characterized by progressive weakness and impaired sensory function in the legs and arms. The disorder, which is sometimes called "chronic relapsing polyneuropathy," is caused by damage to the myelin sheath (the fatty covering that wraps around and protects nerve fibers) of the peripheral nerves. Although it can occur at any age and in both genders, CIDP is more common in young adults, and in men more so than women.

Symptoms

It often presents with symptoms that include tingling or numbness (beginning in the toes and fingers), weakness of the arms and legs, loss of deep tendon reflexes (areflexia), fatigue, and abnormal sensations. CIDP is closely related to Guillain-Barre syndrome, and it is considered the chronic counterpart of that acute disease.

Treatment

Treatment for CIDP includes corticosteroids, such as prednisone, which may be prescribed alone or in combination with immunosuppressant drugs. Plasmapheresis (plasma exchange) and intravenous immunoglobulin (IVIg) therapy are effective. IVIg may be used even as first-line therapy. Physiotherapy may improve muscle strength, function, and mobility, and minimize the shrinkage of muscles and tendons and distortions of the joints.

Prognosis

The course of CIDP varies widely among individuals. Some may have a bout of CIDP followed by spontaneous recovery, while others may have many bouts with partial recovery in between relapses. The disease is a treatable cause of acquired neuropathy, and initiation of early treatment to prevent loss of nerve axons is recommended. However, some individuals are left with some residual numbness or weakness.

Section 9.2

Neuromyelitis Optica

This section includes text excerpted from "Neuromyelitis Optica," Genetic and Rare Diseases Information Center (GARD), National Center for Advancing Translational Sciences (NCATS), November 7, 2017.

Neuromyelitis optica (NMO) is an autoimmune disease that affects the spinal cord and optic nerves (nerves that carry visual messages to and from the brain). In neuromyelitis optica, the body's immune system mistakenly attacks healthy cells and a substance called "myelin" in the spinal cord and eyes.

Symptoms may begin in childhood or adulthood. Spinal cord involvement results in transverse myelitis, which may cause pain, paralysis, and abnormal sensations in the spine and limbs. Bladder and bowel problems may also develop. Symptoms from optic nerve involvement include eye pain and vision loss from optic neuritis. Other symptoms of neuromyelitis optica may include episodes of nausea, vomiting, and hiccups. Some people have episodes of symptoms months or years apart (the relapsing form), while others have a single episode lasting several months (the monophasic form). In either form, people with neuromyelitis optica often develop permanent muscle weakness and vision loss.

The cause of the immune system dysfunction leading to neuromyelitis optica is not known. It usually occurs in only one person in a family. There is no cure, but there are therapies to reduce symptoms during episodes and to prevent relapses.

Symptoms

The most common signs and symptoms of neuromyelitis optica are optic neuritis (inflammation of the optic nerve) and transverse myelitis (inflammation of the spinal cord).

Optic neuritis tends to occur suddenly and causes eye pain and varying degrees of vision loss. In most cases, only one eye is affected. Some people develop optic neuritis in both eyes at the same time.

Transverse myelitis develops over hours or days. It may cause pain in the spine or limbs, mild to severe paralysis of the limbs, abnormal sensations in the legs, and loss of bowel or bladder control. Depending on which part of the spinal cord is involved, breathing problems may be present. Some people also have muscle spasms in the upper body or limbs. Transverse myelitis often eventually causes full paralysis of the legs, requiring the use of a wheelchair.

Neuromyelitis optica can also affect the brain stem (the part of the brain connected to the spinal cord). This can lead to severe nausea, vomiting, and/or hiccups.

Causes

Neuromyelitis optica is considered an autoimmune disease in which the immune system mistakenly attacks cells and proteins in the spinal cord and optic nerves. Unfortunately, the reason that the immune system functions abnormally is not known.

In rare cases, more than one person in a family may have neuromyelitis optica. Additionally, many people with neuromyelitis optica have another autoimmune disease or have family members with an autoimmune disease. While this suggests that genes play a role in predisposing a person to the disease, no responsible genes have been found.

There have been a few cases of neuromyelitis optica occurring in association with certain viruses (e.g., syphilis, human immunodeficiency virus (HIV), chlamydia, varicella, cytomegalovirus (CMV), and Epstein Barr virus (EBV)). The nature of this link is not clear. It is possible that certain infections may trigger neuromyelitis optica in people who are predisposed to the condition.

Inheritance

Neuromyelitis optica usually is not inherited. The disease typically occurs in only one person in a family. However, about three percent of people with neuromyelitis optica report having a family member with the disease. It is possible that some people have a genetic predisposition (or susceptibility) to developing neuromyelitis optica. However, it is likely that unknown environmental factors are also involved.

Diagnosis

A diagnosis of NMO is based upon the presence of characteristic symptoms, and imaging studies of the brain, spinal cord, and eyes, as well as results of laboratory tests. Additionally, other more common conditions (particularly multiple sclerosis) must be ruled out.

Imaging studies may include magnetic resonance imaging (MRI scan) of the brain, spinal cord, and orbits (eyes), and optical coherence tomography (specialized pictures of the retina).

Laboratory tests may include:

- A blood test for aquaporin-4 (also known as "NMO-IgG")— this test detects the aquaporin-4 antibody, which specifically indicates the diagnosis when characteristic symptoms are present. It also helps to distinguish the disease from multiple sclerosis (in which this antibody is not present). However, the absence of this antibody does not mean that a person does not have NMO.

- Examination of the cerebrospinal fluid—this may show high levels of white blood cells and proteins.

Treatment

There is no cure for neuromyelitis optica, but there are therapies aimed at treating episodes in progress, reducing symptoms, and preventing relapses.

Sudden episodes and relapses are usually treated with intravenous corticosteroids. If this does not relieve symptoms, a plasma exchange may be effective. Low doses of carbamazepine may be used to control painful muscle spasms during an episode. Muscle relaxants may be used for spasticity that develops in those with permanent muscle dysfunction.

For prevention of recurrent episodes, the main treatment is long-term use of medication that suppresses the immune system (systemic immunosuppressive therapy). There are no controlled trials evaluating this treatment, so recommendations are generally based on data from observational studies and by the experience of experts who have treated the disease.

People with severe, permanent symptoms may benefit from collaborating with occupational therapists, physical therapists, and social service professionals to address their rehabilitation needs.

Prognosis

The severity of impairment and life expectancy may depend on the severity of the first (or only) episode, the number of relapses within the first two years, and a person's age when the disease begins. In general, the outlook (prognosis) is thought to be worse for people who have severe symptoms during the first episode, have many relapses within a shorter amount of time, and/or are older when the disease begins.

For people with the relapsing form (90 percent of those with the disease), each episode causes more damage to the nervous system. Often, this eventually leads to permanent muscle weakness, paralysis, and/or vision loss within five years. People with the monophasic form (those who experience one episode) can also have lasting impairment of muscle function and vision.

The disease reportedly may ultimately be fatal in 25 to 50 percent of people, with loss of life most commonly due to respiratory failure. However, life expectancy varies from person to person.

Chapter 10

Multiple Sclerosis: Yesterday, Today, and Tomorrow

Yesterday

Multiple sclerosis (MS) was first recognized as a disorder in the late nineteenth century, but only by the 1960s did researchers first begin to understand some of the disease processes that cause symptoms and long-term disability. These processes seemed to involve inflammation and the loss of myelin, a protective covering around nerve fibers.

The first standard guidelines for the diagnosis of MS and a disability rating scale were also established in the 1960s, setting the stage for clinical research to test new therapies.

In the late 1960s, the first controlled clinical trials for MS therapy showed that treatment with adrenocorticotropic hormone (ACTH) could speed recovery from an attack. While this therapy helped to reduce inflammation during the acute symptoms of an attack, it did not slow progression of the disease.

Today

MS is recognized as a chronic inflammatory and autoimmune disease of the central nervous system. It is among the most common

This chapter includes text excerpted from "Multiple Sclerosis," Research Portfolio Online Reporting Tools (RePORT), National Institutes of Health (NIH), June 30, 2018.

causes of neurological disability in young adults and occurs at least twice as frequently in women as in men.

Research has now shown that MS not only damages the myelin covering of nerve fibers but also causes degeneration of the nerve fibers themselves. Depending on which nerve fibers in the brain and spinal cord are affected, MS can impair movement, coordination, sensation, and thinking. For most people with MS, episodes of worsening function (relapses) are initially followed by recovery periods (remissions). Over time, recovery may be incomplete, leading to progressive decline.

Magnetic resonance imaging (MRI), first used in patients with MS in the 1980s, has shown that damage to nerve fibers may be present at very early stages of the disease and may remain when symptoms subside. MRI has also revolutionized the diagnosis of MS, reducing the average time from first symptoms to diagnosis from several years to months.

Several U.S. Food and Drug Administration (FDA)-approved therapies are now available to ameliorate the symptoms of MS and to, in some cases, slow disease progression. National Institutes of Health (NIH)-supported research contributed to the development of many of these treatments, which include the beta interferons (Betaseron®, Rebif®, Avonex®, Extavia®), copolymer 1 (Copaxone®, also called "glatiramer acetate"), the immunosuppressant mitoxantrone (Novantrone®), and most recently, natalizumab (Tysabri®), an antibody-based therapy that represents a new class of immunomodulatory agents for treating MS.

Although the direct causes of MS remain unknown, studies in an animal model of MS have significantly advanced scientists' understanding of the immune and inflammatory processes that cause damage to myelin and nerve fibers. NIH-supported scientists recently reported the first genes linked to MS since the 1970s, and ongoing studies continue to search for additional genetic and nongenetic risk factors, including exposure to viruses, cigarette smoking, vitamin D levels, and reproductive history.

Tomorrow

Treatments will be available to more effectively slow or halt the progression of MS. Combination therapy with existing treatments may improve care in the near term, and NIH supports a Phase III clinical trial (CombiRx) to determine if treatment combining beta-interferon and glatiramer acetate offers an improvement over the partial efficacy of either common medication alone. NIH is also conducting a trial to test the safety and efficacy of the drug idebenone as a treatment for primary progressive MS, for which therapies are currently lacking. Idebenone is similar to the natural compound coenzyme Q10 and may protect against tissue damage.

Researchers will identify brain imaging and molecular biomarkers associated with MS susceptibility, disease progression, and treatment response profiles. NIH intramural investigators are collaborating with the CombiRx trial to identify biomarkers associated with clinical features and responses to different treatments. Such biomarkers will facilitate early diagnosis and therapy development research, and they could also inform predictions about which treatment regime will most likely benefit a given patient.

Further advances in understanding the genetic and environmental causes of MS will help identify those at higher risk for the disease. Along with growing knowledge about the mechanisms that lead to symptoms, these advances will point to new targets for developing treatments and preventive strategies.

Research on neuroimmune interactions and the processes of neurodegeneration and repair will lead to a new generation of neuroprotective therapies that will complement current MS treatments. These neuroprotective agents will help to prevent, reduce, or even repair the damage to nerve fibers that can cause long-term, progressive impairments.

Part Two

Symptoms of Multiple Sclerosis

Chapter 11

Overview of Multiple Sclerosis Symptoms

The symptoms of multiple sclerosis (MS) usually begin over one to several days, but in some forms, they may develop more slowly. They may be mild or severe and may go away quickly or last for months. Sometimes, the initial symptoms of MS are overlooked because they disappear in a day or so and normal function returns. Because symptoms come and go in the majority of people with MS, the presence of symptoms is called an "attack," or, in medical terms, an "exacerbation." Recovery from symptoms is referred to as "remission," while a return of symptoms is called a "relapse." This form of MS is, therefore, called "relapsing-remitting MS," in contrast to a more slowly developing form called "primary progressive MS." Progressive MS can also be a second stage of the illness that occurs years after relapsing-remitting symptoms.

A diagnosis of MS is often delayed because MS shares symptoms with other neurological conditions and diseases.

The first symptoms of MS often include:

- Vision problems, such as blurred or double vision or optic neuritis, which causes pain in the eye and a rapid loss of vision

This chapter includes text excerpted from "Multiple Sclerosis: Hope through Research," National Institute of Neurological Disorders and Stroke (NINDS), July 6, 2018.

- Weak, stiff muscles, often with painful muscle spasms

- Tingling or numbness in the arms, legs, trunk of the body, or face

- Clumsiness, particularly difficulty staying balanced when walking

- Bladder-control problems, either inability to control the bladder or urgency

- Dizziness that doesn't go away

  MS may also cause later symptoms such as:

- Mental or physical fatigue, which accompanies the above symptoms during an attack

- Mood changes, such as depression or euphoria (inappropriate episodes of high spirits)

- Changes in the ability to concentrate or multitask effectively

- Difficulty making decisions, planning, or prioritizing at work or in private life

Some people with MS develop transverse myelitis, a condition caused by inflammation in the spinal cord. Transverse myelitis causes loss of spinal cord function over a period of time and lasts for several hours to several weeks. It usually begins as a sudden onset of lower back pain, muscle weakness, or abnormal sensations in the toes and feet, and can rapidly progress to more severe symptoms, including paralysis. In most cases of transverse myelitis, people recover at least some function within the first 12 weeks after an attack begins. Transverse myelitis can also result from viral infections, arteriovenous malformations, or neuroinflammatory problems unrelated to MS. In such instances, there are no plaques (scar tissue) in the brain that suggest previous MS attacks.

Neuromyelitis optica (NMO) is a disorder associated with transverse myelitis, as well as optic nerve inflammation. Patients with this disorder usually have antibodies that are against a particular protein in their spinal cord, called the "aquaporin channel." These patients respond differently to treatment than most people with MS.

Most individuals with MS have muscle weakness, often in their hands and legs. Muscle stiffness and spasms can also be a problem. These symptoms may be severe enough to affect walking or standing.

In some cases, MS leads to partial or complete paralysis. Many people with MS find that weakness and fatigue are worse when they have a fever or when they are exposed to heat. MS exacerbations may occur following common infections.

Tingling and burning sensations are common, as well as the numbness and loss of sensations. Moving the neck from side to side or flexing it back and forth may cause "Lhermitte's sign," a characteristic sensation of MS that feels like a sharp spike of electricity coursing down the spine.

While it is rare for pain to be the first sign of MS, pain often occurs with optic neuritis and trigeminal neuralgia, a neurological disorder that affects one of the nerves that runs across the jaw, cheek, and face. Painful spasms of the limbs and sharp pain shooting down the legs or around the abdomen can also be symptoms of MS.

Most individuals with MS experience difficulties with coordination and balance at some time during the course of the disease. Some individuals may have a continuous trembling of the head, limbs, and body, especially during movement; although, such trembling is more common with other disorders, such as Parkinson disease.

Fatigue is common, especially during exacerbations of MS. A person with MS may be tired all the time or may be easily fatigued from mental or physical exertion.

Urinary symptoms, including loss of bladder control and sudden attacks of urgency, are common as MS progresses. People with MS sometimes also develop constipation or sexual problems.

Depression is a common feature of MS. A small number of individuals with MS may develop more severe psychiatric disorders, such as bipolar disorder and paranoia, or experience euphoria.

People with MS, especially those who have had the disease for a long time, can experience difficulty with thinking, learning, memory, and judgment. The first signs of what doctors call "cognitive dysfunction" may be subtle. The person may have problems finding the right word to say or trouble remembering how to do routine tasks on the job or at home. Day-to-day decisions that once came easily may now be made more slowly and show poor judgment. Changes may be so small or happen so slowly that it takes a family member or friend to point them out.

Chapter 12

Spasticity in Multiple Sclerosis

Spasticity is a common symptom affecting many people with multiple sclerosis (MS). Although the stiffness associated with spasticity can sometimes be helpful for performing daily activities, such as getting in and out of a wheelchair or walking, it can also be a nuisance and lead to serious health concerns, such as pain, wounds, or loss of function. The good news is that there are a growing number of treatments available to help ease the burden of troublesome spasticity. To prevent good spasticity from turning into bad spasticity, all people with MS, their caregivers, and/or loved ones should have a basic understanding of the signs of spasticity and the various options to keep it in check.

Is This Spasticity?

Generally, spasticity shows up as increased tightness, resistance to movement, or an involuntary movement of a body part. For some, spasticity means one or both legs make uncontrolled bouncing or jumping motions. For others, spasticity may be a tight arm that makes it difficult to wash the underarm area during showers or a feeling of tightness that makes a stretching program painful or difficult. When

This chapter includes text excerpted from "VA Multiple Sclerosis Centers of Excellence—MS Changed My Life," U.S. Department of Veterans Affairs (VA), 2014. Reviewed March 2019.

in doubt, it is helpful to ask a therapist, neurologist, or rehabilitation provider to evaluate suspicious symptoms and tease out spasticity from other conditions.

Why Is Spasticity Acting Up Now?

Many issues can actually trigger a sudden increase in spasticity. Therefore, it's important to consider whether any of these causes are behind a sudden change in symptoms before "covering up" the symptoms with medication or other treatment. Common triggers for increased spasticity include a bladder or urinary tract infection (UTI), a skin wound, or kidney/bladder stones. Before starting treatment for spasticity, your healthcare provider might recommend a physical exam, blood or urine tests, or imaging studies to look for one of these spasticity triggers.

Are There Treatment Options for Spasticity?

A wide variety of possible treatments for spasticity exist. These allow the healthcare provider to match the treatment to the severity of the symptoms and the preferences of the person with MS.

Stretching and Therapies

In all cases, overactive muscles causing tightness or spasticity should be regularly stretched multiple times a day to maintain range of motion and minimize the symptoms of spasticity. Prolonged stretches (at least 20 to 30 seconds at a time) are the most effective in treating spasticity. When needed, physical or occupational therapists can help set up a stretching program, evaluate for and provide splints to provide a longer lasting stretch (over hours rather than minutes), and also offer useful tricks to quiet spasticity and permit more stretching. Many of these tricks or "modalities"—such as using ice, vibration, or electrical stimulation—have been used for over half a century to treat spasticity and are still commonly used today. While the results from these treatments might not last a long time (less than an hour), the positive side is that most of these treatments can be done at home, can be controlled by the person with MS or their caregiver, and have little to no side effects.

Medications

Medications to relax overactive muscles provide another mean to address spasticity that is out of control. These medications—such as baclofen, tizanidine, diazepam, gabapentin, and others—can provide longer-lasting relief of spasticity (for hours). Side effects, such as drowsiness or weakness, may be experienced with these medications. Most of these medications are taken several times per day, every day, in order to prevent or suppress spasticity.

Injections

Overactive muscles from spasticity can also be treated with local injections with medications, such as botulinum toxin, phenol, or alcohol. These medications are injected directly into the overactive muscles and block the communication between the overactive muscle and the nerve controlling it. These injections can be a good option for individuals with spasticity affecting a few individual muscles (rather than the whole body). The advantage to this treatment is that one round of injections can have effects lasting for several months. One possible disadvantage is that these treatments work by weakening the muscle, so the risk of too much weakness needs to be considered before the injections are performed.

Intrathecal Baclofen Pump

When spasticity affects a larger region of the body, particularly in the legs, an intrathecal baclofen pump is another possible option for treatment. This device delivers small amounts of an antispasticity medication directly to the spinal canal. The benefit of this intervention is that the medication is delivered directly to the place it needs to go to (without having to take pills), and the treatment is adjustable to meet an individual's needs over time. The drawback of this treatment is that it involves a surgery to implant the pump and routine clinic visits to adjust and refill the pump as needed.

Chapter 13

Tremors

Tremor is an involuntary, rhythmic muscle contraction that leads to shaking movements in one or more parts of the body. It is a common movement disorder that most often affects the hands, but it can also occur in the arms, head, vocal cords, torso, and legs. Tremor may be intermittent (occurring at separate times, with breaks) or constant. It can occur sporadically (on its own) or happen as a result of another disorder.

Tremor is most common among middle-aged and older adults, although it can occur at any age. The disorder generally affects men and women equally.

Tremor is not life-threatening. However, it can be embarrassing and even disabling, making it difficult or impossible to perform work and daily life tasks.

What Causes Tremor

Generally, tremor is caused by a problem in the deep parts of the brain that control movements. Most types of tremor have no known cause, although there are some forms that appear to be inherited and run in families.

Tremor can occur on its own or be a symptom associated with a number of neurological disorders, including:

This chapter includes text excerpted from "Tremor Fact Sheet," National Institute of Neurological Disorders and Stroke (NINDS), July 6, 2018.

- Multiple sclerosis (MS)
- Stroke
- Traumatic brain injury (TBI)
- Neurodegenerative diseases that affect parts of the brain (e.g., Parkinson disease)

Some other known causes can include:

- The use of certain medicines (Particular asthma medication, amphetamines, caffeine, corticosteroids, and drugs used for certain psychiatric and neurological disorders)
- Alcohol abuse or withdrawal
- Mercury poisoning
- Overactive thyroid
- Liver or kidney failure
- Anxiety or panic

What Are the Symptoms of Tremor?

Symptoms of tremor may include:

- A rhythmic shaking in the hands, arms, head, legs, or torso
- Shaky voice
- Difficulty writing or drawing
- Problems holding and controlling utensils, such as a spoon

Some tremor may be triggered by, or become worse, during times of stress or strong emotion, when an individual is physically exhausted, or when a person is in certain postures or makes certain movements.

How Is Tremor Classified?

Tremor can be classified into two main categories:

Resting tremor occurs when the muscle is relaxed, such as when the hands are resting on the lap. With this disorder, a person's hands, arms, or legs may shake even when they are at rest. Often, the tremor only affects the hand or fingers. This type of tremor is often seen in people with Parkinson disease and is called a "pillrolling" tremor because the circular finger and hand movements resemble the rolling of small objects or pills in the hand.

Action tremor occurs with the voluntary movement of a muscle. Most types of tremor are considered action tremor. There are several subclassifications of action tremor, many of which overlap.

- **Postural tremor** occurs when a person maintains a position against gravity, such as holding the arms outstretched.

- **Kinetic tremor** is associated with any voluntary movement, such as moving the wrists up and down or closing and opening the eyes.

- **Intention tremor** is produced with purposeful movement toward a target, such as lifting a finger to touch the nose. Typically the tremor will become worse as an individual gets closer to their target.

- **Task-specific tremor** only appears when performing highly-skilled, goal-oriented tasks, such as handwriting or speaking.

- **Isometric tremor** occurs during a voluntary muscle contraction that is not accompanied by any movement, such as holding a heavy book or a dumbbell in the same position.

What Are the Different Categories or Types of Tremor?

Tremor is most commonly classified by its appearance and cause or origin. There are more than 20 types of tremor. Some of the most common forms of tremor include:

Essential Tremor

Essential tremor (previously called "benign essential tremor" or "familial tremor") is one of the most common movement disorders. The exact cause of essential tremor is unknown. For some people, this tremor is mild and remains stable for many years. The tremor usually appears on both sides of the body, but is often noticed more in the dominant hand because it is an action tremor.

The key feature of essential tremor is a tremor in both hands and arms, which is present during action and when standing still. Additional symptoms may include head tremor (e.g., a "yes" or "no" motion) without abnormal posturing of the head and a shaking or quivering sound to the voice if the tremor affects the voice box. The action tremor in both hands with essential tremor can lead to problems with writing, drawing, drinking from a cup, or using tools or a computer.

Tremor frequency (how fast the tremor shakes) may decrease as the person ages, but the severity may increase, affecting the person's ability to perform certain tasks or activities of daily living. Heightened emotion, stress, fever, physical exhaustion, or low blood sugar may trigger tremor and/or increase its severity. Though the tremor can start at any age, it most often appears for the first time during adolescence or in middle age (between the ages of 40 and 50). Small amounts of alcohol may help decrease essential tremor, but the mechanism behind this is unknown.

About 50 percent of the cases of essential tremor are thought to be caused by a genetic risk factor (referred to as "familial tremor"). Children of a parent who has familial tremor have a greater risk of inheriting the condition. Familial forms of essential tremor often appear early in life.

For many years, essential tremor was not associated with any known disease. However, some scientists think essential tremor is accompanied by a mild degeneration of certain areas of the brain that control movement. This is an ongoing debate in the research field.

Dystonic Tremor

Dystonic tremor occurs in people who are affected by dystonia—a movement disorder where incorrect messages from the brain cause muscles to be overactive, resulting in abnormal postures or sustained, unwanted movements. Dystonic tremor usually appears in young or middle-aged adults and can affect any muscle in the body. Symptoms may sometimes be relieved by complete relaxation.

Although some of the symptoms are similar, dystonic tremor differs from essential tremor in some ways. The dystonic tremor:

- Is associated with abnormal body postures, due to forceful muscle spasms or cramps

- Can affect the same parts of the body as essential tremor, but it can also—and more often than essential tremor—affect the head, without any other movement in the hands or arms

- Can also mimic resting tremor, such as the one seen in Parkinson disease

* May be reduced by touching the affected body part or muscle, and tremor movements are "jerky" or irregular instead of rhythmic

Cerebellar Tremor

Cerebellar tremor is typically a slow, high amplitude (easily visible) tremor of the extremities (e.g., arm, leg) that occurs at the end of a purposeful movement, such as trying to press a button. It is caused by damage to the cerebellum and its pathways to other brain regions, resulting from a stroke or tumor. Damage also may be caused by a disease, such as multiple sclerosis, or an inherited degenerative disorder, such as ataxia (in which people lose muscle control in the arms and legs) and Fragile X syndrome (FXS) (a disorder marked by a range of intellectual and developmental problems). It can also result from chronic damage to the cerebellum, due to alcoholism.

Psychogenic Tremor

Psychogenic tremor (also called "functional tremor") can appear as any form of tremor. Its symptoms may vary but often start abruptly and may affect all body parts. The tremor increases in times of stress and decreases or disappears when distracted. Many individuals with psychogenic tremor have an underlying psychiatric disorder, such as depression or posttraumatic stress disorder (PTSD).

Physiologic Tremor

Physiologic tremor occurs in all healthy individuals. It is rarely visible to the eye and typically involves a fine shaking of both of the hands and also the fingers. It is not considered a disease but is a normal human phenomenon that is the result of physical properties in the body (for example, rhythmical activities, such as heartbeat and muscle activation).

Enhanced Physiologic Tremor

Enhanced physiological tremor is a more noticeable case of physiologic tremor that can be easily seen. It is generally not caused by a neurological disease but by a reaction to certain drugs, alcohol withdrawal, or medical conditions, including an overactive thyroid and hypoglycemia. It is usually reversible once the cause is corrected.

Parkinsonian Tremor

Parkinsonian tremor is a common symptom of Parkinson disease, although not all people with Parkinson disease have tremor. Generally, symptoms include shaking in one or both hands at rest. It may also affect the chin, lips, face, and legs. The tremor may initially appear in only one limb or on just one side of the body. As the disease progresses, it may spread to both sides of the body. The tremor is often made worse by stress or strong emotions. More than 25 percent of people with Parkinson disease also have an associated action tremor.

Orthostatic Tremor

Orthostatic tremor is a rare disorder characterized by rapid muscle contractions in the legs that occur when standing. People typically experience feelings of unsteadiness or imbalance, causing them to immediately attempt to sit or walk. Because the tremor has such a high frequency (very fast shaking), it may not visible to the naked eye. However, the tremor can be felt by touching the thighs or calves, or it can be detected by a doctor examining the muscles with a stethoscope. In some cases, the tremor can become more severe over time. The cause of orthostatic tremor is unknown.

How Is Tremor Diagnosed?

Tremor is diagnosed based on a physical and neurological examination and an individual's medical history. During the physical evaluation, a doctor will assess the tremor based on:

- Whether the tremor occurs when the muscles are at rest or in action

- The location of the tremor on the body (and if it occurs on one or both sides of the body)

- The appearance of the tremor (tremor frequency and amplitude)

The doctor will also check other neurological findings, such as impaired balance, speech abnormalities, or increased muscle stiffness. Blood or urine tests can rule out metabolic causes, such as thyroid malfunction and certain medications, that can cause tremor. These tests may also help to identify contributing causes, such as drug interactions, chronic alcoholism, or other conditions or diseases. Diagnostic imaging may help determine if the tremor is the result of damage in the brain.

Additional tests may be administered to determine functional limitations, such as difficulty with handwriting or the ability to hold a fork or cup. Individuals may be asked to perform a series of tasks or exercises, such as placing a finger on the tip of their nose or drawing a spiral.

The doctor may order an electromyogram (EMG) to diagnose muscle or nerve problems. This test measures involuntary muscle activity and muscle response to nerve stimulation.

How Is Tremor Treated?

Although there is no cure for most forms of tremor, treatment options are available to help manage symptoms. In some cases, a person's symptoms may be mild enough that they do not require treatment.

Finding an appropriate treatment depends on an accurate diagnosis of the cause. Tremor caused by underlying health problems can sometimes be improved or eliminated entirely with treatment. For example, tremor due to thyroid hyperactivity will improve or even resolve (return to the normal state) after treating the thyroid malfunction. Also, if tremor is caused by medication, discontinuing the tremor-causing drug may reduce or eliminate this tremor.

If there is no underlying cause for tremor that can be modified, available treatment options include:

Medication

- Beta blocking drugs, such as propranolol, are normally used to treat high blood pressure, but they also help treat essential tremor. Propranolol can also be used in some people with other types of action tremor. Other beta-blockers that may be used include atenolol, metoprolol, nadolol, and sotalol.

- Antiseizure medications, such as primidone, can be effective in people with essential tremor who do not respond to beta-blockers. Other medications that may be prescribed include gabapentin and topiramate. However, it is important to note that some antiseizure medications can cause tremor.

- Tranquilizers (also known as "benzodiazepines"), such as alprazolam and clonazepam, may temporarily help some people with tremor. However, their use is limited due to unwanted side effects that include sleepiness, poor concentration, and poor coordination. This can affect an individual's ability of performing daily activities, such as driving, going to school, and working. Also, when taken regularly, tranquilizers can cause physical dependence, and when stopped abruptly, they can cause several withdrawal symptoms.

- Parkinson disease medications (levodopa, carbidopa) are used to treat tremor associated with Parkinson disease.

- Botulinum toxin injections can treat almost all types of tremor. It is especially useful for head tremor, which generally does not respond to medications. Botulinum toxin is widely used to control dystonic tremor. Although botulinum toxin injections can improve tremor for roughly three months at a time, they can also cause muscle weakness. While this treatment is effective and usually well tolerated for head tremor, botulinum toxin treatment in the hands can cause weakness in the fingers, a hoarse voice, and difficulty swallowing when used to treat voice tremor.

Focused Ultrasound

A new treatment for essential tremor uses magnetic resonance images to deliver focused ultrasound to create a lesion in tiny areas of the brain's thalamus thought to be responsible for causing the tremors. The treatment is approved only for those individuals with essential tremor who do not respond well to anticonvulsant or beta blocking drugs.

Surgery

When people do not respond to drug therapies or have a severe tremor that significantly impacts their daily life, a doctor may recommend surgical interventions, such as deep brain stimulation (DBS) or, very rarely, thalamotomy. While DBS is usually well tolerated, the most common side effects of tremor surgery include dysarthria (trouble speaking) and balance problems.

- Deep brain stimulation is the most common form of surgical treatment of tremor. This method is preferred because it is effective, low risk, and treats a broader range of symptoms than thalamotomy. The treatment uses surgically implanted electrodes to send high frequency electrical signals to the thalamus, the deep structure of the brain that coordinates and controls some involuntary movements. A small pulse-generating device placed under the skin in the upper chest (similar to a pacemaker) sends electrical stimuli to the brain and temporarily disables the tremor. DBS is currently used to treat parkinsonian tremor, essential tremor, and dystonia.

- Thalamotomy is a surgical procedure that involves the precise, permanent destruction of a tiny area in the thalamus. Currently, surgery is replaced by radiofrequency ablation to treat severe tremor when deep brain surgery is contraindicated—meaning it is unwise as a treatment option or has undesirable side effects. Radiofrequency ablation uses a radio wave to generate an electric current that heats up a nerve and disrupts its signaling ability for typically six months or more. It is usually performed on only one side of the brain to improve tremor on the opposite side of the body. Surgery on both sides is not recommended as it can cause problems with speech.

Lifestyle Changes

- Physical, speech-language, and occupational therapy may help to control tremor and daily challenges caused by the tremor. A physical therapist can help people improve their muscle control, functioning, and strength through coordination, balancing, and other exercises. Some therapists recommend the use of weights, splints, other adaptive equipment, and special plates and utensils for eating. Speech-language pathologists can evaluate and treat speech, language, communication, and swallowing disorders. Occupational therapists can teach individuals new ways of performing activities of daily living that may be affected by tremor.

- Eliminating or reducing tremor-inducing substances, such as caffeine and other medication (such as stimulants), can help improve tremor. Though small amounts of alcohol can improve tremor for some people, tremor can become worse once the effects of the alcohol wear off.

What Is the Prognosis?

Tremor is not considered a life-threatening condition. Although many cases of tremor are mild, tremor can be very disabling for other people. It can be difficult for individuals with tremor to perform normal daily activities, such as working, bathing, dressing, and eating. Tremor can also cause "social disability." People may limit their physical activity, travel, and social engagements to avoid embarrassment or other consequences.

The symptoms of essential tremor usually worsen with age. Additionally, there is some evidence that people with essential tremor are more likely than average to develop other neurodegenerative conditions, such as Parkinson disease or Alzheimer disease, especially in individuals whose tremor first appears after the age of 65.

Unlike essential tremor, the symptoms of physiologic and drug-induced tremor do not generally worsen over time and can often be improved or eliminated once the underlying causes are treated.

What Research Is Being Done?

The mission of the National Institute of Neurological Disorders and Stroke (NINDS) is to seek fundamental knowledge about the brain and nervous system and use that knowledge to reduce the burden of neurological disease. The NINDS is a component of the National Institutes of Health (NIH), the leading supporter of biomedical research in the world.

Researchers are working to better understand the underlying brain functions that cause tremor, identify the genetic factors that make individuals more susceptible to the disorder, and develop new and better treatment options.

Brain Functioning

It can be difficult to distinguish between movement disorders, such as Parkinson disease, and essential tremor. These debilitating movement disorders have different prognoses and can respond very differently to available therapies. NINDS researchers are working to identify structural and functional changes in the brain using non-invasive neuroimaging techniques to develop sensitive and specific markers for each of these diseases and then track how they change as each disease progresses.

Other researchers are using functional magnetic resonance imaging technology to better understand normal and diseased brain circuit functions and associated motor behaviors. Scientists hope to design therapies that can restore normal brain circuit function in diseases such as Parkinson disease and tremor.

Genetics

Research has shown that essential tremor may have a strong genetic component affecting multiple generations of families. NINDS researchers are building on previous genetics work to identify susceptibility genes for familial early-onset (before the age of 40) essential tremor. Researchers are focusing on multigenerational, early-onset families to better detect linkages.

Additionally, NINDS scientists are researching the impact of genetic abnormalities on the development of essential tremor. Previous research has shown a link between essential tremor and possible genetic variants on chromosome 6 and 11; ongoing research is targeting the impact of other genetic variations in families.

Medications and Other Treatment Methods

While drugs can be effective for some people, approximately 50 percent of individuals do not respond to medication. In order to develop assistive and rehabilitative tremor-suppressing devices for people with essential tremor, researchers are exploring where and how to minimize or suppress tremor while still allowing for voluntary movements.

Many people with essential tremor respond to ethanol (alcohol); however, it is not clear why or how. NINDS researchers are studying the impact of ethanol on tremor to determine the correct dosage amount and its physiological impact on the brain and whether other medications, without the side effects of ethanol, can be effective.

Other NIH researchers hope to identify the source of essential tremor, study the effects of currently available tremor-suppressant drugs on the brain, and develop more targeted and effective therapies.

Chapter 14

Fatigue in People with Multiple Sclerosis

Symptoms of multiple sclerosis (MS) are varied and numerous. Among them, fatigue is one of the most common and important problems. It is associated with a reduced quality of life (QOL) and interferes with the ability to function both at home and at work. It is one of the most important reasons why many people with MS have to leave the workforce early.

People with MS who struggle with fatigue are far from alone. About 75 to 95 percent of people with MS report fatigue as a problem, and half of these people say that fatigue is their single worst problem. There is a need to better understand the causes of fatigue in MS and to develop better strategies for coping with this problem.

What Is Fatigue in Multiple Sclerosis?

Fatigue in MS is defined as an overwhelming sense of tiredness, lack of energy, or a feeling of exhaustion. It is distinct from weakness, and it is different than depression. Fatigue alone, even in the apparent absence of other physical symptoms, may significantly slow people with MS, who otherwise have no physical impairments or disabilities,

This chapter includes text excerpted from "VA Multiple Sclerosis Centers of Excellence—Living with MS," U.S. Department of Veterans Affairs (VA), 2009. Reviewed March 2019.

simply by limiting their ability to participate. For those without MS, it can be described as the feeling of fatigue we feel when we get the flu.

What Causes Fatigue in Multiple Sclerosis

The causes for fatigue in MS are not fully understood; a specific, affected location of the brain that could explain the fatigue in MS has not yet been identified. Imaging studies have not shown a significant association between lesion size or number with the severity of fatigue in MS.

Depression may contribute to fatigue and should be evaluated and treated if it is a problem. However, depression alone cannot fully explain the extent of fatigue experienced by so many, particularly those who do not experience any depression.

Some hypothesize that the fatigue in MS may result from the direct effects of inflammatory enzymes released in the blood and nervous tissue. These chemicals may be released as a part of the chronic inflammation that occurs in MS. Another hallmark of MS is the injury to the myelin covering the nerves. Without this myelin covering, signals are not transmitted as efficiently. An increased energy demand of conducting signals down these injured, demyelinated axons may also contribute to fatigue. Possible abnormalities in hormonal regulation have also been linked to fatigue in MS. The control of certain hormonal responses to physical stress may contribute to how fatigue affects people. In the end, it is likely that there are different contributions from multiple causes of fatigue in MS.

How Can Fatigue in Multiple Sclerosis Be Treated?

Goals of treatment are to reduce fatigue severity, improve QOL, and help people reach their goals. This is first done by addressing contributing factors of fatigue, such as depression. If someone is depressed, that must be treated first. No progress will be made toward reducing MS fatigue while significant depression is present. If someone has impaired sleep, this should also be evaluated and treated. If someone is inactive, deconditioned, or taking medications that are responsible for fatigue, each must be addressed to reduce fatigue. These factors should be evaluated by a healthcare provider.

Keep in mind that physical therapy and exercise can be beneficial for someone trying to battle fatigue. For example, yoga and aerobic exercise have been shown to positively impact fatigue in clinical trials. Keeping cool, sometimes by using a cooling vest, can be helpful since fatigue is made worse by heat. Other good strategies include taking rest periods, doing endurance training, and having a regular sleep schedule. It is also important to reassure people that this fatigue is a part of MS. Fatigue in MS is not a product of being lazy. It is a part of MS, and it can improve. There are a number of different medications that have been used successfully for fatigue in MS. One of the first was amantadine, which is actually an antiflu agent. Its benefit was discovered by accident.

A physician in Canada (who happened to have MS) was taking amantadine for the flu and noticed that, while he was taking the medication, his fatigue was less prominent. This led to several research studies that showed it was an effective treatment for many people with MS.

Another frequently used medication that may be helpful for fatigue in MS is modafinil. Although it is not universally effective for all people with MS, many people have benefitted. In some cases, a stimulant called "methylphenidate" has also been tried. However, it has not been studied in an MS clinical trial, and it can be addicting in some circumstances. The VA also recently completed a clinical trial of ginseng for fatigue in MS. Although the study did not show a significant benefit overall, many people in the study reported some improvement in their fatigue while on ginseng.

In the end, fatigue can be treated. Please share your concerns with your healthcare provider. There are a variety of medications and rehabilitation strategies that are available to address fatigue and other MS symptoms.

Chapter 15

Speech and Swallowing Problems Associated with Multiple Sclerosis

Approximately 40 percent of people with multiple sclerosis (MS) will experience speech and/or swallowing problems. MS can damage the nerves that aid in speech and swallowing. Depending upon the area that is damaged, MS lesions can impact the lips, tongue, soft palate, vocal cords, and diaphragm muscles that control speech patterns. Damage to the brain can also interfere with the ability to produce or understand words; this is called "aphasia." In addition, because many of the muscles that aid in speech are also part of the swallowing function, MS lesions can impact the ability to swallow. Impairment can impact not only communication, but it can also affect an individual's interactions with others.

Speech

Speech is a highly complex process that depends on finely controlled and coordinated muscles. Speech problems, also called "dysarthrias," can include speech that is slurred, slow, very soft, or nasal sounding.

This chapter includes text excerpted from "VA Multiple Sclerosis Centers of Excellence—A Second Generation Veteran with MS," U.S. Department of Veterans Affairs (VA), 2012. Reviewed March 2019.

Speech that can't seem to keep up with your thoughts, causing long pauses between your thoughts and words (scanned speech), is a common occurrence with people who have MS. For a thorough evaluation of your speech disorder, it is important to see a speech and language pathologist (SLP). They can help you develop skills and techniques to manage your speech impairment such as:

- **Exercise your speech muscles.** Your SLP can provide you with exercises that can be practiced daily to improve function and strengthen the muscles that support breath control and speech production. These exercises will also promote relaxation of these muscles.

- **Practice speech techniques.** Your SLP can teach you techniques that can slow down your speech, help with your phrasing and pausing to help make speech more clear, and can demonstrate how to over articulate words to make your speech more understandable.

- **Self-monitor your speech patterns.** Use a recording device to capture how you speak. This allows you to correct some of your speech issues by adjusting your volume or phrasing.

- **Use new devices and current technology to assist with your speech.** Devices, such as voice amplification, electronic aids, and other computer-assisted communication systems, are readily available and easy to use. Many programs can be downloaded for free on the Internet.

- **Practice speech in group settings.** Involving supportive friends and family who can provide you with feedback on your speech patterns will be helpful.

- **Consider medications.** Check with your healthcare provider about medications that can improve speech by helping the affected muscles.

Swallowing

As MS progresses, swallowing problems, also called "dysphagia," can increase. These problems include difficulty with chewing or starting the swallowing process, a feeling of a sticking sensation, frequent throat clearing, or a choking sensation when you eat or drink. Some people might also experience an unintentional inhaling of food or liquid into the airways. This is called "aspiration" and sometimes referred to as "going down the wrong pipe."

Difficulty with swallowing interferes with eating and the desire to eat, which can lead to poor nutrition and dehydration. The overall goal of treating swallowing problems is to maximize the safety and efficiency of eating. To create a safe-eating environment, the swallowing techniques listed below should be routinely practiced.

1. Sit upright when eating or drinking.

2. Take smaller bites of food, eat slowly, and do not speak when food is in your mouth.

3. Sip drinks, do not gulp.

4. Double swallows might be needed. Double swallows refers to swallowing once to send liquids or food down then doing a dry swallow to clear any leftover particles.

5. Add moisture/liquid to foods. Foods with moisture are easier to swallow.

6. Eat smaller portions. If you are experiencing fatigue, which can interfere with swallowing, try to consume smaller meals throughout the day instead of one or two large meals.

It is very important that a multidisciplinary healthcare team be involved in managing speech and swallowing problems. This team should include patients, family members, and caregivers who can provide essential feedback to providers as to what is working in the home environment and when modifications are needed to address these problems.

Improved speech can increase your ability to communicate with others, as well as improve relationships. It is important to have a SLP complete a full evaluation so specific treatment recommendations can be made.

Chapter 16

Vocal Fold Paralysis

What Is Vocal Fold Paralysis?

Vocal fold paralysis (also known as "vocal cord paralysis") is a voice disorder that occurs when one or both of the vocal folds don't open or close properly. Single vocal fold paralysis is a common disorder. Paralysis of both vocal folds is rare and can be life threatening.

The vocal folds are two elastic bands of muscle tissue located in the larynx (voice box) directly above the trachea (windpipe) (see figure 16.1). When you breathe, your vocal folds remain apart, and when you swallow, they are tightly closed. When you use your voice, however, air from the lungs causes your vocal folds to vibrate between open and closed positions.

If you have vocal fold paralysis, the paralyzed fold or folds may remain open, leaving the air passages and lungs unprotected. You could have difficulty swallowing, or food or liquids could accidentally enter the trachea and lungs, causing serious health problems.

What Causes Vocal Fold Paralysis

Vocal fold paralysis may be caused by injury to the head, neck, or chest; lung or thyroid cancer; tumors of the skull base, neck, or chest; or infection (for example, Lyme disease). People with certain neurologic

This chapter includes text excerpted from "Vocal Fold Paralysis," National Institute on Deafness and Other Communication Disorders (NIDCD), March 6, 2017.

conditions, such as multiple sclerosis (MS) or Parkinson disease, or who have sustained a stroke, may experience vocal fold paralysis. In many cases, however, the cause is unknown.

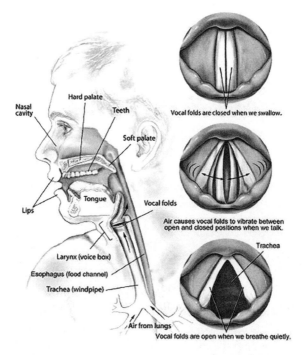

Figure 16.1. *Structures Involved in Speech and Voice Production*

What Are the Symptoms?

Symptoms of vocal fold paralysis include changes in the voice, such as hoarseness or a breathy voice; difficulties with breathing, such as shortness of breath or noisy breathing; and swallowing problems, such as choking or coughing when you eat because food accidentally enters the windpipe instead of the esophagus (the muscular tube that connects the throat to the stomach). Changes in voice quality, such as loss of volume or pitch, also may occur. Damage to both vocal folds, although rare, usually causes serious problems with breathing.

How Is Vocal Fold Paralysis Diagnosed?

Vocal fold paralysis is usually diagnosed by an otolaryngologist—a doctor who specializes in ear, nose, and throat disorders. He or she will ask you about your symptoms and when the problems began in order to help determine their cause. The otolaryngologist will also listen to your voice to identify breathiness or hoarseness. Using an endoscope—a tube with a light at the end—your doctor will look directly into the throat at the vocal folds. Some doctors also use a procedure called "laryngeal electromyography," which measures the electrical impulses of the nerves in the larynx, to better understand the areas of paralysis.

How Is Vocal Fold Paralysis Treated?

The most common treatments for vocal fold paralysis are voice therapy and surgery. Some people's voices will naturally recover sometime during the first year after diagnosis, which is why doctors often delay surgery for at least a year. During this time, your doctor will likely refer you to a speech-language pathologist for voice therapy, which may involve exercises to strengthen the vocal folds or improve breath control while speaking. You might also learn how to use your voice differently, for example, by speaking more slowly or opening your mouth wider when you speak. Several surgical procedures are available, depending on whether one or both of your vocal folds are paralyzed. The most common procedures change the position of the vocal fold. These may involve inserting a structural implant or stitches to reposition the laryngeal cartilage and bringing the vocal folds closer together. These procedures usually result in a stronger voice. Surgery is followed by additional voice therapy to help fine-tune the voice.

When both vocal folds are paralyzed, a tracheotomy may be required to help breathing. In a tracheotomy, an incision is made in the front of the neck and a breathing tube is inserted through an opening, called a "stoma," into the trachea. Rather than occurring through the nose and mouth, breathing now happens through the tube. Following surgery, therapy with a speech-language pathologist helps you learn how to use the voice and how to properly care for the breathing tube.

What Research Is Being Done on Vocal Fold Paralysis?

The National Institute on Deafness and Other Communication Disorders (NIDCD) supports research studies that explore the causes of vocal fold paralysis, as well as better ways to treat the disorder. One surgical procedure, called "medialization laryngoplasty," inserts a structural implant into the larynx to return voice quality. However, close to a quarter of the people who receive this treatment must return for repositioning surgery to fine-tune the placement of the implant. An NIDCD-supported researcher currently is developing a preoperative planning system that uses three dimensional (3-D) computer modeling to determine the best location for, and configuration of, the implant. The surgery also uses an image-guided system that allows the surgeon to visualize the precise location of the vocal fold to ensure exact placement of the implant. Researchers hope this new system will reduce the need for repeated surgeries and lower the cost and risk of surgical complications from the procedure.

The NIDCD also has been supporting a decades-long project to develop an electrical stimulation technology to help people avoid having a tracheotomy when both vocal folds are paralyzed. The device, which currently is being tested in animals and people, uses an implanted pacemaker to stimulate laryngeal nerves. This returns mobility to the vocal folds so that they can open to allow breathing and close to allow speaking and swallowing.

Where Can I Get Help?

If you notice any unexplained voice changes or discomfort, you should consult an otolaryngologist or a speech-language pathologist for evaluation and possible treatment.

Chapter 17

Vision Problem and Multiple Sclerosis

Eye and vision problems are common in people with multiple sclerosis (MS) but rarely result in permanent blindness. Inflammation of the optic nerve or damage to the myelin that covers the optic nerve and other nerve fibers can cause a number of symptoms, including blurring or graying of vision, blindness in one eye, loss of normal color vision, depth perception, or a dark spot in the center of the visual field (scotoma).

Uncontrolled horizontal or vertical eye movements (nystagmus) and "jumping vision" (opsoclonus) are common to MS, and can be either mild or severe enough to impair vision.

Double vision (diplopia) occurs when both eyes are not perfectly aligned. This occurs commonly in MS when a pair of muscles that control a specific eye movement aren't coordinated due to weakness in one or both muscles. Double vision may increase with fatigue or

This chapter contains text excerpted from the following sources: Text in this chapter begins with excerpts from "Multiple Sclerosis: Hope through Research," National Institute of Neurological Disorders and Stroke (NINDS), July 6, 2018; Text under the heading "Multiple Sclerosis-Associated Optic Neuritis" is excerpted from "VA Multiple Sclerosis Centers of Excellence—We Keep Going... and Going..." U.S. Department of Veterans Affairs (VA), 2012. Reviewed March 2019; Text under the heading "Multiple Sclerosis-Associated Uveitis" is excerpted from "Facts about Uveitis," National Eye Institute (NEI), August 2011. Reviewed March 2019.

as the result of spending too much time reading or on the computer. Periodically resting the eyes may be helpful.

Multiple Sclerosis-Associated Optic Neuritis

Vision is very important in almost everything we do, including watching television, reading a book, driving, and many other activities. When MS disturbs vision, it can have a significant impact on an individual's quality of life (QOL). People with MS can have many different kinds of vision problems, one of the most common being optic neuritis (ON).

Optic neuritis is caused by inflammation or demyelination of the optic nerve, the nerve that connects the eye to the brain. People with optic neuritis generally complain of blurry vision or hazy vision affecting one eye. Often the center of vision is most affected, making it difficult to see people's faces or creating a "line" in the center of vision. Some people with optic neuritis describe the blur as a film over their eye. Color perception is usually affected as well, with colors seeming faded or less intense in the eye that is affected by optic neuritis. Optic neuritis is often associated with some eye pain or discomfort, especially with eye movements, which may be described as an ache or sticking sensation behind the eye.

Treating Optic Neuritis

In optic neuritis, the blurring of vision may gradually worsen over the course of a week or so. Afterward, there is usually a gradual recovery of vision, occurring over a four to six week period. Intravenous (IV) methylprednisolone (a type of steroid known as "Solu-Medrol®") is often given to treat optic neuritis. IV steroids do not appear to improve the ultimate visual outcome, but they do seem to speed up vision recovery. With or without steroid treatment, optic neuritis almost always gets better, though the vision in the affected eye may not return 100 percent. Vision in the optic neuritis eye might not be as clear as before, and colors may remain faded or washed out. Depth perception, or 3-D vision, is often not as good after an episode of optic neuritis, making it more difficult to judge distances, as when climbing stairs or reaching for objects.

Predicting Multiple Sclerosis Risk with Brain Magnetic Resonance Imaging

More than half of all people with MS will experience optic neuritis at some point in their lives. In fact, for 15 to 20 percent of people with

MS, optic neuritis will be the first sign of the disease. Not all people who get optic neuritis, however, will go on to develop MS. Many studies have examined the relationship between optic neuritis and MS over time. Depending on the study, the risk of developing MS after an episode of optic neuritis varies from 42 to 63 percent, which roughly equates to 50/50 odds.

Brain magnetic resonance imaging (MRI) can be very useful in predicting which person with optic neuritis will go on to develop MS. People with optic neuritis who have a normal brain MRI scan have a relatively low risk of going on to develop MS, ranging from 8 to 25 percent, depending on the study. People with optic neuritis who have demyelination (also called "spots," "plaques," or "lesions") on their brain MRI have a much higher risk of developing MS, possibly as high as 80 percent.

Though this risk is significant, and much greater than the risk of MS in people who start out with a normal brain MRI, it should be noted that 20 to 40 percent of the high-risk individuals in these studies who had an episode of optic neuritis did not go on to develop MS, even after many years of follow-up.

Though optic neuritis generally goes away on its own, with or without treatment, it is still important for people with optic neuritis to be seen by a neurologist to find out if a development of MS is likely. For people who already have a diagnosis of MS, it may still be important to see a neurologist after an episode of optic neuritis to review MS treatment options.

Multiple Sclerosis-Associated Uveitis

Uveitis is a general term describing a group of inflammatory diseases that produces swelling and destroys eye tissues. These diseases can slightly reduce vision or lead to severe vision loss. The term "uveitis" is used because the diseases often affect a part of the eye called the "uvea." Nevertheless, uveitis is not limited to the uvea. These diseases also affect the lens, retina, optic nerve, and vitreous, and produce reduced vision or blindness. Uveitis may be caused by problems or diseases occurring in the eye, or it can be part of an inflammatory disease affecting other parts of the body.

What Is the Uvea and What Parts of the Eye Are Most Affected by Uveitis?

The uvea is the middle layer of the eye which contains much of the eye's blood vessels. This is one way that inflammatory cells can enter the eye. Located between the sclera (the eye's white outer coat) and the inner layer of the eye (called the "retina"), the uvea consists of the iris, ciliary body, and choroid.

- **Iris:** The colored circle at the front of the eye. It defines eye color, secretes nutrients to keep the lens healthy, and controls the amount of light that enters the eye by adjusting the size of the pupil.

- **Ciliary body:** It is located between the iris and the choroid. It helps the eye focus by controlling the shape of the lens, and it provides nutrients to keep the lens healthy.

- **Choroid:** A thin, spongy network of blood vessels, which primarily provides nutrients to the retina.

Uveitis disrupts vision by primarily causing problems with the lens, retina, optic nerve, and vitreous.

- **Lens:** A transparent tissue that allows light into the eye.

- **Retina:** The layer of cells on the back, inside part of the eye that converts light into electrical signals sent to the brain.

- **Optic nerve:** A bundle of nerve fibers that transmits electrical signals from the retina to the brain.

- **Vitreous:** The fluid-filled space inside the eye.

What Causes Uveitis

Uveitis is caused by inflammatory responses inside the eye. Inflammation is the body's natural response to tissue damage, germs, or toxins. It produces swelling, redness, heat, and destroys tissues as certain white blood cells rush to the affected part of the body to contain or eliminate the insult. Intermediate uveitis has been linked to several disorders, such as sarcoidosis and multiple sclerosis (MS). The center of the inflammation often appears in the vitreous.

Uveitis can affect one or both eyes. Anyone suffering severe light sensitivity and experiencing any change in vision should immediately be examined by an ophthalmologist. The signs and symptoms of uveitis depend on the type of inflammation. Intermediate uveitis causes blurred vision and floaters. Usually, it is not associated with pain.

How Is Uveitis Detected?

Diagnosis of uveitis includes a thorough examination and the recording of the patient's complete medical history. Laboratory tests may be done to rule out an infection or an autoimmune disorder.

A central nervous system (CNS) evaluation will often be performed on patients with a subgroup of intermediate uveitis, called "pars planitis," to determine whether they have multiple sclerosis, which is often associated with pars planitis.

The eye exams used include:

- **An eye chart or visual acuity test:** This test measures whether a patient's vision has decreased.

- **A funduscopic exam:** The pupil is widened (dilated) with eye drops, and a light is shown through with an instrument called an "ophthalmoscope" to noninvasively inspect the back, inside part of the eye.

- **Ocular pressure:** An instrument, such a tonometer or a tonopen, measures the pressure inside the eye. Drops that numb the eye may be used for this test.

- **A slit lamp exam:** A slit lamp exam noninvasively inspects a large portion of the eye. It can inspect the front and back parts of the eye, and some lamps may be equipped with a tonometer to measure eye pressure. A dye called "fluorescein," which makes blood vessels easier to see, may be added to the eye during the examination. The dye only temporarily stains the eye.

Chapter 18

Bladder Changes in Multiple Sclerosis

Changes in bladder function are common after developing multiple sclerosis (MS), and they often occur early after the onset. Between 50 to 90 percent of people with MS will develop bladder problems at some point. The big question is—why does this occur?

The symptoms of bladder problems are wide ranging and can include:

- Urgency—barely getting to the bathroom in a timely manner

- Frequency—feeling the need to urinate more than every two to three hours

- Hesitancy—being unable to easily start a flow of urine

- Incontinence—a loss of control of urine

- Nocturia—being awakened from a restful state by a need to urinate

- Double voiding—needing to urinate again a few minutes after voiding

---

This chapter includes text excerpted from "VA Multiple Sclerosis Centers of Excellence—Never Give Up!" U.S. Department of Veterans Affairs (VA), 2011. Reviewed March 2019.

Other symptoms may include feeling as if the bladder isn't empty after urinating, an involuntary leaking of urine, a difficult or painful discharge of urine, and urinary tract infections (UTIs).

Bladder symptoms are broken down into three basic types of problems: emptying problems (hypoactive bladder), storage problems (hyperactive bladder), and a combination of the previous two problems (combined dysfunction). Each of these types of problems has a different treatment approach.

Hypoactive Bladder

Approximately 20 percent of people with MS have a hypoactive bladder. A hypoactive bladder overfills and stretches the bladder wall, causing the sensors that trigger bladder contractions to stop working. Additionally, the sphincter that allows urine to leave the bladder often doesn't release, and the urge to urinate doesn't occur until after a large volume of urine has collected. The danger with this type of bladder problem is that when the bladder becomes overfilled, urine can back up into the kidneys, causing kidney damage or infection.

The methods used to treat this condition are abdominal tapping (tapping on your lower abdomen to trigger a urination reflex), double voiding, adequate fluid intake, good bowel management, catheterization (intermittent catheterization or indwelling Foley/suprapubic urinary catheter) and, for males, good prostate care. Medications, such as bethanechol, to stimulate bladder contractions or prostate/antihypertension medications to reduce prostate swelling have been successfully used.

Hyperactive Bladder

The majority of people with MS (60%) have the opposite type of bladder—a hyperactive bladder. A hyperactive bladder doesn't hold the normal amount of urine before the urge to urinate occurs. Instead of triggering urination when it fills to 350 to 400 ml (normal), the urge occurs at 150 to 200 ml (or less), making it important to always know where every bathroom is located.

Treatments for this type of problem include decreasing irritants that trigger bladder spasms (caffeine, artificial sweeteners, alcohol, tobacco, spicy foods), reducing excessive weight, practicing good bowel care (to reduce the amount of abdominal pressure on the bladder), pelvic-muscle exercises (especially with women), and learning to manage when and where urination occurs.

Managing urine output can involve a number of strategies, such as wearing easily removable lower garments, using external urinary-drainage devices or protective pads/garments, and determining what the best time and amount of fluid intake should be. Changing the volume or time at which fluids are consumed will help make sure the need to urinate doesn't occur at inopportune times.

The last common treatment strategy is the use of medications. Common medications used include antispasmodics (such as baclofen), bladder-relaxing medications (such as oxybutynin and tolterodine), or botulinum toxin (Botox) injections into the bladder sphincter.

Combined Dysfunction

The third type of problem is a combination of these first two problems and may be more difficult to treat. With this type of bladder dysfunction, the bladder wall spasms, but the sphincter releasing urine won't relax and open. Finding the correct balance of the above treatments that work best can be a trial-and-error process. Most people are able to find a combination of treatment strategies that work well for them by working with their healthcare provider.

Chapter 19

Cognitive Deficits in People with Multiple Sclerosis

Cognition refers to a person's ability to perform high-level brain functions and includes tasks such as thinking, learning, remembering, and understanding. Approximately 50 percent of individuals with multiple sclerosis (MS) will develop cognitive dysfunction over the course of their disease. For some people, cognitive dysfunction can be very mild and not easily noticed by those around them. For others, it can be significant and make it difficult to work or take care of things at home. When a person has cognitive dysfunction, there may be feelings of depression, anxiety, or insecurity. Three areas that are commonly affected by cognitive dysfunction in MS are information processing, learning and memory, and executive functioning.

Information processing includes working memory and processing speed. We use working memory when we need to remember something but cannot write it down, such as remembering a phone number for a few moments before dialing it. While this can be difficult for most people, those with working memory problems find it even more challenging. Processing speed refers to how quickly we can deal with

This chapter contains text excerpted from the following sources: Text in this chapter begins with excerpts from "VA Multiple Sclerosis Centers of Excellence— Competition Brings out the Best in Me!" U.S. Department of Veterans Affairs (VA), 2013. Reviewed March 2019; Text beginning with the heading "What to Do If You Have Concerns about Thinking Skills" is excerpted from "Multiple Sclerosis and Cognition: Patient Fact Sheet," U.S. Department of Veterans Affairs (VA), n.d.

information that we see or hear. A person with slowed processing speed might have difficulty keeping up with conversations and feel as if others are talking too quickly. If processing speed is particularly slow, it is important for that individual to not be placed in danger, such as driving a vehicle. Problems with information processing can also make other cognitive functions difficult, such as problem-solving or memory.

People with MS can have problems with certain aspects of **learning and memory**. Remembering the name of your third-grade teacher or what you ate for breakfast are two examples of what is called "episodic memory." People with MS can usually remember things from their childhood, but may have difficulty remembering things that happened yesterday. Studies have shown that people with memory problems because of MS tend to remember more when information is repeated or when they have reminders.

Executive functioning is a broad term that refers to things such as organizing an event, multitasking, and problem-solving. An individual with such problems might find it difficult to plan a party for a large group of friends or to "let go" of a topic in a conversation and move on to a new one. This can be even more noticeable if the person also has a slowed processing speed and these tasks have to happen quickly.

Although there is no cure for cognitive dysfunction because of MS, there are things that people can do to try to lessen the effects.

Working memory tools: It can be helpful to write down phone numbers, addresses, directions, shopping needs, etc. as soon as you learn them. A calendar, organizer, or application on a computer or smartphone are good for tracking appointments and activities for you and your family. These can also be used to remember names, as well as conversations. If you tend to lose things, pick a designated place for objects. Using visual reminders is a great way to keep on track. For example, place the laundry basket upside down in an obvious location when laundry is being washed.

Processing speed tools: If you find that you can't keep up with a conversation, ask people to slow down when talking to you or ask them to repeat themselves. Allow yourself extra time to complete tasks, and plan your most challenging tasks at a time of day when you feel your best. If you feel like something is taking too long to complete, take a short breather and come back to it with a fresh mind.

Executive functioning tools: Give your full attention to the task at hand, and reduce the noise and distractions around you. Trying to do too many things at once can be difficult and overwhelming. Get organized, or have someone help you get organized. Reducing clutter can improve your focus. If you run into a problem you just can't solve, ask for some advice or find someone that can help.

Getting enough sleep, maintaining adequate nutrition, and taking care of your physical and emotional needs can also be useful. While it can take time and practice to get used to doing these things, many people find them helpful, and studies have shown that using such strategies can make someone feel less depressed or anxious.

If you have any concerns about cognitive dysfunction, talk to a medical provider. Early assessment and treatment are important, as cognitive dysfunction may affect quality of life (QOL). In some cases, it might be helpful to see a neuropsychologist who is a doctor with specialized training in cognitive problems. This type of doctor can do specific testing to see if there are problems and, if so, how severe they are. Once a person knows if she/he is having cognitive problems and what type, the individual can work with a doctor or therapist to come up with strategies to help manage the cognitive challenges.

What to Do If You Have Concerns about Thinking Skills

- The first step is to discuss this with your medical or mental-health care providers. They will assist you in addressing your concerns and may refer you to a specialist for further evaluation.

- Your healthcare provider may ask questions to better understand your symptoms. For example:

  - When did these symptoms start?

  - What are some examples?

  - How do they affect your daily life?

- You may be referred for a neuropsychological evaluation. This may include an interview and taking standardized paper-and-pencil tests designed to assess thinking skills.

- You may be referred for a treatment called "cognitive rehabilitation (CR)." This is a treatment designed to help with thinking difficulties. Your healthcare provider can refer you to a clinical specialist (e.g., neuropsychologist, speech-language pathologist, and occupational therapist) for this treatment.

Some Ways to Improve Thinking Skills
Cognitive Strategies

- **Memory:** set alarms and reminders to prompt you to complete tasks, attend appointments, or take your medication

- **Attention/concentration:** when you need to concentrate, reduce distractions (turn off the TV, go to a quiet room, wear earplugs, etc.)

Positive Health Behaviors

- Plan and organize your day by prioritizing your to-do list and focus on the most important tasks first.

- Practice good sleep hygiene (e.g., set sleep and wake times, avoid screen time in bed).

- Follow medical- and mental-health treatment recommendations.

- Use relaxation strategies (e.g., deep breathing, meditation) to reduce stress.

- Exercise, as it may improve thinking skills, mood, and physical health.

Common Myths about Thinking Skills in People with Multiple Sclerosis

Below are some of the common myths about thinking difficulties in the people who are affected by MS.

Myth: Thinking difficulties are rare in people with MS.

Truth: People with MS commonly have problems with thinking skills, with >50% of people reporting cognitive difficulties.

Myth: Thinking difficulties are only due to MS.

Truth: MS affects brain function and can lead to difficulties with thinking. These problems may be worse in people with other cognitive risk factors (e.g., depression, high blood pressure, alcohol/drug use, sleep problems).

Myth: Thinking difficulties are always a sign of Alzheimer disease (AD).

Truth: Most people with MS do not meet criteria for dementia and do not display the primary symptoms of AD.

Chapter 20

Depression and Anxiety in People with Multiple Sclerosis

Multiple sclerosis (MS) is often experienced as a debilitating illness that creates many hardships for the millions of people with this disease. MS causes a wide range of symptoms, including physical and, sometimes, psychological problems. MS can affect the person's self-image and identity: how they look, behave, think, feel, and how others see them.

Since MS has no clear cause or cure, people with MS often wonder, "Why me?" and struggle with existential questions after receiving this diagnosis. Questions such as "What does my life mean now?" and "Is there any hope?" are common. The difficulty with not knowing how this occurred and how they will deal with it can trigger a sense of hopelessness, unfairness, and even victimization—as if life itself has done them "dirty." Some people experience MS as trauma in their lives. This is especially true given that the attack of symptoms themselves are unpredictable. Dealing with disability associated with MS can trigger strong feelings of anxiety and depression. In addition, MS can cause depression directly, likely because of lesions in the brain and the inflammation associated with the disease.

This chapter includes text excerpted from "VA Multiple Sclerosis Centers of Excellence—Do It Yourself," U.S. Department of Veterans Affairs (VA), 2018.

Depression and anxiety in people with MS can go less noticed than the physical symptoms. But depression and anxiety are common with MS and can have more impact on the person's daily functioning than the physical symptoms. They can linger in the shadows, influencing the person to see themselves in a negative fashion. And, by the time the person recognizes the depression and anxiety, it may already have a significant amount of power and influence in their lives, shaping almost every decision they make on a day-to-day basis.

MS can cause a profound sense of fear that can shake a person's most fundamental beliefs (e.g., belief in a "just world"). And at the root of this fear is an internalized feeling of helplessness, which can lead the person to feel as if they always need to be "on guard" from future MS attacks and increased disability. This "on guard" behavior can lead people to develop coping mechanisms rooted in avoidance. To cope, people with MS will often avoid going out in public, being in crowds, or being around others (including family and friends)—preferring to isolate. Isolation can have devastating impacts on a person's life and is one of the main symptoms of both depression and anxiety. Isolation cuts people off from things they used to do for fun, people they love, and those who support them. Isolation stops people from participating in things that make life feel good to them. Over time, isolation also magnifies feelings of anger, as life may begin to feel more and more unfair. Trust and intimacy problems are also common, as the person is likely to see herself/himself as a "burden" and feel as if others cannot understand what they are going through.

There are several telltale signs of depression and anxiety. Depression is referred to as "the absence or decrease of positive emotionality." The hallmark sign of depression is a pronounced decrease in the amount of positive emotions the person experiences (e.g., pride, joy, happiness, satisfaction). Depression is the absence of the "spark" in the person's life and may be a by-product of the isolation and the physical limitations imposed by MS. With depression, as the person loses their "spark," they may begin to feel as if their life has no meaning or is not worth living. Anxiety, on the other hand, is an increase of negative emotions. Unlike depression, with anxiety everything "ramps up too fast"—the heart beats faster, thoughts "race," you sweat more, etc. People with MS often experience both depression and anxiety; in general, it will impact their sleep, interest, guilt, energy, concentration, appetite, psychomotor (i.e., how fast they move/think), and degree of suicidal ideation. If you or your loved one is experiencing changes in these areas, it is possible that you/they have depression and/or anxiety.

In addition to antidepressant and antianxiety medications, there are things you can do to help with depression and anxiety associated with MS. There are four main protective factors, grounded in solid research, that can help with depression and anxiety: diet, exercise, social support, and an emphasis on posttraumatic growth. Specific to diet, eating a balanced, healthy diet can promote healthy brain function. Although exercise may be difficult, it is important to stay as active as you can for as long as you can. Social support is also key as it lessens the feelings of "aloneness" you or your loved one might be feeling. Try to set a target to find five really solid people you can learn to trust with what you are going through. Having a few good people in your life can greatly impact your mood.

Lastly, remember that growth is possible. Many people report positive changes in their lives after traumas, even including a diagnosis of MS. Find out what others did, how they approached redefining meaning in their lives, and what their secrets to success were. Therapy or counseling that focuses on these factors can be a "gamechanger" in a person's experience of depression and anxiety related to MS. Do not be afraid to reach out to improve the quality of you or your loved one's life.

Part Three

Diagnostic Tests, Treatments, and Therapies for Multiple Sclerosis

Chapter 21

Diagnosing Multiple Sclerosis

Chapter Contents

Section 21.1

Magnetic Resonance Imaging for Diagnosing Multiple Sclerosis

This section contains text excerpted from the following sources: Text in this section begins with excerpts from "Multiple Sclerosis Centers of Excellence," U.S. Department of Veterans Affairs (VA), October 9, 2018; Text under the heading "Understanding Your Magnetic Resonance Imaging Report" is excerpted from "VA Multiple Sclerosis Centers of Excellence—I Am Not My MS," U.S. Department of Veterans Affairs (VA), 2014. Reviewed March 2019.

Multiple sclerosis (MS) is a condition involving damage to nerve cells and is characterized by damage (lesions) on the brain and spinal cord.

The basis of MS diagnosis is determined by "lesions disseminated in space and time." In other words, an MS diagnosis is based on plaques occurring in multiple parts of the central nervous system (CNS) over a specific amount of time. The diagnosis is further determined by clinical criteria, with support from magnetic resonance imaging (MRI) and spinal fluid analysis when necessary. The criteria have evolved over time to allow a more rapid diagnosis of MS, permitting earlier treatment of MS. The diagnosis of MS can be challenging and is focused on excluding other disorders that are similar to MS but have alternative treatments. Given that MS is a clinical diagnosis that can evolve over time, careful follow-up of patients is necessary to confirm that MS, once diagnosed, remains the best possible diagnosis.

Diagnostic Criteria

Diagnostic criteria have evolved over time from the Schumacher Criteria (1965), to the Poser Criteria (1983), and, finally, to the McDonald Criteria (2001). The McDonald Criteria were developed by an international panel in association with the National MS Society of America, modified in 2005, and revised again in 2010 and 2017. The McDonald Criteria revisions enable a more rapid diagnosis of MS, allowing for an earlier treatment of MS. For clinical research trials, the McDonald Criteria ensure that those without a definite diagnosis of MS are not enrolled.

Diagnosis of Multiple Sclerosis

The clinical diagnosis of MS is made after a thorough evaluation, usually executed by a neurologist or other provider with experience in

MS, and is not based on one specific physical finding, laboratory test, or symptom. Notably, the diagnosis of MS also relies on the exclusion of other causes of symptoms and signs that might suggest MS, but are accompanied by red flags that point to an alternative and unifying diagnosis (Toledano 2015). In addition, it is important to understand what is typical to find, in relation to MS, in imaging tests to avoid misattributing lesions found with MRI screenings. The diagnosis of MS takes time and can be challenging.

The symptoms of MS can come and go, and they are not the same for every person. Since the diagnosis of MS is a clinical diagnosis, MRI and laboratory testing are not required. However, given the high sensitivity and specificity of MRI findings in MS, and the utility for monitoring disease and the body's response to therapy, MRI is universally conducted when possible.

An MRI has the ability to show dissemination in space with lesions in typical locations and dissemination in time with the presence of simultaneous enhancing and nonenhancing lesions, or new lesion formations on a subsequent MRI. Consensus recommendations are to use brain MRI with and without contrast for the initial diagnosis (Filippi 2016). Spinal cord imaging is suggested if the clinical exam localizes to the spinal cord or the brain MRI does not demonstrate dissemination in space. Spinal cord imaging of the whole chord (cervical through lumbar) is advised with and without contrast; however, the bulk of the cord lesions occur in the cervical and thoracic cord.

Additional testing for the diagnosis of MS may be necessary, and these additional tests may include blood tests and spinal fluid analysis. Elevated cerebrospinal fluid (CSF) oligoclonal bands, an elevated immunoglobulin G (IgG) index, and/or IgG synthetic rate is found in about 75 percent of people with MS. In patients with one clinical attack and evidence of two or more typical lesions with MRI, oligoclonal bands can establish dissemination over time (and thus a diagnosis of MS). There is no one laboratory, MRI, or clinical test that definitively points to MS.

Diagnosis Requirements

Relapsing multiple sclerosis: 85 percent of people with MS have a relapsing form of MS at onset. A relapsing MS diagnosis requires objective clinical evidence of two or more CNS lesions (dissemination in space) that have occurred at different times (dissemination in time) or objective clinical evidence of one lesion with reasonable historical evidence of a prior attack. The reasonable historical evidence can be documentation, from a prior provider, of symptoms and signs attributable to an acute CNS attack. A good patient historian can also give a description of symptoms that are typical for MS, thus acting as the historical event. Descriptions of fully or partially reversible symptoms that describe optic neuritis, transverse myelitis, a brainstem syndrome, or other symptoms clearly referable to the CNS represent good historical evidence of a prior attack. Although they could be a result of MS, symptoms such as headache, poor cognition, fatigue, and generalized weakness are not specific for MS or a CNS event and should not count as a historical attack. An MS attack should last at least 24 hours, usually lasting no more than 1 to 2 months, and resolves fully or partially with residual symptoms. Dissemination of attacks in space and time is the cornerstone of an MS diagnosis.

Primary progressive multiple sclerosis: 15 percent of people with MS have a progressive form of the disease at onset, which is defined as a gradual worsening of neurological symptoms and signs related to the CNS for at least one year. Diagnosis of primary progressive MS can be more challenging and relies heavily on ruling out other causes of symptoms. The MRI and spinal fluid evaluation are used more often in primary progressive MS to support the diagnosis. It is important to distinguish relapsing from primary progressive MS, as the treatments can be different.

Secondary progressive multiple sclerosis: After approximately 15 to 20 years, about half of the people initially diagnosed with relapsing MS transition to secondary progressive MS. In this phase, there is a gradual worsening of neurological symptoms and signs in the time between MS attacks. In many, MS attacks eventually stop altogether, but some have both relapses and progression. It is important to recognize if a relapsing patient also has a progressive component between attacks, as current MS therapies do not effectively slow the progressive aspect of MS. Secondary progressive MS does not have set criteria and is not part of any MS diagnostic criteria.

Clinically isolated syndrome: Clinically isolated syndrome (CIS) is a term that describes an isolated episode of neurological symptoms caused by inflammatory disease of the brain or spinal cord that does not align with MS (Brownlee 2014). CIS can be monofocal, meaning a single symptom, such as vision loss from optic neuritis, or multifocal due to lesions in several locations.

In diagnosing CIS, the physician faces two challenges: first, to determine whether the person's symptoms are caused by CNS inflammation or are a result of a different problem, and second, to determine the likelihood that a person experiencing this type of demyelinating event is going to develop MS. A person with CIS has a higher risk (70 to 80%) of developing MS when the CIS is accompanied by MRI-detected brain lesions that are similar to those seen in MS (i.e., typical lesions). Conversely, there is a lower risk (20 to 30%) for MS when the MRI does not show brain lesions. A radiologist or neurologist trained in examining lesions is helpful in determining if lesions, if present, are typical of MS.

An accurate diagnosis of high- or low-risk CIS is important because people with a high-risk CIS are encouraged to begin treatment with a disease-modifying medication to delay or prevent a second neurologic episode and, therefore, the onset of MS. In addition, early treatment may minimize future disability caused by MS. Several medications are now approved by the U.S. Food and Drug Administration (FDA) for CIS.

Abnormal Brain Magnetic Resonance Imaging

Occasionally, people get brain MRIs for reasons other than suspected MS, such as a car accident or migraines. Sometimes these MRIs look similar to ones from people with MS. MRI mimics of MS are numerous, and not all radiologists are familiar with current MRI criteria (Aliaga 2014). It is important to remember that the radiologist cannot make the diagnosis of MS, as it is a clinical diagnosis based on historical and neurological examination. Patients with abnormal MRIs that are at risk of obtaining MS should be evaluated for a history of events typical of MS or neurological findings related to the CNS. Usually, a neurologist is best able to perform this evaluation.

Patients diagnosed prior to MRIs, or by another provider, deserve to have their original diagnosis reviewed in light of the McDonald Criteria. This is important as MS treatment comes with risks to the patient, which can be avoided with a correct diagnosis.

Understanding Your Magnetic Resonance Imaging Report

MRI is a wonderful tool to help diagnose and monitor people with MS. MRI is safe and relatively noninvasive, yet can provide very detailed images of the brain and spinal cord, which can reveal MS lesions (also known as "demyelination," "spots," or "plaques") and changes in MS activity over time. With advances in information technology, people have increased access to their own medical records through computerized medical records, meaning that it is now possible for people to read their own MRI reports, sometimes even before discussing them with their healthcare provider. Reviewing an MRI report is best-accomplished face-to-face or over the phone with a healthcare provider who can explain the language of the report, the significance of any MRI findings, and interpret the report in a broader context of your overall condition. If you choose to review your MRI report on your own, you should be prepared to encounter a great deal of radiological jargon. MRI can show the brain and spinal cord in many different orientations. Commonly, the brain is "sliced" into sections in one of three possible ways. Axial slices are horizontal slices taken from top to bottom or from bottom to top. Sagittal slices are side-view slices taken from left to right or from right to left. Coronal slices are face-forward slices taken from front to back or from back to front. Using these different orientations allows MS lesions to be seen from different points of view, giving a better sense of where the lesions are located in relation to other brain or spinal cord structures. MRI scans are obtained using different physical parameters that create a variety of different types of images, known as "sequences." Each sequence has its advantages and disadvantages. T1 sequences are used to show the anatomy of the brain and spinal cord. MS lesions may not be very noticeable on T1 sequences unless they are very old. Old lesions, which have resulted in atrophy, may appear as dark spots or "black holes" on T1 sequences.

T2 sequences highlight MS lesions, areas of demyelination, or edema (abnormal accumulation of fluid). T2 sequences may be used to count the total number of MS lesions or the "MS lesion burden." MS lesions look like white spots on T2 sequences. Fluid attenuation inversion recovery (FLAIR) sequences are special T2 scans in which signals from the cerebrospinal fluid (CSF—fluid surrounding the brain tissue) has been removed. This makes MS lesions easier to identify. Contrast-enhanced sequences (also known as "T1+ sequences") are special T1 scans taken after a person has been injected with gadolinium (naturally occurring rare earth metal) solution.

Gadolinium highlights or "enhances" any activate MS lesions, which are characterized by inflammation or breakdown of the blood-brain barrier (the semipermeable barrier around the brain).

In other words, T2 and FLAIR sequences help show the overall number of MS lesions in the brain or spinal cord. T1 sequences show any old areas of atrophy, and contrast-enhanced sequences show any new and active MS lesions. Just as looking at MS lesions using different orientations gives you a better sense of the anatomy of the lesions, using multiple MRI sequences gives a more complete picture of the age and activity of the MS lesions. Sometimes, MRI reports describe lesions as hyperintense, hypointense, or isointense. Hyperintense lesions are bright or white. In general, MS lesions are hyperintense or bright on T2 or FLAIR sequences. Hypointense lesions are dark or black. In general, old MS lesions are hypointense or dark on T1 sequences. Isointense lesions are gray, the color of the surrounding brain tissue. Some MS lesions that are hyperintense on T2 or FLAIR may be isointense (difficult to see) on T1 sequences.

Is It Multiple Sclerosis or Not?

MRI scans are an important way to help healthcare providers figure out if a person has MS or not, but MRI scans cannot diagnose MS by themselves. While it is true that almost all people with MS will have lesions on MRI, not all people with MRI lesions have MS. This is one of the many challenges faced by a healthcare provider in trying to make an MS diagnosis. MRI lesions can occur in MS, but can also be seen as a result of strokes and migraines or even rarer conditions, such as vasculitis, lupus, and sarcoid.

MRI reports are created by radiologists who might know very little about a given person's clinical history and examination. In order to be thorough, radiologists must provide a list of all possible explanations that could be compatible with the MRI appearance. The long list of possibilities or "differential diagnosis" must be evaluated by the person's healthcare provider and interpreted in the context of the broader picture.

Is My Multiple Sclerosis Getting Worse?

By itself, an MRI report cannot tell whether or not a person with MS is doing well. Some people have a lot of MS lesions but are doing very well clinically. Some people with just a few MS lesions can be significantly disabled. In general, though, the fewer MS lesions a person has, the better. A single MRI may reveal many T1 hyperintensities ("black holes"), suggesting old damage or multiple contrast-enhancing lesions, suggesting active MS. Even more valuable, however, is making a comparison between old and new MRI scans. Comparing a new MRI to an old one can reveal changes over time, which suggest ongoing MS, as opposed to no changes over time (sometimes referred to as "no interval change"), which suggests that the person is stable.

While it is always better to review an MRI report with your healthcare provider, with a little bit of understanding of the terminology, it is possible to make some sense of your MRI report before communicating with your doctor or nurse.

Section 21.2

Neurological Diagnostic Tests and Procedures

This section includes text excerpted from "Neurological Diagnostic
Tests and Procedures Fact Sheet," National Institute of Neurological
Disorders and Stroke (NINDS), July 6, 2018.

Diagnostic tests and procedures are vital tools that help physicians
confirm or rule out the presence of a neurological disorder or other medical condition. A century ago, the only way to make a positive diagnosis
for many neurological disorders was by performing an autopsy after a
patient had died. But decades of basic research into the characteristics
of the disease, and the development of techniques that allow scientists
to see inside the living brain and monitor nervous system activity as
it occurs have given doctors powerful and accurate tools to diagnose
disease and to test how well a particular therapy may be working.

Perhaps the most significant changes in diagnostic imaging over the
past 20 years are improvements in spatial resolution (size, intensity,
and clarity) of anatomical images and reductions in the time needed
to send signals to and receive data from the area being imaged. These
advances allow physicians to simultaneously see the structure of the
brain and the changes in brain activity as they occur. Scientists continue to improve methods that will provide sharper anatomical images
and more detailed functional information.

Researchers and physicians use a variety of diagnostic imaging techniques and chemical and metabolic analyses to detect, manage, and
treat neurological disease. Some procedures are performed in specialized
settings, conducted to determine the presence of a particular disorder or
abnormality. Many tests that were previously conducted in a hospital
are now performed in a physician's office or at an outpatient testing
facility with little, if any, a risk to the patient. Depending on the type
of procedure, results are either immediate or may take several hours
to process.

What Are Some of the More Common Screening Tests?

Laboratory screening tests of blood, urine, or other substances
are used to help diagnose disease, better understand the disease process, and monitor levels of therapeutic drugs. Certain tests, ordered
by the physician as part of a regular checkup, provide general

information, while others are used to identify specific health concerns. For example, blood and blood-product tests can detect brain and/or spinal cord infection, bone marrow disease, hemorrhage, blood vessel damage, toxins that affect the nervous system, and the presence of antibodies that signal the presence of an autoimmune disease. Blood tests are also used to monitor levels of therapeutic drugs used to treat epilepsy and other neurological disorders. Genetic testing of deoxyribonucleic acid (DNA) extracted from white cells in the blood can help diagnose Huntington disease and other congenital diseases. Analysis of the fluid that surrounds the brain and spinal cord can detect meningitis, acute and chronic inflammation, rare infections, and some cases of multiple sclerosis. Chemical and metabolic testing of the blood can indicate protein disorders, some forms of muscular dystrophy and other muscle disorders, and diabetes. Urinalysis can reveal abnormal substances in the urine or the presence or absence of certain proteins that cause diseases, including the mucopolysaccharidoses.

Genetic testing or counseling can help parents who have a family history of a neurological disease determine if they are carrying one of the known genes that cause the disorder or find out if their child is affected. Genetic testing can identify many neurological disorders, including spina bifida, in utero (while the fetus is inside the mother's womb). Genetic tests include the following:

- **Amniocentesis**, usually done at 14 to 16 weeks of pregnancy, tests a sample of the amniotic fluid in the womb for genetic defects (the fluid and the fetus have the same DNA). Under local anesthesia, a thin needle is inserted through the woman's abdomen and into the womb. About 20 milliliters of fluid (roughly 4 teaspoons) is withdrawn and sent to a lab for evaluation. Test results often take 1 to 2 weeks.

- **Chorionic villus sampling**, or CVS, is performed by removing and testing a very small sample of the placenta during early pregnancy. The sample, which contains the same DNA as the fetus, is removed by a catheter or fine needle inserted through the cervix or by a fine needle inserted through the abdomen. It is tested for genetic abnormalities and results are usually available within two weeks. CVS should not be performed after the tenth week of pregnancy.

- **Uterine ultrasound** is performed using a surface probe with gel. This noninvasive test can suggest the diagnosis of conditions, such as chromosomal disorders.

What Is a Neurological Examination?

A neurological examination assesses motor and sensory skills, the functioning of one or more cranial nerves, hearing and speech, vision, coordination and balance, mental status, and changes in mood or behavior, among other abilities. Items including a tuning fork, flashlight, reflex hammer, ophthalmoscope, and needles are used to help diagnose brain tumors; infections, such as encephalitis and meningitis; and diseases, such as Parkinson disease, Huntington disease, amyotrophic lateral sclerosis (ALS), and epilepsy. Some tests require the services of a specialist to perform and analyze results.

X-rays of the patient's chest and skull are often taken as part of a neurological workup. X-rays can be used to view any part of the body, such as a joint or major organ system. In a conventional X-ray, also called a "radiograph," a technician passes a concentrated burst of low-dose ionized radiation through the body and onto a photographic plate. Since calcium in bones absorbs X-rays more easily than soft tissue or muscle, the bony structure appears white on the film. Any vertebral misalignment or fractures can be seen within minutes. Tissue masses, such as injured ligaments or a bulging disc, are not visible on conventional X-rays. This fast, noninvasive, and painless procedure is usually performed in a doctor's office or at a clinic.

Fluoroscopy is a type of X-ray that uses a continuous or pulsed beam of low-dose radiation to produce continuous images of a body part in motion. The fluoroscope (X-ray tube) is focused on the area of interest, and pictures are either videotaped or sent to a monitor for viewing. A contrast medium may be used to highlight the images. Fluoroscopy can be used to evaluate the flow of blood through arteries.

What Are Some Diagnostic Tests Used to Diagnose Neurological Disorders?

Based on the result of a neurological exam, physical exam, patient history, X-rays of the patient's chest and skull, and any previous screening or testing, physicians may order one or more of the following diagnostic tests to determine the specific nature of a suspected neurological disorder or injury. These diagnostics generally involve either nuclear medicine imaging, in which very small amounts of radioactive materials are used to study organ function and structure or diagnostic imaging, which uses magnets and electrical charges to study human anatomy.

The following list of available procedures—in alphabetical rather than sequential order—includes some of the more common tests used to help diagnose a neurological condition.

Angiography is a test used to detect blockages of the arteries or veins. A cerebral angiogram can detect the degree of narrowing or obstruction of an artery or blood vessel in the brain, head, or neck. It is used to diagnose stroke and to determine the location and size of a brain tumor, aneurysm, or vascular malformation. This test is usually performed in a hospital outpatient setting and takes up to three hours, followed by a six- to eight-hour resting period. The patient, wearing a hospital or imaging gown, lies on a table that is wheeled into the imaging area. While the patient is awake, a physician anesthetizes a small area of the leg near the groin and then inserts a catheter into a major artery located there. The catheter is threaded through the body and into an artery in the neck. Once the catheter is in place, the needle is removed and a guide wire is inserted. A small capsule containing a radiopaque dye (one that is highlighted on X-rays) is passed over the guide wire to the site of release. The dye is released and travels through the bloodstream into the head and neck. A series of X-rays are taken, and any obstruction is noted. Patients may feel a warm to hot sensation or slight discomfort as the dye is released.

A **biopsy** involves the removal and examination of a small piece of tissue from the body. Muscle or nerve biopsies are used to diagnose neuromuscular disorders and may also reveal if a person is a carrier of a defective gene that could be passed on to children. A small sample of muscle or nerve is removed under local anesthetic and studied under a microscope. The sample may be removed either surgically, through a slit made in the skin, or by needle biopsy, in which a thin, hollow needle is inserted through the skin and into the muscle. A small piece of muscle or nerve remains in the hollow needle when it is removed from the body. The biopsy is usually performed at an outpatient testing facility. A brain biopsy used to determine tumor type requires surgery to remove a small piece of the brain or tumor. Performed in a hospital, this operation is riskier than a muscle biopsy and involves a longer recovery period.

Brain scans are imaging techniques used to diagnose tumors, blood vessel malformations, or hemorrhage in the brain. These scans are used to study organ function, injury, or disease to tissue or muscle. Types of brain scans include computed tomography (CT), magnetic resonance imaging (MRI), and positron emission tomography (PET).

121

Cerebrospinal fluid analysis involves the removal of a small amount of the fluid that protects the brain and spinal cord. The fluid is tested to detect any bleeding or brain hemorrhage, diagnose infection to the brain and/or spinal cord, identify some cases of multiple sclerosis and other neurological conditions, and measure intracranial pressure.

The procedure is usually done in a hospital. The sample of fluid is commonly removed by a procedure known as a "lumbar puncture" or "spinal tap." The patient is asked to either lie on one side, in a ball position with knees close to the chest or lean forward while sitting on a table or bed. The doctor will locate a puncture site in the lower back, between two vertebrae, then clean the area and inject a local anesthetic. The patient may feel a slight stinging sensation from this injection. Once the anesthetic has taken effect, the doctor will insert a special needle into the spinal sac and remove a small amount of fluid (usually about three teaspoons) for testing. Most patients will feel a sensation of pressure only as the needle is inserted.

A common aftereffect of a lumbar puncture is a headache, which can be lessened by having the patient lie flat. Risk of nerve-root injury or infection from the puncture can occur, but it is rare. The entire procedure takes about 45 minutes.

Computed tomography, also known as a "CT scan," is a noninvasive, painless process used to produce rapid, clear two-dimensional (2D) images of organs, bones, and tissues. Neurological CT scans are used to view the brain and spine. They can detect bone and vascular irregularities, certain brain tumors and cysts, herniated discs, epilepsy, encephalitis, spinal stenosis (narrowing of the spinal canal), a blood clot or intracranial bleeding in patients with stroke, brain damage from a head injury, and other disorders. Many neurological disorders share certain characteristics, and a CT scan can aid in proper diagnosis by differentiating the area of the brain affected by the disorder.

Scanning takes about 20 minutes (a CT of the brain or head may take slightly longer) and is usually done at an imaging center or hospital on an outpatient basis. The patient lies on a special table that slides into a narrow chamber. A sound system built into the chamber allows the patient to communicate with the physician or technician. As the patient lies still, X-rays are passed through the body at various angles and are detected by a computerized scanner. The data is processed and displayed as cross-sectional images, or "slices," of the internal structure of the body or organ. A light sedative may be given to patients who are unable to lie still and pillows may be used to support and stabilize the head and body. Persons who are claustrophobic may have difficulty taking this imaging test.

Occasionally, a contrast dye is injected into the bloodstream to highlight the different tissues in the brain. Patients may feel a warm or cool sensation as the dye circulates through the bloodstream or they may experience a slight metallic taste.

Although very little radiation is used in CT, pregnant women should avoid the test because of potential harm to the fetus from ionizing radiation.

Discography is often suggested for patients who are considering lumbar surgery or whose lower back pain has not responded to conventional treatments. This outpatient procedure is usually performed at a testing facility or a hospital. The patient is asked to put on a metal-free hospital gown and lie on an imaging table. The physician numbs the skin with anesthetic and inserts a thin needle, using X-ray guidance, into the spinal disc. Once the needle is in place, a small amount of contrast dye is injected, and CT scans are taken. The contrast dye outlines any damaged areas. More than one disc may be imaged at the same time. Patient recovery usually takes about an hour. Pain medicine may be prescribed for any resulting discomfort.

An **intrathecal contrast-enhanced CT scan** (also called "cisternography") is used to detect problems with the spine and spinal nerve roots. This test is most often performed at an imaging center. The patient is asked to put on a hospital or imaging gown. Following the application of a topical anesthetic, the physician removes a small sample of the spinal fluid via lumbar puncture. The sample is mixed with a contrast dye and injected into the spinal sac located at the base of the lower back. The patient is then asked to move to a position that will allow the contrast fluid to travel to the area to be studied. The dye allows the spinal canal and nerve roots to be seen more clearly on a CT scan. The scan may take up to an hour to complete. Following the test, patients may experience some discomfort and/or headache that may be caused by the removal of spinal fluid.

Electroencephalography, or EEG, monitors brain activity through the skull. EEG is used to help diagnose certain seizure disorders, brain tumors, brain damage from head injuries, inflammation of the brain and/or spinal cord, alcoholism, certain psychiatric disorders, and metabolic and degenerative disorders that affect the brain. EEGs are also used to evaluate sleep disorders, monitor brain activity when a patient has been fully anesthetized or loses consciousness, and confirm brain death.

This painless, risk-free test can be performed in a doctor's office or at a hospital or testing facility. Prior to taking an EEG, the person must avoid caffeine intake and prescription drugs that affect the nervous system. A series of cup-like electrodes are attached to the patient's scalp, either with a special conducting paste or with extremely fine needles. The electrodes (also called "leads") are small devices that are attached to wires and carry the electrical energy of the brain to a machine for reading. A very low electrical current is sent through the electrodes, and the baseline brain energy is recorded. Patients are then exposed to a variety of external stimuli—including bright or flashing light, noise, or certain drugs—or are asked to open and close the eyes or to change breathing patterns. The electrodes transmit the resulting changes in brain wave patterns. Since movement and nervousness can change brain wave patterns, patients usually recline in a chair or on a bed during the test, which takes up to an hour. Testing for certain disorders requires performing an EEG during sleep, which takes at least three hours.

In order to explore more about brain wave activity, electrodes may be inserted through a surgical opening in the skull and into the brain to reduce signal interference from the skull.

Electromyography, or EMG, is used to diagnose nerve and muscle dysfunction and spinal cord disease. It records the electrical activity from the brain and/or spinal cord to a peripheral nerve root (found in the arms and legs) that controls muscles during contraction and at rest.

During an EMG, very fine wire electrodes are inserted into a muscle to assess changes in electrical voltage that occur during movement and when the muscle is at rest. The electrodes are attached through a series of wires to a recording instrument. Testing usually takes place at a testing facility and lasts about an hour but may take longer, depending on the number of muscles and nerves to be tested. Most patients find this test to be somewhat uncomfortable.

An EMG is usually done in conjunction with a nerve conduction velocity (NCV) test, which measures electrical energy by assessing the nerve's ability to send a signal. This 2-part test is conducted most often in a hospital. A technician tapes 2 sets of flat electrodes on the skin over the muscles. The first set of electrodes is used to send small pulses of electricity (similar to the sensation of static electricity) to stimulate the nerve that directs a particular muscle. The second set of electrodes transmits the responding electrical signal to a recording machine. The physician then reviews the response to verify any nerve damage or muscle disease. Patients who are preparing to take an EMG or NCV test may be asked to avoid caffeine and not smoke for 2 to 3 hours prior to the test, as well as to avoid aspirin and nonsteroidal anti-inflammatory drugs (NSAIDs) for 24 hours before the EMG. There is no discomfort or risk associated with this test.

Electronystagmography (ENG) describes a group of tests used to diagnose involuntary eye movement, dizziness, balance disorders, and to evaluate some brain functions. The test is performed at an imaging center. Small electrodes are taped around the eyes to record eye movements. If infrared photography is used in place of electrodes, the patient wears special goggles that help record the information. Both versions of the test are painless and risk-free.

Evoked potentials (also called "evoked response") measure the electrical signals to the brain generated by hearing, touch, or sight. These tests are used to assess sensory-nerve problems and confirm neurological conditions including multiple sclerosis, brain tumor, acoustic neuroma (small tumors of the inner ear), and spinal cord injury. Evoked potentials are also used to test sight and hearing (especially in infants and young children), monitor brain activity among coma patients, and confirm brain death.

Testing may take place in a doctor's office or hospital setting. It is painless and risk-free. Two sets of needle electrodes are used to test for nerve damage. One set of electrodes, which will be used to measure the electrophysiological response to stimuli, is attached to the patient's scalp using conducting paste. The second set of electrodes is attached to the part of the body to be tested. The physician then records the amount of time it takes for the impulse generated by stimuli to reach the brain. Under normal circumstances, the process of signal transmission is instantaneous.

Auditory evoked potentials (also called "brain stem auditory-evoked response") are used to assess high-frequency hearing loss, diagnose any damage to the acoustic nerve and auditory pathways in the brainstem, and detect acoustic neuromas. The patient sits in a soundproof room and wears headphones. Clicking sounds are delivered one at a time to one ear while a masking sound is sent to the other ear. Each ear is usually tested twice, and the entire procedure takes about 45 minutes.

Visual evoked potentials detect loss of vision from optic nerve damage (in particular, damage caused by multiple sclerosis). The patient sits close to a screen and is asked to focus on the center of a shifting checkerboard pattern. Only one eye is tested at a time; the other eye is either kept closed or covered with a patch. Each eye is usually tested twice. Testing takes 30 to 45 minutes.

Somatosensory evoked potentials measure response from stimuli to the peripheral nerves and can detect nerve or spinal cord damage or nerve degeneration from multiple sclerosis and other degenerating diseases. Tiny electrical shocks are delivered by an electrode to a nerve in an arm or leg. Responses to the shocks, which may be delivered for more than a minute at a time, are recorded. This test usually lasts less than an hour.

Magnetic resonance imaging (MRI) uses computer-generated radio waves and a powerful magnetic field to produce detailed images of body structures including tissues, organs, bones, and nerves. Neurological uses include the diagnosis of brain and spinal cord tumors, eye disease, inflammation, infection, and vascular irregularities that may lead to stroke. MRI can also detect and monitor degenerative disorders, such as multiple sclerosis, and can document brain injury from trauma.

The equipment houses a hollow tube that is surrounded by a very large cylindrical magnet. The patient, who must remain still during the test, lies on a special table that is slid into the tube. The patient will be asked to remove jewelry, eyeglasses, removable dental work, or other items that might interfere with the magnetic imaging. The patient should wear a sweatshirt and sweatpants or other clothing free of metal eyelets or buckles. MRI scanning equipment creates a magnetic field around the body strong enough to temporarily realign water molecules in the tissues. Radio waves are then passed through the body to detect the "relaxation" of the molecules back to a random alignment and trigger a resonance signal at different angles within the body. A computer processes this resonance into either a three-dimensional (3D) picture or a two-dimensional (2D) "slice" of the tissue being scanned and differentiates between bone, soft tissues and fluid-filled spaces by their water content and structural properties. A contrast dye may be used to enhance the visibility of certain areas or tissues. The patient may hear some grating or knocking noises when the magnetic field is turned on and off. (Patients may wear special earphones to block out the sounds.) Unlike CT scanning, MRI does not use ionizing radiation to produce images. Depending on the part(s) of the body to be scanned, MRI can take up to an hour to complete. The test is painless and risk-free, although persons who are obese or claustrophobic may find it somewhat uncomfortable. (Some centers also use open MRI machines that do not completely surround the person being tested and are less confining. However, open MRI does not currently provide the same picture quality as standard MRI, and some tests may not be available using this equipment). Due to the incredibly strong magnetic field generated by an MRI, patients with implanted medical devices, such as a pacemaker, should avoid the test.

Functional MRI (fMRI) uses the blood's magnetic properties to produce real-time images of blood flow to particular areas of the brain. An fMRI can pinpoint areas of the brain that become active and note how long they stay active. It can also tell if brain activity within a region occurs simultaneously or sequentially. This imaging process is used to assess brain damage from head injury or degenerative disorders, such as Alzheimer disease, and to identify and monitor other neurological disorders, including multiple sclerosis, stroke, and brain tumors.

Myelography involves the injection of water- or oil-based contrast dye into the spinal canal to enhance X-ray imaging of the spine. Myelograms are used to diagnose spinal nerve injury, herniated discs, fractures, back or leg pain, and spinal tumors.

The procedure takes about 30 minutes and is usually performed in a hospital. Following injection of anesthesia to a site between 2 vertebrae in the lower back, a small amount of the cerebrospinal fluid is removed by a spinal tap, and the contrast dye is injected into the spinal canal. After a series of X-rays are taken, most or all of the contrast dye is removed by aspiration. Patients may experience some pain during the spinal tap and when the dye is injected and removed. Patients may also experience headache following the spinal tap. The risk of fluid leakage or allergic reaction to the dye is slight.

Positron emission tomography (PET) scans provide two- and three-dimensional pictures of brain activity by measuring radioactive isotopes that are injected into the bloodstream. PET scans of the brain are used to detect or highlight tumors and diseased tissue, measure cellular and/or tissue metabolism, show blood flow, evaluate patients who have seizure disorders that do not respond to medical therapy and patients with certain memory disorders, and determine brain changes following injury or drug abuse, among other uses. PET may be ordered as a follow-up to a CT or MRI scan to give the physician a greater understanding of specific areas of the brain that may be involved with certain problems. Scans are conducted in a hospital or at a testing facility on an outpatient basis. A low-level radioactive isotope, which binds to chemicals that flow to the brain, is injected into the bloodstream and can be traced as the brain performs different functions. The patient lies still while overhead sensors detect gamma rays in the body's tissues. A computer processes the information and displays it on a video monitor or on film. Using different compounds, more than one brain function can be traced simultaneously. PET is painless and relatively risk-free. The length of test time depends on the part of the body to be scanned. PET scans are performed by skilled technicians at highly sophisticated medical facilities.

A **polysomnogram** measures brain and body activity during sleep. It is performed over one or more nights at a sleep center. Electrodes are pasted or taped to the patient's scalp, eyelids, and/or chin. Throughout the night and during the various wake/sleep cycles, the electrodes record brain waves, eye movement, breathing, leg, and skeletal muscle activity, blood pressure, and heart rate. The patient may be videotaped to note any movement during sleep. Results are then used to identify any characteristic patterns of sleep disorders, including restless legs syndrome, periodic limb movement disorder, insomnia, and breathing disorders, such as obstructive sleep apnea. Polysomnograms are non-invasive, painless, and risk-free.

Single photon emission computed tomography (SPECT), a nuclear imaging test involving blood flow to tissue, is used to evaluate certain brain functions. The test may be ordered as a follow-up to an MRI to diagnose tumors, infections, degenerative spinal disease, and stress fractures. As with a PET scan, a radioactive isotope, which binds to chemicals that flow to the brain, is injected intravenously into the body. Areas of increased blood flow will collect more of the isotope. As the patient lies on a table, a gamma camera rotates around the head and records where the radioisotope has traveled. That information is converted by a computer into cross-sectional slices that are stacked to produce a detailed three-dimensional (3D) image of blood flow and activity within the brain. The test is performed at either an imaging center or a hospital.

Thermography uses infrared-sensing devices to measure small temperature changes between the two sides of the body or within a specific organ. Also known as "digital infrared thermal imaging," thermography may be used to detect vascular disease of the head and neck, soft tissue injury, various neuromusculoskeletal disorders, and the presence or absence of nerve root compression. It is performed at an imaging center, using infrared light recorders to take thousands of pictures of the body from a distance of five to eight feet. The information is converted into electrical signals which results in a computer-generated two-dimensional (2D) picture of abnormally cold or hot areas indicated by color or shades of black and white. Thermography does not use radiation and is safe, risk-free, and noninvasive.

Ultrasound imaging, also called "ultrasound scanning" or "sonography," uses high-frequency sound waves to obtain images inside the body. Neurosonography (ultrasound of the brain and spinal column) analyzes blood flow in the brain and can diagnose stroke, brain tumors, hydrocephalus (buildup of cerebrospinal fluid in the brain), and vascular problems. It can also identify or rule out inflammatory processes causing pain. It is more effective than an X-ray in displaying soft tissue masses and can show tears in ligaments, muscles, tendons, and other soft tissue masses in the back. Transcranial Doppler ultrasound is used to view arteries and blood vessels in the neck and determine blood flow and risk of stroke.

During the ultrasound, the patient lies on an imaging table and removes clothing around the area of the body to be scanned. A jelly-like lubricant is applied and a transducer, which both sends and receives high-frequency sound waves, is passed over the body. The sound wave echoes are recorded and displayed as a computer-generated real-time visual image of the structure or tissue being examined. Ultrasound is painless, noninvasive, and risk-free. The test is performed on an outpatient basis and takes between 15 and 30 minutes to complete.

725073884
COM9338182A
9780780816978

REFERENCE

R 616.834 MUL

Multiple sclerosis sourcebook.
9780780816978

LINDENHURST MEMORIAL LIBRARY
One Lee Avenue
Lindenhurst, New York 11757

31801006132231

For Reference

Not to be taken from this room

REFERENCE

Chapter 22

The Multiple Sclerosis Healthcare Team

As a person with multiple sclerosis (MS), you will get to know more about the condition than anybody else. It is common to experience a variety of symptoms before your actual MS diagnosis. Symptoms of MS often mimic those of other diseases. Ruling out any other condition is part of the diagnostic process. Sometimes this process is long or confusing. It is understandable if you may have felt worried or frustrated. You understand how your symptoms affect you, both physically and mentally. You can monitor any changes in your condition and learn what triggers to avoid that may make your symptoms worse. Remember, too, that having the right information about MS will mean you will be in a better position to make informed decisions for yourself. Management of MS involves the following healthcare professionals:

- **Neurologists** are physicians that specialize in the treatment of disorders that affect the brain, spinal cord, and nerves. They provide testing and assessment for the diagnosis of MS, as well as ongoing care and management for symptoms and disease activity or progression.

This chapter includes text excerpted from "Overview of Multiple Sclerosis for Veterans," U.S. Department of Veterans Affairs (VA), March 2017.

- **Physiatrists** (Physical medicine and rehabilitation physicians (PM and R)) manage symptoms that limit function in day-to-day life or your ability to participate in work and the community. Your rehabilitation provider may be involved with your care for a specific issue or for long-term management of your MS.

- **Primary care physicians** (PCPs) focus on preventive health and chronic disease management. They coordinate care with other specialty care providers and programs and are able to manage some chronic MS symptoms without the help of MS specialists.

- **Nurse practitioners and physician assistants** (NPs and PAs) provide a wide range of healthcare services, including establishing plans of care, diagnosis, medication management, addressing complex medical issues, education, training, and collaborating with other specialists.

- **Nurses** provide direct care in addition to coordinating services, promoting health and wellness, and providing advice and education about your specific symptoms and various health conditions.

- **Psychologists** assist with mental, emotional, or behavior challenges; evaluate psychological testing to identify cognitive strengths and weaknesses; and provide clinical and counseling services.

- **Social workers** assist to resolve emotional, psychosocial, and economic problems. Assistance includes counseling and planning for care after the patient leaves the medical center.

- **Physical therapists** assist with injuries and disabilities to improve an individual's movement, restore function, reduce and manage their pain, and help with the appropriate selection for adaptive mobility devices.

- **Occupational therapists** (OTs) assist in developing, recovering, and improving the skills needed for activities that occur in daily life. They also help with energy conservation for fatigue and with the selection and use of assistive technology.

- **Speech therapists** assist with speech, language, swallowing, and voice issues involving communication. They can provide evaluation and treatment options if needed.

- **Recreational therapists** assist to engage in recreation-based treatment programs, which can include arts and crafts, sports, and community outings to help maintain or improve physical, social, and emotional well-being.

Chapter 23

Working with a Neurologist

Neurologists are medical doctors who specialize in diagnosing, treating, and managing disorders of the brain and nervous system, including the peripheral nerves that connect the brain to organs and muscles throughout the body. Their extensive training includes an undergraduate degree, four years of medical school, a one-year internship, and a minimum of three years of specialty training. In addition, many neurologists train in subspecialties, such as specific diseases or disorders that affect particular body systems. Because of the complexity of the brain and nervous system, which influence and control many bodily functions, neurologists must be extremely detail-oriented and attuned to even the smallest signs of neurological problems.

What Do Neurologists Do?

Neurologists do not perform surgery but rather treat disorders through the use of medication, physical therapy, and rehabilitation. However, the neurosurgeons who do perform surgeries always work with neurologists to ensure the best possible outcome for the patient, so consulting is another important role for a neurologist. And when patients require ongoing treatment, the neurologist is often the principal care provider. Some of the disorders treated by neurologists include:

- Headaches

- Pain

"Working with a Neurologist," © 2017 Omnigraphics. Reviewed March 2019.

- Stroke

- Brain tumors

- Sleep disorders

- Epilepsy

- Brain and spinal-cord injuries

- Parkinson disease

- Seizure disorders

- Alzheimer disease

- Multiple sclerosis

- Amyotrophic lateral sclerosis (ALS or Lou Gehrig disease)

How Do Neurologists Diagnose Disorders?

As is the case with most doctors, the first thing a neurologist will do is perform an examination of the patient. This includes a review of the person's medical history and a discussion of the current condition, followed by a neurological exam. This will generally include an assessment of the patient's vision, hearing, reflexes, strength, and coordination. Often, additional tests will be required, such as:

- **Magnetic resonance imaging (MRI)**. This test uses a magnetic field and radio waves to get an accurate picture of the brain.

- **Computer-assisted tomography (CAT scan)**. X-rays and a computer are used to create 3-D images of various body parts.

- **Electroencephalogram (EEG)**. This records electrical activity in the brain and is used to diagnose physical brain disorders.

- **Electromyogram (EMG)**. An EMG records electrical activity in muscles and nerves to help determine the cause of pain, numbness, or weakness.

- **Transcranial Doppler (TCD)**. This test measures blood flow in the vessels in the brain using sound waves. It can detect blockages or constrictions that may be causing symptoms.

- **Neurosonography**. Ultra-high-frequency sound waves analyze the flow of blood in the vessels in or leading to the brain.

- **Cerebrospinal fluid analysis.** Also called a "lumbar puncture" or "spinal tap," this procedure tests for blood, infection, or other abnormalities in the brain, spinal cord, and nerves.

- **Evoked potentials.** These tests record the brain's response to various types of stimulation in order to diagnose problems with eyesight, hearing, dizziness, or numbness.

- **Sleep studies.** The patient usually spends the night in a sleep lab with sensors placed on the scalp. These record brain waves and electrical activity, as well as functions such as heart rate, blood oxygen levels, and breathing, to help determine the cause of sleep disorders.

How Do Neurologists Treat Disorders?

Because of the wide range of neurological disorders, treatments can vary considerably depending on the nature of the disease and the parts of the body that are affected. In the case of stroke, treatment options depend on whether the diagnosis is ischemic stroke or hemorrhagic stroke.

Ischemic strokes result from an obstruction (clot) in a vessel supplying blood to the brain. Treatment options for ischemic stroke generally include:

- **Medication.** A drug called a "tissue plasminogen activator" (tPA) is injected into a vein in the arm to dissolve the clot that is restricting blood flow to the brain. For this treatment to be most effective, it's important for the medication to be given as soon as possible after the stroke occurs. In addition, an anticoagulant, such as heparin, may be administered to help prevent more blood clots from forming.

- **Mechanical thrombectomy.** Here, a catheter is inserted into an artery leading to the brain, and a wire-cage device called a "stent retriever" is used to capture and remove the clot and restore blood flow to the brain. The procedure is most beneficial if it is performed within six hours of the onset of stroke symptoms, and it can only be used on patients who have a clot in one of the large arteries in the brain.

Hemorrhagic strokes occur when a vessel ruptures and allows blood to flow into the brain where it compresses the brain tissue. Treatment options for hemorrhagic stroke usually include:

- **Emergency treatment.** Emergency care is vital for a patient with hemorrhagic stroke in order to control bleeding and reduce pressure in the brain. Medication can be used to reduce blood pressure or slow the bleeding. Patients who are taking blood thinners will likely be given drugs to counteract their effects.

- **Mechanical repair.** A catheter may be inserted through an artery in the arm or leg and guided to site of the rupture in the brain. Then the doctor places a coil or other device through the catheter to help repair the problem. In some cases, though, surgery may be required to repair the problem.

How to Choose a Neurologist

Obviously, in an emergency situation, patients don't get to choose their doctors, but often there's time to consider which neurologist might be the best physician to work with. Here are some tips:

- **Referrals.** Your primary care doctor will likely recommend a neurologist that she or he works with and knows to be good. Family and friends might also have recommendations.

- **Research.** Make the effort to research the neurologist's credentials, experience, and patient satisfaction surveys and ratings. This information is generally available online, as are records of malpractice claims and disciplinary actions.

- **Meet.** Request an introductory visit with the neurologist. Discuss your case, and ask about his or her experience treating your condition, as well as possible treatment plans.

- **Consider.** Think about what you've learned, and take into account your impressions of the neurologist at your meeting. It's important not only that the doctor is qualified, but also that you feel comfortable with her or him.

- **Don't forget the hospital.** In addition to researching the neurologist, be sure to do your homework about the hospital or treatment facility. Again, get recommendations when possible and research the facility online, paying special attention to its neurology unit.

- **Insurance.** It's also important to be sure the neurologist, facility, and expected treatment are compatible with your insurance plan in order to incur the least out-of-pocket expense.

References

1. Caplan, Louis. "Stroke Is Best Managed by Neurologists," Stroke, November 6, 2003.

2. "How Is Stroke Treated?" National Institutes of Health (NIH), January 27, 2017.

3. "Neurologists and Neurosurgeons Explained," Lifenph.com, n.d.

4. "Quick Stroke Treatment for Saving the Brain," American Stroke Association, n.d.

5. "What Does a Neurologist Do?" Sokanu.com, n.d.

6. "Working with Your Doctor," American Academy of Neurology (AAN), n.d.

Chapter 24

Treatment Options for Multiple Sclerosis

The goals of multiple sclerosis (MS) therapies are to reduce the frequency of relapses, slow the progression of the disease, manage symptoms, and improve quality of life (QOL). Medications for MS focus on controlling the immune system and managing symptoms. People with MS should work with their MS Multidisciplinary Care Team to find the best approach to address their MS symptoms.

Disease Modifying Therapies

Over 16 different disease-modifying therapies (DMTs) have been approved by the U.S. Food and Drug Administration (FDA) for the treatment of MS. These include injectable, oral, and infused medications. DMTs have been shown to reduce relapses and neurologic disability, but be aware that DMTs do not treat chronic symptoms or restore lost function.

People with MS who are good candidates for a DMT should start treatment as soon as possible. Research shows that early treatment with DMTs can reduce long-term disability from MS. The use of DMTs is not limited by the frequency of relapses, age, or level of disability. Treatment is not stopped unless it is clearly no longer effective, there are intolerable side effects, or a better treatment becomes available.

This chapter includes text excerpted from "Treatment Options for Multiple Sclerosis," U.S. Department of Veterans Affairs (VA), October 26, 2018.

As with all medications, there can be side effects. Your healthcare provider will discuss these with you and help you to select the most appropriate medication. If your condition changes or you experience bothersome medication side effects, your healthcare team will work with you to find solutions.

Choosing the Best Disease Modifying Therapies for You

- Discuss your MS disease course with your healthcare provider, as well as the benefits and risks of therapies.

- Contemplate the route of the therapy—oral, self-injection by needle, or clinic appointment infusion (into the vein)—and your ability to take the therapy as prescribed.

- Understand how often you will need to be seen for exams, labs, infusions, and follow-up care.

- Consider your overall health and family planning.

Symptomatic Therapies

People with MS may suffer from a variety of symptoms, including bladder problems, bowel dysfunction, depression, dizziness, walking difficulties, sexual dysfunction, pain, and fatigue. Fortunately, there are a number of medications, interventions, and therapies that can effectively manage these symptoms. Therapies and interventions can include physical therapy for walking difficulties and muscle stiffness, occupational therapy for tremor, or a cooling vest for heat sensitivity. Other lifestyle changes, such as a healthy diet and safe exercise plan, can significantly help with symptoms and improve overall health. These treatment approaches may not always make the symptom go away completely, but can often make symptoms easier to manage.

If the first treatment does not work or has too many side effects, there are others you can try. It may be important to address the most bothersome symptom first. Discuss your options with your healthcare team to create an individualized treatment plan for you.

Relapse Management

An MS relapse (also known as an "MS exacerbation" or "MS flare") is when inflammation in the brain and/or spinal cord causes a new symptom or worsening of an old symptom. Symptoms from an MS relapse must last over 24 hours; most relapses last from a few days to several weeks or months. Symptoms with a relapse can range from mild to severe. Occasionally, infection, stress, and heat can make old symptoms worse, also called a "pseudo-relapse." Unlike an MS relapse, a pseudo-relapse does not reflect new inflammation or MS progression. Your MS specialist can help determine whether worsening symptoms are from an MS relapse or a pseudo-relapse.

Steroid medications may help speed up recovery from a severe relapse, though milder relapses may not require steroids. You and your healthcare team should make the decision together whether steroids are a good option for you. During and after a relapse, you may need to work with a rehabilitation therapist to help with any changes to your ability to perform activities of daily living. If you think you may be experiencing a relapse, contact your MS specialist right away.

Complementary Therapies and Integrative Medicine

The term "complementary and alternative medicine" (CAM) generally refers to products and practices that are not currently part of "mainstream" medicine. Complementary medicine is used with standard care, whereas alternative medicine is used instead of standard care. The term "integrative medicine" refers to care that blends both mainstream and complementary practices.

Some CAM approaches include nutritional supplements; lifestyle changes, such as stress reduction techniques, mindfulness meditation, physical programs (such as yoga or chiropractic manipulation); and pain management. The use of appropriate integrative medicine, which combines the practices of complementary and standard care is supported by healthcare professionals. Always check with your healthcare provider before trying complementary therapy; some may not be helpful for people with MS or can make the symptoms of MS worse.

Chapter 25

Drug Treatments and Therapies for Multiple Sclerosis

Chapter Contents

145

Section 25.1

Multiple Sclerosis Agents

This section includes text excerpted from "Multiple Sclerosis Agents," LiverTox®, National Institutes of Health (NIH), October 30, 2018.

Multiple sclerosis (MS) is a chronic demyelinating disorder of the central nervous system of unknown etiology. It is most likely caused by a gradual, intermittent autoimmune destruction of myelin. The disorder is characterized by a relapsing-remitting course, but in a small proportion of patients, it is unremittingly progressive even from the onset. The disease typically presents itself between the ages of 20 and 40 and is more common in women than men. Rates of multiple sclerosis vary geographically, being highest in northern parts of Europe and the United States and in Canada. Multiple sclerosis affects an estimated 400,000 persons in the United States and is the most common cause of neurologic disability in young adulthood.

Therapies of multiple sclerosis can be divided into disease-modifying agents and symptomatic therapies. The disease-modifying agents are largely immunomodulatory drugs, and includes interferon beta-1a (Avonex, 1994 and Rebif, 2003), interferon beta-1b (Betaseron, 1993 and Extavia, 2008), peginterferon beta-1a (Plegridy, 2014), glatiramer acetate (Copaxone, 1996), alemtuzumab (Lemtrada, 2001), fingolimod (Gilenya, 2010), teriflunomide (Aubagio, 2012), and dimethyl fumarate (Tecfidera, 2013). Disease-modifying agents that are used in resistant cases of multiple sclerosis, some of which are not specifically approved for this use (off-label use), include methotrexate, cyclophosphamide, intravenous immunoglobulins, mitoxantrone (Novantrone), and natalizumab (Tysabri [now withdrawn]). The disease-modifying agents are more effective in relapsing-remitting forms of disease than in the more severe and intractable progressive forms. Symptomatic therapies developed for multiple sclerosis include dalfampridine (4-aminopyrine, Ampyra: 2010), a potassium channel blocker that improves mobility and walking speed in patients with relapsing-remitting forms of multiple sclerosis.

While transient, asymptomatic and mild-to-moderate serum aminotransferase elevations occur not uncommonly with most of the drugs used to treat multiple sclerosis, clinically apparent hepatotoxicity is rare. Nevertheless, several convincing instances of acute liver injury have been reported for the various forms of interferon beta and glatiramer acetate. Importantly, clinically apparent liver injury was usually first attributed to these two agents several years after their introduction, and initially they were not believed to be hepatotoxic.

Thus, the more recently introduced agents (fingolimod, teriflunomide, and dimethyl fumarate) have not had wide enough general use to state that they do not cause clinically apparent liver injury, and all three have been associated occasionally with marked but transient increases in serum aminotransferase levels. The following agents are discussed individually:

Disease-Modifying Agents
Alemtuzumab

Alemtuzumab was approved in the United States in 2004 for use in chronic lymphocytic leukemia. It has also been used extensively off-label as a part of induction therapy for prevention of rejection after solid organ transplantation. It is currently under evaluation in several autoimmune diseases, including resistant or relapsing multiple sclerosis. Alemtuzumab is available in single use vials of 30 mg/mL under the brand name "Campath." The typical dose and regimen varies with indication. Alemtuzumab has significant adverse side effects, largely due to the profound immunosuppression. Common adverse events include epistaxis, headache, hypertension, rhinitis, dry skin, back pain, excessive bleeding, and skin rash. Uncommon, but serious complications include severe infusions reactions, cytopenias (including fatal autoimmune anemia and thrombocytopenia), and opportunistic infections.

Dimethyl Fumarate

Dimethyl fumarate was approved for use in relapsing multiple sclerosis in the United States in 2013 and is now available in delayed-release capsules of 120 and 240 mg under the brand name "Tecfidera." The recommended dose is 120 mg twice daily for 7 days, followed by a maintenance dose of 240 mg twice daily. Common side effects are flushing (25 to 50%); gastrointestinal symptoms of nausea, diarrhea or abdominal pain (10 to 60%); dizziness; erythema (5%); and skin rash (9%).

Fingolimod

Fingolimod in several large, randomized controlled trials, fingolimod was shown to reduce relapse rates and improve neuro-radiologic outcomes in adult patients with relapsing-remitting multiple sclerosis. Fingolimod was approved for use in relapsing multiple sclerosis in the United States in 2010 and was the first oral disease-modifying agent approved in this condition. Fingolimod is available in capsules of 0.5 mg under the brand name "Gilenya." The recommended dose in adults is 0.5 mg orally once daily. Common side effects are lymphopenia, headache, diarrhea, cough, rhinorrhea, and back and abdominal pain. Rare, but potentially severe adverse events include viral infections, atrial arrhythmias, macular edema, progressive multifocal leukoencephalopathy (PML), posterior reversible encephalopathy syndrome (PRES), and acute hypersensitivity reactions.

Glatiramer Acetate

Glatiramer acetate was shown to reduce relapse rates and improve neuroradiologic outcomes in adult patients with relapsing-remitting multiple sclerosis. Glatiramer was approved for use for multiple sclerosis in the United States in 1996 and is available in prefilled syringes of 20 mg and 40 mg generically and under the brand names "Copaxone" and "Glatopa." The recommended dose is 20 mg subcutaneously once daily or 40 mg 3 times weekly. Common side effects are injection site reactions (pain, erythema, pruritus, induration), as well as mild and transient hypersensitivity reactions of flushing, chest tightness, dyspnea, and anxiety occurring within minutes of the injection in about 10 percent of patients.

Interferon Beta

Interferon beta was developed largely as an immunomodulatory agent and showed evidence of benefit in relapsing multiple sclerosis for which it was first approved for use in the United States in 1993. Its major indication is to reduce the frequency of clinical exacerbations. Currently, five forms of interferon beta are available:

- Betaseron—interferon ß-1b, subcutaneous injection (250 mcg) every other day. Approved in 1993.

- Extavia—interferon ß-1b, subcutaneous injection (250 mcg) every other day. Approved in 1993.

- Avonex—interferon ß-1a, intramuscular injection (30 mcg) once weekly. Approved in 1996.

- Rebif—interferon ß-1a, subcutaneous injection (8.8 mcg, 22 mcg, 44 mcg) thrice weekly. Approved in 2003.

- Plegridy—peginterferon ß-1a, subcutaneous injection (63, 94, 125 mcg) every 14 days. Approved in 2014.

The various forms of beta interferon are provided as a lyophilized powder for reconstitution or as a solution in single dose vials or in pre-filled syringes, pens, or autoinjectors. All five forms of beta interferon are produced by recombinant DNA techniques.

Mitoxantrone

Mitoxantrone evaluation in patients with progressive forms of multiple sclerosis was shown to have activity in decreasing the rates of relapse and development of new lesions. Mitoxantrone was approved for use in the United States in 1987 and current indications include acute nonlymphocytic leukemia and advanced prostate cancer. Mitoxantrone is also approved for use in relapsing and progressive multiple sclerosis. Mitoxantrone is available in several generic formulations as a solution for injection (usually 2 mg/mL). Mitoxantrone is administered intravenously in varying doses typically ranging from 12 to 14 mg/m^2 at intervals of every 3 months (multiple sclerosis) or in monthly cycles (prostate cancer and leukemia). Side effects of mitoxantrone include bone marrow suppression, nausea, vomiting, abdominal discomfort, diarrhea, alopecia, headache, dizziness, and rash. Serious side effects include febrile neutropenia, cardiac toxicity (similar to that caused by doxorubicin) and secondary leukemia (in patients with multiple sclerosis).

Natalizumab

Natalizumab is used in the therapy of severe inflammatory bowel disease and relapsing multiple sclerosis and is available in 15 mL vials of 300 mg under the brand name "Tysabri." The recommended dose is 300 mg intravenously every 4 weeks. Common side effects include headache, fatigue, and infusion reactions. Natalizumab is also capable of causing immune suppression, resulting in an increased susceptibility to severe viral and bacterial infections.

Ocrelizumab

Ocrelizumab was found to be beneficial in multiple sclerosis, decreasing rates of relapse as well as slowing progression. Ocrelizumab was approved for use in the United States in 2017 for both progressive and relapsing multiple sclerosis. Ocrelizumab is under evaluation in other autoimmune and malignant conditions but is not approved for these uses. Ocrelizumab is available in liquid solution in single use vials of 300 mg (30 mg/mL) under the brand name "Ocrevus." The recommended dose is 600 mg intravenously every 6 months, the initial dose being given as 2 separate infusions of 300 mg 2 weeks apart. Treatment results in a rapid decline in circulating B cells and decrease in immunoglobulin levels, effects that persist for 6 to 18 months. Common adverse events include infusion reactions, cough, diarrhea, skin rash, and infections, particularly herpes simplex. Rare, but potentially serious adverse events include reactivation of hepatitis B, increased risk of malignancy and progressive multifocal leukoencephalopathy (PMLE).

Teriflunomide

Teriflunomide was found to reduce relapse rates and improve neuroradiologic outcomes in adult patients with relapsing-remitting multiple sclerosis. Teriflunomide was approved for use for multiple sclerosis in the United States in 2012 and is now available in tablets of 7 and 14 mg under the brand name "Aubagio." The recommended dose in adults is 7 or 14 mg orally once daily. Common side effects are headache, diarrhea, nausea, and hair loss (alopecia). Rare, but potentially serious adverse events include increased risk of severe infections, reactivation of tuberculosis and peripheral neuropathy.

Symptomatic Therapies
Dalfampridine

Dalfampridine was approved for use in the United States in 2010 and current indications are for symptomatic treatment of motor weakness in relapsing multiple sclerosis. Dalfampridine is available in tablets of 10 mg under the brand name "Ampyra." The typical dose in adults is 10 mg twice daily. Side effects may include insomnia, dizziness, headache, nausea, fatigue, back pain, and ataxia. Uncommon, but serious side effects include seizures, delirium, and stupor. Actually, 4-aminopyridine is a well known neurotoxin and is used as an avicide. Overdoses in humans can cause seizures, stupor, coma, and death.

Section 25.2

Multiple Sclerosis: Therapeutics under Research

This section includes text excerpted from "How Drugs Could Repair Damage from Multiple Sclerosis," National Institutes of Health (NIH), August 14, 2018.

Multiple sclerosis (MS) is an autoimmune disease in which the body's own immune system mistakenly attacks the lining of the nerves in the brain and spinal cord. When this insulating lining, called "myelin," is damaged, communication between nerve cells can be interrupted. This leads to muscle weakness, problems with coordination and vision, and other symptoms of the disease.

Experts estimate that almost half a million people nationwide live with multiple sclerosis. Existing drugs can relieve symptoms for a while by calming the immune system. But in most people, the disease gets worse over time. If scientists can develop drugs that promote myelin repair in people, the damage caused by multiple sclerosis could potentially be reversed.

In previous research, a team led by Dr. Paul Tesar at Case Western Reserve University and Dr. Robert Miller at George Washington University found that miconazole, an antifungal drug, activated stem cells and repaired myelin damage in mice. The researchers, joined by Dr. Drew Adams from Case Western Reserve, wanted to understand exactly how this drug—and others that have been discovered—encourage myelin repair. The study was funded by the National Institutes of Health's (NIH) National Institute of Neurological Diseases and Stroke (NINDS) and other NIH components. Results were published on July 25, 2018, in *Nature,* along with a companion methods paper in *Nature Methods.*

The team used a series of laboratory techniques to examine how drugs interact with the molecules in the body that are involved in myelin production. They found that miconazole and eight other related drugs all blocked an enzyme called "CYP51." Blocking CYP51 encouraged stem cells to form new oligodendrocytes. These are the cells that create myelin coatings around nerve cells.

CYP51 is part of the molecular pathway that produces cholesterol. The researchers discovered that blocking two other enzymes in that pathway also promoted oligodendrocyte production.

The boost in oligodendrocyte production appeared to be due to the buildup of a specific type of cholesterol precursor (called "8,9-unsaturated sterols") when any of the three enzymes was blocked. When the researchers treated stem cells with 8,9-unsaturated sterols, they saw oligodendrocyte production rise.

The team next screened over 3,000 approved drugs and other small molecules for their ability to promote oligodendrocyte production. The top 10 all caused a buildup of 8,9-unsaturated sterols.

When tested on human stem cells grown in the laboratory, drugs or genetic manipulations that targeted any one of the three enzymes caused oligodendrocytes to form and start laying down myelin. In mice with damage to myelin in their spinal cords, injection of drugs that targeted one of the enzymes caused restoration of myelin in the damaged tissue.

"We were shocked to find that almost all of these previously identified molecules share the ability to inhibit specific enzymes that help to make cholesterol. This insight reorients drug discovery efforts onto this novel, druggable targets," Adams says.

The researchers have formed a company to build on these findings and develop therapeutics to promote myelin repair.

Section 25.3

New Drugs for Treating Multiple Sclerosis

This section contains text excerpted from the following sources: Text under the heading "Ocrevus (Ocrelizumab) to Treat Adult Patients with Relapsing Forms of Multiple Sclerosis" is excerpted from "FDA Approves New Drug to Treat Multiple Sclerosis," U.S. Food and Drug Administration (FDA), March 28, 2018; Text under the heading "U.S. Food and Drug Administration Approves Zinbryta to Treat Multiple Sclerosis" is excerpted from "U.S. Food and Drug Administration Approves Zinbryta to Treat Multiple Sclerosis," U.S. Food and Drug Administration (FDA), May 31, 2016.

Ocrevus (Ocrelizumab) to Treat Adult Patients with Relapsing Forms of Multiple Sclerosis

The U.S. Food and Drug Administration (FDA) has approved Ocrevus (ocrelizumab) to treat adult patients with relapsing forms of multiple sclerosis (MS) and primary progressive multiple sclerosis (PPMS). This is the first drug approved by the FDA for PPMS. Ocrevus is an intravenous infusion given by a healthcare professional.

"Multiple sclerosis (MS) can have a profound impact on a person's life," said Billy Dunn, M.D., director of the Division of Neurology Products in the FDA's Center for Drug Evaluation and Research (CDER). "This therapy not only provides another treatment option for those with relapsing MS, but for the first time provides an approved therapy for those with primary progressive MS."

MS is a chronic, inflammatory, autoimmune disease of the central nervous system that disrupts communication between the brain and other parts of the body. It is among the most common causes of neurological disability in young adults and occurs more frequently in women than men. For most people with MS, episodes of worsening function (relapses) are initially followed by recovery periods (remissions). Over time, recovery may be incomplete, leading to progressive decline in function and increased disability. Most people experience their first symptoms of MS between the ages of 20 and 40.

PPMS is characterized by steadily worsening function from the onset of symptoms, often without early relapses or remissions. The U.S. Centers for Disease Control and Prevention (CDC) estimates that approximately 15 percent of patients with MS have PPMS.

The efficacy of Ocrevus for the treatment of relapsing forms of MS was shown in 2 clinical trials in 1,656 participants treated for 96 weeks. Both studies compared Ocrevus to another MS drug, Rebif (interferon beta-1a). In both studies, the patients receiving Ocrevus had reduced relapse rates and reduced worsening of disability compared to Rebif.

In a study of PPMS in 732 participants treated for at least 120 weeks, those receiving Ocrevus showed a longer time to the worsening of disability compared to placebo.

Ocrevus should not be used in patients with hepatitis B infection or a history of life-threatening infusion-related reactions to Ocrevus. Ocrevus must be dispensed with a patient medication guide that describes important information about the drug's uses and risks. Ocrevus can cause infusion-related reactions, which can be serious. These reactions include, but are not limited to, itchy skin, rash, hives, skin redness, flushing, low blood pressure, fever, tiredness, dizziness, headache, throat irritation, shortness of breath, swelling of the throat, nausea, and fast heartbeat. Additionally, Ocrevus may increase the risk for malignancies, particularly breast cancer. Ocrevus treatment should be delayed for patients with active infections. Vaccination with live or live attenuated vaccines is not recommended in patients receiving Ocrevus.

In addition to the infusion-related reactions, the most common side effect of Ocrevus seen in the clinical trials for relapsing forms of MS was upper respiratory tract infection. The most common side effects in the study of PPMS were upper respiratory tract infection, skin infection, and lower respiratory tract infection.

The FDA granted this application breakthrough therapy designation, fast track designation, and priority review. The FDA granted approval of Ocrevus to Genentech, Inc.

The FDA, an agency within the U.S. Department of Health and Human Services (HHS), protects the public health by assuring the safety, effectiveness, and security of human and veterinary drugs, vaccines and other biological products for human use, and medical devices. The agency also is responsible for the safety and security of our nation's food supply, cosmetics, dietary supplements, products that give off electronic radiation, and for regulating tobacco products.

The U.S. Food and Drug Administration Approves Zinbryta to Treat Multiple Sclerosis

The U.S. Food and Drug Administration (FDA) on May 27, 2016 approved Zinbryta (daclizumab) for the treatment of adults with relapsing forms of multiple sclerosis (MS). Zinbryta is a long-acting injection that is self-administered by the patient monthly.

"Zinbryta provides an additional choice to patients who may require a new option for treatment," said Billy Dunn, M.D., director of the Division of Neurology Products in the FDA's Center for Drug Evaluation and Research (CDER).

MS is a chronic, inflammatory, autoimmune disease of the central nervous system that disrupts communication between the brain and other parts of the body. It is among the most common causes of neurological disability in young adults and occurs more frequently in women than men. For most people with MS, episodes of worsening function (relapses) are initially followed by recovery periods (remissions). Over time, recovery may be incomplete, leading to progressive decline in function and increased disability. Most people experience their first symptoms of MS between the ages of 20 and 40.

The effectiveness of Zinbryta was shown in 2 clinical trials. One trial compared Zinbryta and Avonex in 1,841 participants who were studied for 144 weeks. Patients on Zinbryta had fewer clinical relapses than patients taking Avonex. The second trial compared Zinbryta with placebo and included 412 participants who were treated for 52 weeks. In that study, those receiving Zinbryta had fewer relapses compared to those receiving placebo.

Zinbryta should generally be used only in patients who have had an inadequate response to two or more MS drugs because Zinbryta has serious safety risks, including liver injury and immune conditions. Because of the risks, Zinbryta has a boxed warning and is available only through a restricted distribution program under a risk evaluation and mitigation strategy.

The boxed warning tells prescribers that the drug can cause severe liver injury, including life-threatening and fatal events. Healthcare professionals should perform blood tests to monitor the patient's liver function prior to starting Zinbryta, monthly before each dose, and for up to six months after the last dose.

- The boxed warning also highlights other important risks of Zinbryta treatment including immune conditions, such as inflammation of the colon (noninfectious colitis), skin reactions, and enlargement of lymph nodes (lymphadenopathy).

- Additional highlighted warnings include hypersensitivity reactions (anaphylaxis or angioedema), increased risk of infections, and symptoms of depression and/or suicidal ideation.

- The most common adverse reactions reported by patients receiving Zinbryta in the clinical trial that compared it to

Avonex include cold symptoms (nasopharyngitis), upper respiratory tract infection, rash, influenza, dermatitis, throat (oropharyngeal) pain, eczema, and enlargement of lymph nodes. The most common adverse reactions reported by patients receiving Zinbryta when compared to the placebo are depression, rash, and increased alanine aminotransferase.

• Zinbryta is manufactured by Biogen, Inc. of Cambridge, Massachusetts.

• The FDA, an agency within the U.S. Department of Health and Human Services (HHS), protects the public health by assuring the safety, effectiveness, and security of human and veterinary drugs, vaccines and other biological products for human use, and medical devices. The agency also is responsible for the safety and security of our nation's food supply, cosmetics, dietary supplements, products that give off electronic radiation, and for regulating tobacco products.

Section 25.4

The U.S. Food and Drug Administration Warns about Worsening of Multiple Sclerosis after Stopping the Medicine Gilenya

This section includes text excerpted from "FDA Warns about Severe Worsening of Multiple Sclerosis after Stopping the Medicine Gilenya (Fingolimod)," U.S. Food and Drug Administration (FDA), December 20, 2018.

The U.S. Food and Drug Administration (FDA) has warned that when the multiple sclerosis (MS) medicine Gilenya (fingolimod) is stopped, the disease can become much worse than before the medicine was started or while it was being taken. This MS worsening is rare but can result in permanent disability. As a result, the FDA has added a new warning about this risk to the prescribing information of the Gilenya drug label and in the patient medication guide.

Gilenya is one of several medicines approved to treat a form of MS called "relapsing MS," which are periods of time when MS symptoms get worse. The medicine was approved in the United States in 2010.

Healthcare professionals should inform patients before starting treatment about the potential risk of a severe increase in disability after stopping Gilenya. When Gilenya is stopped, patients should be carefully observed for evidence of an exacerbation of their MS and treated appropriately. Patients should be advised to seek immediate medical attention if they experience new or worsened symptoms of MS after Gilenya is stopped.

Patients should contact their healthcare professional immediately if they experience new or worsened symptoms of MS after Gilenya treatment is stopped. These symptoms vary and include new or worsened weakness; increased trouble using arms or legs; or changes in thinking, eyesight, or balance. Gilenya treatment may have to be stopped for reasons such as adverse drug reactions, planned or unplanned pregnancy, or because the medicine is not working. However, patients should not stop taking it without first talking to their prescribers, as stopping treatment can lead to worsening MS symptoms.

By 2018, the FDA identified 35 cases of severely increased disability accompanied by the presence of multiple new lesions on magnetic resonance imaging (MRI) that occurred 2 to 24 weeks after Gilenya was stopped. Most patients experienced this worsening in the first 12 weeks after stopping. The analyses include only reports submitted to the FDA and those found in the medical literature, so there may be additional cases about which the FDA are unaware. The severe increase in disability in these patients was more severe than typical MS relapses, and in cases where baseline disability was known, appeared unrelated to the patients' prior disease state. Several patients who were able to walk without assistance prior to discontinuing Gilenya progressed to needing wheelchairs or becoming totally bedbound. In patients experiencing worsening of their disability after stopping Gilenya, recovery varied. 17 patients had partial recovery, 8 experienced permanent disability or no recovery, and 6 eventually returned to the level of disability they had before or during Gilenya treatment.

The FDA previously communicated safety information about Gilenya in August 2015 and August 2013 (rare brain infection), May 2012 (revised cardiovascular monitoring recommendations), and December 2011 (safety review of reported death).

To help FDA track safety issues with medicines, healthcare professionals and patients are urged to report side effects involving Gilenya and other medicines to the FDA MedWatch program.

Facts about Gilenya (Fingolimod)

* Gilenya is one of several medicines used to treat relapsing multiple sclerosis (MS).

* Gilenya is available as 0.5 mg capsules. It is taken once daily by mouth.

* Common side effects include cough, headache, back pain, and diarrhea.

* In addition to the increase in disability that can occur after Gilenya discontinuation, Gilenya can cause a number of other serious adverse reactions that are already included in the prescribing information, such as:

  * Slow heart rate called "bradycardia," or with an abnormal heart rhythm called "bradyarrhythmia"

  * Infections, including a rare brain infection called "progressive multifocal leukoencephalopathy"

  * Swelling in the eye, called "macular edema," which causes vision problems

Information for Patients and Caregivers

* The FDA warns that when Gilenya is discontinued, symptoms of disability and other effects of multiple sclerosis (MS) can become worse than they were before or during Gilenya treatment. This severe disease worsening is rare but can result in permanent disability.

* Gilenya treatment may have to be stopped for reasons such as drug adverse reactions, planned or unplanned pregnancy, or because the medicine is not working.

* Because of this disease worsening, do not stop taking Gilenya without first talking to your healthcare professional.

* Seek medical attention immediately if you experience worsening symptoms after stopping Gilenya, such as:

- New or worsening weakness
- Increased trouble using your arms or legs
- Changes in thinking
- Changes in eyesight
- Changes in strength or balance

Chapter 26

Treating the Symptoms of Multiple Sclerosis

Multiple sclerosis (MS) causes a variety of symptoms that can interfere with daily activities, which can usually be treated or managed to reduce their impact. Many of these issues are best treated by neurologists who have advanced training in the treatment of MS and who can prescribe specific medications to treat the problems.

Vision Problems

Eye and vision problems are common in people with MS but rarely result in permanent blindness. Inflammation of the optic nerve or damage to the myelin that covers the optic nerve and other nerve fibers can cause a number of symptoms, including blurring or graying of vision, blindness in one eye, loss of normal color vision, depth perception, or a dark spot in the center of the visual field (scotoma).

Uncontrolled horizontal or vertical eye movements (nystagmus) and "jumping vision" (opsoclonus) are common with MS and can be either mild or severe enough to impair vision.

Double vision (diplopia) occurs when the two eyes are not perfectly aligned. This occurs commonly in MS when a pair of muscles that control a specific eye movement aren't coordinated due to weakness

This chapter includes text excerpted from "Multiple Sclerosis: Hope through Research," National Institute of Neurological Disorders and Stroke (NINDS), July 6, 2018.

in one or both muscles. Double vision may increase with fatigue or as the result of spending too much time reading or on the computer. Periodically resting the eyes may be helpful.

Weak Muscles, Stiff Muscles, Painful Muscle Spasms, and Weak Reflexes

Muscle weakness is common in MS, along with muscle spasticity. Spasticity refers to muscles that are stiff or that go into spasms without any warning. Spasticity in MS can be as mild as a feeling of tightness in the muscles or so severe that it causes painful, uncontrolled spasms. It can also cause pain or tightness in and around the joints. It also frequently affects walking, reducing the normal flexibility, or "bounce," involved in taking steps.

Tremor

People with MS sometimes develop tremor, or uncontrollable shaking, often triggered by movement. Tremor can be very disabling. Assistive devices and weights attached to the limbs are sometimes helpful for people with tremor. Deep brain stimulation and drugs, such as clonazepam, also may be useful.

Problems with Walking and Balance

Many people with MS experience difficulty walking. In fact, studies indicate that half of those with relapsing-remitting MS will need some kind of help walking within 15 years of their diagnosis if they remain untreated. The most common walking problem in people with MS experience is ataxia—unsteady, uncoordinated movements—due to damage to the areas of the brain that coordinate the movement of muscles. People with severe ataxia generally benefit from the use of a cane, walker, or other assistive devices. Physical therapy can also reduce walking problems in many cases.

In 2010, the U.S. Food and Drug Administration (FDA) approved the drug dalfampridine to improve walking in patients with MS. It is the first drug approved for this use. Clinical trials showed that patients treated with dalfampridine had faster walking speeds than those treated with a placebo pill.

Fatigue

Fatigue is a common symptom of MS and may be both physical (for example, tiredness in the legs) and psychological (due to depression).

Probably the most important measures people with MS can take to counter physical fatigue are to avoid excessive activity and to stay out of the heat, which often aggravates MS symptoms. On the other hand, daily physical activity programs of mild to moderate intensity can significantly reduce fatigue. An antidepressant, such as fluoxetine, may be prescribed if the fatigue is caused by depression. Other drugs that may reduce fatigue in some individuals include amantadine and modafinil.

Fatigue may be reduced if the person receives occupational therapy to simplify tasks and/or physical therapy to learn how to walk in a way that saves physical energy or that takes advantage of an assistive device. Some people benefit from stress management programs, relaxation training, membership in an MS support group, or individual psychotherapy. Treating sleep problems and MS symptoms that interfere with sleep (such as spastic muscles) may also help.

Pain

People with MS may experience several types of pain during the course of the disease.

Trigeminal neuralgia is a sharp, stabbing, facial pain caused by MS affecting the trigeminal nerve as it exits the brainstem on its way to the jaw and cheek. It can be treated with anticonvulsant or antispasmodic drugs, alcohol injections, or surgery.

People with MS occasionally develop central pain, a syndrome caused by damage to the brain and/or spinal cord. Drugs, such as gabapentin and nortriptyline, sometimes help to reduce central pain.

Burning, tingling, and prickling (commonly called "pins and needles") are sensations that happen in the absence of any stimulation. The medical term for them is "dysesthesias." They are often chronic and hard to treat.

Chronic back or other musculoskeletal pain may be caused by walking problems or by using assistive aids incorrectly. Treatments may include heat, massage, ultrasound treatments, and physical therapy to correct faulty posture and strengthen and stretch muscles.

Problems with Bladder Control and Constipation

The most common bladder-control problems encountered by people with MS are urinary frequency, urgency, or the loss of bladder control. The same spasticity that causes spasms in legs can also affect the bladder. A small number of individuals will have the opposite

163

problem—retaining large amounts of urine. Urologists can help with treatment of bladder-related problems. A number of medical treatments are available. Constipation is also common and can be treated with a high-fiber diet, laxatives, and other measures.

Sexual Problems

People with MS sometimes experience sexual problems. Sexual arousal begins in the central nervous system, as the brain sends messages to the sex organs along nerves running through the spinal cord. If MS damages these nerve pathways, sexual response—including arousal and orgasm—can be directly affected. Sexual problems may also stem from MS symptoms, such as fatigue, cramped or spastic muscles, and psychological factors related to lowered self-esteem or depression. Some of these problems can be corrected with medications. Psychological counseling also may be helpful.

Depression

Studies indicate that clinical depression is more frequent among people with MS than it is in the general population or in persons with many other chronic, disabling conditions. MS may cause depression as part of the disease process since it damages myelin and nerve fibers inside the brain. If the plaques are in parts of the brain that are involved in emotional expression and control, a variety of behavioral changes can result, including depression. Depression can intensify symptoms of fatigue, pain, and sexual dysfunction. It is most often treated with selective serotonin reuptake inhibitor (SSRI) antidepressant medications, which are less likely than other antidepressant medications to cause fatigue.

Inappropriate Laughing or Crying

MS is sometimes associated with a condition called "pseudobulbar affect" that causes inappropriate and involuntary expressions of laughter, crying, or anger. These expressions are often unrelated to mood; for example, the person may cry when they are actually very happy, or laugh when they are not especially happy. In 2010, the FDA approved the first treatment specifically for pseudobulbar affect, which is a combination of the drugs dextromethorphan and quinidine. The condition can also be treated with other drugs, such as amitriptyline or citalopram.

Cognitive Changes

Half to three-quarters of people with MS experience cognitive impairment, which is a phrase doctors use to describe a decline in the ability to think quickly and clearly and to remember easily. These cognitive changes may appear at the same time as the physical symptoms, or they may develop gradually over time. Some individuals with MS may feel as if they are thinking more slowly, are easily distracted, have trouble remembering, or are losing their way with words. The right word may often seem to be on the tip of their tongue.

Some experts believe that it is more likely to be the cognitive decline, rather than physical impairment, that causes people with MS to eventually withdraw from the workforce. A number of neuropsychological tests have been developed to evaluate the cognitive status of individuals with MS. Based on the outcomes of these tests, a neuropsychologist can determine the extent of strengths and weaknesses in different cognitive areas. Drugs, such as donepezil, which is usually used for Alzheimer disease, may be helpful in some cases.

Chapter 27

Treating Exacerbations and Relapses

What Is an Exacerbation or Attack of Multiple Sclerosis?

An exacerbation—which is also called a "relapse," "flare-up," or "attack"—is a sudden worsening of multiple sclerosis (MS) symptoms or the appearance of new symptoms that lasts for at least 24 hours. MS relapses are thought to be associated with the development of new areas of damage in the brain. Exacerbations are characteristic of relapsing-remitting MS, in which attacks are followed by periods of complete or partial recovery with no apparent worsening of symptoms.

An attack may be mild, or its symptoms may be severe enough to significantly interfere with life's daily activities. Most exacerbations last from several days to several weeks, although some have been known to last for months.

This chapter contains text excerpted from the following sources: Text beginning with the heading "What Is an Exacerbation or Attack of Multiple Sclerosis?" is excerpted from "Multiple Sclerosis: Hope through Research," National Institute of Neurological Disorders and Stroke (NINDS), July 6, 2018; Text under the heading "Treatments for Multiple Sclerosis Relapses" is excerpted from "Treatments for Multiple Sclerosis Relapses," U.S. Department of Veterans Affairs (VA), August 3, 2018; Text under the heading "Information on Natalizumab (Marketed as Tysabri)" is excerpted from "Information on Natalizumab (Marketed as Tysabri)," U.S. Food and Drug Administration (FDA), July 17, 2015. Reviewed March 2019.

When the symptoms of the attack subside, an individual with MS is said to be in remission. However, magnetic resonance imaging (MRI) data have shown that this is somewhat misleading because MS lesions continue to appear during these remission periods. Patients do not experience symptoms during remission because the inflammation may not be severe, or it may occur in areas of the brain that do not produce obvious symptoms. Research suggests that only about 1 out of every 10 MS lesion is perceived by a person with MS. Therefore, MRI examination plays a very important role in establishing an MS diagnosis, deciding when the disease should be treated and determining whether treatments work effectively or not. It also has been a valuable tool to test whether an experimental new therapy is effective at reducing exacerbations.

Treatments for Attacks

The usual treatment for an initial MS attack is to inject high doses of a steroid drug, such as methylprednisolone, intravenously (into a vein) over the course of three to five days. It may sometimes be followed by a tapered dose of oral steroids. Intravenous steroids quickly and potently suppress the immune system and reduce inflammation. Clinical trials have shown that these drugs hasten recovery.

The American Academy of Neurology (AAN) recommends using plasma exchange as a secondary treatment for severe flare-ups in relapsing forms of MS when the patient does not have a good response to methylprednisolone. Plasma exchange, also known as "plasmapheresis," involves taking blood out of the body and removing components in the blood's plasma that are thought to be harmful. The rest of the blood, plus replacement plasma, is then transfused back into the body. This treatment has not been shown to be effective for secondary progressive or chronic progressive forms of MS.

Treatments for Multiple Sclerosis Relapses

MS relapse symptoms generally appear over hours to a couple of days and can affect anything controlled by the brain, spinal cord, or optic nerves. MS relapses often cause changes in sensation, bladder or bowel symptoms, muscle strength, or vision. Most people with MS experience relapses, and the timing of these relapses is unpredictable. People with MS should contact their healthcare provider promptly, if they suspect they are experiencing a relapse.

Corticosteroids

The standard treatment for MS relapses associated with significant disability is high-dose corticosteroids for 3 to 5 days. This is usually 1,000 mg of intravenous methylprednisolone (IVMP) in 100cc of normal saline over 1 hour daily for 3 to 5 days. Intravenous dexamethasone at 140 to 200 mg/day for 3 to 5 days is occasionally used in place of IVMP in cases of allergy or intolerance of methylprednisolone. Oral prednisone at 1250 mg/day for 3 to 5 days is used if intravenous treatment is not practical. The high-dose corticosteroids may be followed by a short taper of oral prednisone, but this oral steroid taper has unclear benefits. Intravenous steroids may be administered in several clinical settings.

High-dose corticosteroids given early in a relapse generally shortens the duration of the relapse to a few weeks. However, the treatment of relapses with corticosteroids does not affect the long-term course of MS. Mild relapses, therefore, do not necessarily require treatment. The decision to treat with corticosteroids often depends on how bothersome the symptoms are to the patient and their tolerance of corticosteroids.

Side Effects of Corticosteroids

- Metallic taste in the mouth during the infusion

- Stomach irritation—may be managed with antacids and H2 blockers

- Difficulty sleeping, restlessness, anxiety, or mood change—may be managed with hypnotics

- Increased appetite, resulting in weight gain

- Increased blood sugar in people with diabetes—may need to cover with insulin

- Fluid retention

- Excessive sweating

- Acne

- Aseptic necrosis of the hips, moon face, or swelling between the shoulder blades and osteoporosis can occur with corticosteroid use, but are not usually an issue with short courses of corticosteroids

Plasma Exchange

For severe MS relapses that do not respond to high-dose corticosteroids, plasma exchange may be considered. The side effects of plasma exchange must be balanced against the severity of symptoms. This treatment usually requires hospitalization. A course of treatment consists of plasma exchange every other day for five treatments. Others use daily plasma exchange for five treatments.

Side Effects of Plasma Exchange

- Bleeding, due to the placement of the intravenous lines or due to thrombocytopenia (slow blood clotting)

- Infection, due to the placement of the intravenous lines

- Damage to lungs or other tissues, due to the placement of the intravenous lines

- Episodes of low blood pressure during treatments

- Episodes of irregular heartbeats during treatment

- Allergic reactions to portions of the blood plasma

- Electrolyte abnormalities during treatment

- Thrombocytopenia, due to heparin used during the treatment

- A hypercoagulable state with the risk of thrombosis (clotting of blood)

Rehabilitation

Relapse management may also include rehabilitation, such as physical, occupational, or speech therapy, to help with symptom management and potentially lessen the overall effects of the acute neurological event and any problems remaining after the relapse.

Information on Natalizumab (Marketed as Tysabri)

Natalizumab is used to prevent episodes of symptoms and slow the worsening of disability in patients with relapsing forms (course of a disease where symptoms flare up from time to time) of multiple sclerosis.

Natalizumab is also used to treat and prevent episodes of symptoms in people who have Crohn disease (a condition in which the body attacks the lining of the digestive tract, causing pain, diarrhea, weight loss, and fever) who have not been helped by other medications or who cannot take other medications.

Natalizumab is in a class of medications called "immunomodulators." It works by stopping certain cells of the immune system from reaching the brain and spinal cord and causing damage.

Chapter 28

Treating Involuntary Movement

Chapter Contents

Section 28.1

Controlling Spasticity in Multiple Sclerosis

This section includes text excerpted from "Managing
Spasticity with an Intrathecal Baclofen Pump," U.S.
Department of Veterans Affairs (VA), August 17, 2018.

People living with multiple sclerosis (MS) can experience muscle
stiffness, pain, jerking, weakness, or difficulty coordinating their
movements. This is called "spasticity." Spasticity is a disorder of
the muscles and nerves commonly seen in people living with MS.
Due to MS plaques in the brain and spinal cord, the body's normal
ability to control muscle contractions and muscle relaxation is lost.
Spasticity can be constant or come and go. Spasticity can be triggered
by moving the limbs or irritation, such as a wound or urinary tract
infection. When spasticity is severe, it can limit a person's ability
to walk, get dressed, complete personal hygiene, sit comfortably, or
can cause pain.

How Is Spasticity Treated?

There are many ways to treat spasticity and, frequently, multiple
treatments are used at the same time. Daily stretching and strength-
ening is usually tried first for mild spasticity. Medications, such as
baclofen, tizanidine, gabapentin, clonidine, dantrolene, or in some
instances diazepam, can be used. Botulinum toxin injections can be
used when spasticity only affects a limited area, such as one leg or arm.
Bracing and surgery can also be used in certain cases. Delivering liquid
baclofen into the spinal canal, called "intrathecal baclofen" (ITB), can
also be used if other treatments are unsuccessful.

What Is Intrathecal Baclofen Therapy?

Intrathecal baclofen (ITB) therapy is when liquid baclofen is delivered around the spinal cord. A small, round pump is surgically placed
under the skin in the abdomen. A thin tube (catheter) attaches to the
pump and goes around the abdomen to the back and is inserted into
the spinal canal. Usually, you will be able to see and feel the pump.
You will not be able to see or feel the catheter. The pump generally
holds enough medication to last several months and is refilled in an
office visit. The battery for the pump will last around seven years.

What Are the Benefits of Intrathecal Baclofen?

Medications used to treat spasticity can have side effects, including dizziness, fatigue, or sleepiness. With ITB, since it is going directly to the spinal cord, it uses up to 100 times less medication to get the same effect. Additionally, the medication goes right to the spinal cord and may be more effective.

Who Is the Best Candidate for Intrathecal Baclofen Therapy?

The best candidates for ITB are people whose spasticity or spasms are not well controlled with other treatment options. They will need to be able to come in regularly for management of the pump. ITB therapy can be appropriate for people living with MS and should be considered if people are able to walk or are restricted to their bed.

Goals of ITB therapy could include improving or maintaining the ability to walk, decreasing painful spasms, maintaining joint mobility, protecting the skin, doing personal hygiene activities, or making it easier to sit in a chair.

What Is an Intrathecal Baclofen Screening Test?

Prior to getting a pump, most physicians will perform a screening test or refer you to a physician who does these tests. For the screening test, a dose of baclofen is injected into the spinal canal through a lumbar puncture, also called a "spinal tap." You may have had this when you were diagnosed with MS. The test dose will give you and your doctor an idea if this medication is effective. This screening test may take place in a clinic or during a hospital admission.

During a positive response, the legs may become temporarily weak. This goes away usually in four to eight hours. During this time, you will be monitored by your doctor or physical therapist. They will monitor your blood pressure and heart rate, improvement in your symptoms, and note any negative side effects you may have. When the results of the medication fade, you will be sent home. Usually, this is the same day. Rarely, you may have to spend the night in the hospital. The effects of the ITB therapy are not permanent. Although most doctors do a test dose to see if you are responsive to ITB, the test dose does not always predict exactly what it will be like with an ITB pump.

How Is the Pump Implanted?

After the test dose, you and your doctor will decide if putting an intrathecal baclofen pump in surgically is right for you. The surgery will be scheduled for another admission and will be done by a surgeon who is familiar with this procedure. Most people are sent home the following day after the pump is implanted. Rarely, you may need to stay in the hospital for a couple of days while the dose is adjusted and you receive physical or occupational therapy.

What Is Done to Manage the Intrathecal Baclofen Pump after Implantation?

After the pump is implanted, the dose will be noninvasively adjusted in your doctor's office. Initially, this may be weekly to increase the pump dose and wean off oral spasticity medications. A stable dose is usually reached in several months. The daily dose can continue to be changed as needed. Depending on how much baclofen you use, your pump will need to be refilled every month to every six months. The pump has an alarm that will alert you if the pump runs out of medication or if the battery is no longer functioning. Another surgery will be needed to replace the pump when the battery dies or if there is a problem with the pump or catheter malfunctioning.

Severe consequences are rare, but there is a chance of life-threatening events, such as getting too much baclofen (an overdose) or too little baclofen (withdrawal). Warning signs of an overdose can include drowsiness, lightheadedness, dizziness, difficulty breathing, seizures, lower than normal body temperature, or loss of consciousness. Warning signs of withdrawal can include increase or return of spasticity, itching, low blood pressure, lightheadedness, or a tingling sensation. If you have these symptoms, you will need to seek immediate care, such as seeing your doctor or going to the emergency room.

Spasticity can have a significant negative effect on someone living with MS. An intrathecal baclofen pump is one method for treating spasticity. After the pump is in place, the best treatment for spasticity usually continues to include a variety of treatment options, including daily stretching/strengthening, medications, bracing, or botulinum toxin injections.

Section 28.2

Deep Brain Stimulation for Multiple Sclerosis

This section includes text excerpted from "Deep Brain Stimulation for Movement Disorders Fact Sheet," National Institute of Neurological Disorders and Stroke (NINDS), July 30, 2018.

Deep brain stimulation (DBS) is a surgical procedure used to treat disabling symptoms of neurological disorders, including dystonia, epilepsy, essential tremor, and Parkinson disease. DBS uses a surgically implanted, battery-operated medical device called an "implantable pulse generator" (IPG)—similar to a heart pacemaker and approximately the size of a stopwatch—to deliver electrical stimulation to specific areas in the brain that control movement, which blocks the abnormal nerve signals that cause symptoms.

The DBS system consists of three components: the lead, the extension, and the IPG. The lead (also called an "electrode")—a thin, insulated wire—is inserted through a small opening made in the skull and implanted in the brain. The tip of the electrode is positioned within a specific brain area, depending on the disorder. The extension is an insulated wire that is passed under the skin of the head, neck, and shoulder, connecting the lead to the implantable pulse generator. The IPG (the "battery pack") is usually implanted under the skin near the collarbone. In some cases, it may be implanted lower in the chest or under the skin over the abdomen.

Once the system is in place, and after a period of healing post surgery, the device is programmed to sets of parameters that work best for each person, over several visits with a neurologist. The therapy works by delivering electrical pulses from the IPG along the extension wire and the lead and into the brain. These pulses change the brain's electrical activity pattern at the target site to reduce motor symptoms.

Which Parts of the Brain Are Targeted Using Deep Brain Stimulation for Movement Disorders?

Before the procedure, a neurosurgeon uses noninvasive diagnostic imaging—either magnetic resonance imaging (MRI) or computed tomography (CT) scanning—to identify and locate the exact target in the brain for the surgery. Most surgeons use microelectrode recording—which involves insertion of a tiny wire that monitors the activity of nerve cells—to more specifically identify the precise brain area that will be stimulated.

For treatment of Parkinson disease (PD), DBS targets parts of the brain that play a role in the control of movement—the thalamus (which relays and integrates sensory and motor information), subthalamic nucleus (which helps direct movement preparation), or globus pallidus (which helps regulate intended movement). DBS for dystonia specifically targets the globus pallidus interna (involved in the regulation of voluntary movement), while DBS for essential tremor targets the thalamus. Different areas of the brain may be targeted for individuals with epilepsy who don't respond well to other therapies.

How Is Deep Brain Stimulation Being Used to Treat Movement Disorders?
Parkinson Disease

DBS is used to treat the most commonly debilitating motor symptoms of PD, such as rigidity, slowed movement, stiffness, tremor, and problems walking. It is used only for individuals whose symptoms cannot be adequately controlled with medication. However, only people who improve to some degree after taking medication for Parkinson disease benefit from DBS. A variety of conditions may mimic PD but do not respond to medication or DBS.

Most people with PD still need to take medicine after undergoing DBS, but many people experience considerable reduction of their motor symptoms and may be able to reduce their medications. The degree of reduction varies by individual but can lead to a significant improvement in side effects, such as dyskinesia (involuntary movements caused by long-term use of levodopa). In some cases, the stimulation itself can suppress dyskinesia without a reduction in medication. DBS does not improve cognitive symptoms in PD and may worsen them. Therefore, it is not generally used if there are signs of dementia. DBS does not slow the progression of the neurodegeneration.

Dystonia

For individuals with dystonia, DBS may reduce the disorder-characteristic involuntary muscle contractions that cause such symptoms as abnormal posture, repetitive movements, or twisting. DBS has been shown to reduce both the severity of symptoms caused by dystonia and the level of disability they may cause.

People with dystonia may respond better to DBS than medication; therefore, DBS may be an appropriate option for people who have found little or no improvement of symptoms after botulinum toxin injections (often the most effective treatment for some dystonia). DBS may be quicker to reduce symptoms of dystonia that migrates from place to place in the body than dystonia that remains fixed in a single body site, although both groups are likely to see improvement.

Essential Tremor

DBS targeting the thalamus can improve the involuntary movement of the arms, hands, and head that is associated with essential tremor.

Epilepsy

Brain stimulation for focal epilepsy (seizures that originate in just one part of the brain) may reduce the number of seizures over time. It is not a single therapy but is used along with antiepileptic drugs.

DBS has been approved as add-on therapy for adults with focal epilepsy. Another form of treatment, called "neurostimulation," uses an implanted monitor in the skull and tiny wires to give small pulses of stimulation to the brain when electrical activity in the brain looks like a seizure.

Are There Advantages to Deep Brain Stimulation?

DBS involves minimal permanent surgical changes to the brain. If DBS causes unwanted side effects or more promising treatments develop in the future, the IPG can be removed, and the DBS procedure can be halted. Also, stimulation from the IPG is easily adjustable—without further surgery—if the person's condition changes. Some people describe the pulse generator adjustments as "programming."

What Risks Are Associated with Deep Brain Stimulation?

Although minimally invasive, DBS is a surgical procedure and, therefore, carries some associated risk. There is a low chance that placement of the stimulator may cause bleeding or infection in the brain. Complications of DBS, such as bleeding and swelling of brain tissue, may result from mechanical stress from the device but are generally reversible. Other complications may include headache, seizures, and temporary pain following surgery. Also, the hardware may erode or break down with use, requiring surgery to replace parts of the device.

Side effects of the stimulation may include numbness or tingling sensations, behavioral changes, as well as balance or speech problems.

Section 28.3

Myoclonus

This section includes text excerpted from "Myoclonus Fact Sheet," National Institute of Neurological Disorders and Stroke (NINDS), July 6, 2018.

What Is Myoclonus?

Myoclonus describes a symptom and not a diagnosis of a disease. It refers to sudden, involuntary jerking of a muscle or group of muscles. Myoclonic twitches or jerks usually are caused by sudden muscle contractions, called "positive myoclonus," or by muscle relaxation, called "negative myoclonus." Myoclonic jerks may occur alone or in sequence, in a pattern or without pattern. They may occur infrequently or many times each minute. Myoclonus sometimes occurs in response to an external event or when a person attempts to make a movement. The twitching cannot be controlled by the person experiencing it.

In its simplest form, myoclonus consists of a muscle twitch followed by relaxation. A hiccup is an example of this type of myoclonus. Other familiar examples of myoclonus are the jerks or "sleep starts" that some people experience while drifting off to sleep. These simple forms of myoclonus occur in normal, healthy persons and cause no difficulties. When more widespread, myoclonus may involve persistent, shock-like contractions in a group of muscles. In some cases, myoclonus begins in one region of the body and spreads to muscles in other areas. More severe cases of myoclonus can distort movement and severely limit a person's ability to eat, talk, or walk. These types of myoclonus may indicate an underlying disorder in the brain or nerves.

What Are the Causes of Myoclonus?

Myoclonus may develop in response to an infection, head or spinal cord injury, stroke, brain tumors, kidney or liver failure, lipid storage disease, chemical or drug poisoning, or other disorders. Prolonged oxygen deprivation to the brain, called "hypoxia," may result in post-hypoxic myoclonus. Myoclonus can occur by itself, but most often it is one of several symptoms associated with a wide variety of nervous system disorders. For example, myoclonic jerking may develop in patients with multiple sclerosis, Parkinson disease, Alzheimer disease, or Creutzfeldt-Jakob disease. Myoclonic jerks commonly occur in persons with epilepsy, a disorder in which the electrical activity in the brain becomes disordered and leads to seizures.

What Are the Types of Myoclonus?

Classifying the many different forms of myoclonus is difficult because the causes, effects, and responses to therapy vary widely. Listed below are the types most commonly described.

- **Action myoclonus** is characterized by muscular jerking triggered or intensified by voluntary movement or even the intention to move. It may be made worse by attempts at precise, coordinated movements. Action myoclonus is the most disabling form of myoclonus and can affect the arms, legs, face, and even the voice. This type of myoclonus often is caused by brain damage that results from a lack of oxygen and blood flow to the brain when breathing or heartbeat is temporarily stopped.

- **Cortical reflex myoclonus** is thought to be a type of epilepsy that originates in the cerebral cortex—the outer layer, or "gray matter" of the brain that is responsible for much of the information processing that takes place in the brain. In this type of myoclonus, jerks usually involve only a few muscles in one part of the body, but jerks involving many muscles also may occur. Cortical reflex myoclonus can be intensified when individuals attempt to move in a certain way (action myoclonus) or perceive a particular sensation.

- **Essential myoclonus** occurs in the absence of epilepsy or other apparent abnormalities in the brain or nerves. It can occur randomly in people with no family history of it, but also can appear among members of the same family, indicating that it sometimes may be an inherited disorder. Essential myoclonus tends to be stable without increasing in severity over time. In some families, there is an association of essential myoclonus, essential tremor, and even a form of dystonia, called "myoclonus

181

dystonia." Another form of essential myoclonus may be a type of epilepsy with no known cause.

- **Palatal myoclonus** is a regular, rhythmic contraction of 1 or both sides of the rear of the roof of the mouth, called the "soft palate." These contractions may be accompanied by myoclonus in other muscles, including those in the face, tongue, throat, and diaphragm. The contractions are very rapid, occurring as often as 150 times a minute, and may persist during sleep. The condition usually appears in adults and can last indefinitely. Some people with palatal myoclonus regard it as a minor problem, although some occasionally complain of a "clicking" sound in the ear, a noise made as the muscles in the soft palate contract. The disorder can cause discomfort and severe pain in some individuals.

- **Progressive myoclonus epilepsy (PME)** is a group of diseases characterized by myoclonus, epileptic seizures, and other serious symptoms, such as trouble walking or speaking. These rare disorders often get worse over time and sometimes are fatal. Studies have identified many forms of PME. Lafora body disease is inherited as an autosomal recessive disorder, meaning that the disease occurs only when a child inherits two copies of a defective gene, one from each parent. Lafora body disease is characterized by myoclonus, epileptic seizures, and dementia (progressive loss of memory and other intellectual functions). A second group of PME diseases belonging to the class of cerebral storage diseases usually involves myoclonus, visual problems, dementia, and dystonia (sustained muscle contractions that cause twisting movements or abnormal postures). Another group of PME disorders in the class of system degenerations often is accompanied by action myoclonus, seizures, and problems with balance and walking. Many of these PME diseases begin in childhood or adolescence.

- **Reticular reflex myoclonus** is thought to be a type of generalized epilepsy that originates in the brain stem, the part of the brain that connects to the spinal cord and controls vital functions, such as breathing and heartbeat. Myoclonic jerks usually affect the whole body, with muscles on both sides of the body affected simultaneously. In some people, myoclonic jerks occur in only a part of the body, such as the legs, with all the muscles in that part being involved in each jerk. Reticular reflex myoclonus can be triggered by either a voluntary movement or an external stimulus.

- **Stimulus-sensitive myoclonus** is triggered by a variety of external events, including noise, movement, and light. Surprise may increase the sensitivity of the individual.

- **Sleep myoclonus** occurs during the initial phases of sleep, especially at the moment of dropping off to sleep. Some forms appear to be stimulus-sensitive. Some persons with sleep myoclonus are rarely troubled by, or need treatment for, the condition. However, myoclonus may be a symptom in more complex and disturbing sleep disorders, such as restless legs syndrome, and may require treatment by a doctor.

How Is Myoclonus Treated?

Treatment of myoclonus focuses on medications that may help reduce symptoms. The drug of first choice to treat myoclonus, especially certain types of action myoclonus, is clonazepam, a type of tranquilizer. Dosages of clonazepam usually are increased gradually until the individual improves or side effects become harmful. Drowsiness and loss of coordination are common side effects. The beneficial effects of clonazepam may diminish over time if the individual develops a tolerance for the drug.

Many of the drugs used for myoclonus, such as barbiturates, levetiracetam, phenytoin, and primidone, are also used to treat epilepsy. Barbiturates slow down the central nervous system and cause tranquilizing or antiseizure effects. Phenytoin, levetiracetam, and primidone are effective antiepileptic drugs, although phenytoin can cause liver failure or have other harmful long-term effects in individuals with PME. Sodium valproate is an alternative therapy for myoclonus and can be used either alone or in combination with clonazepam. Although clonazepam and/or sodium valproate are effective in the majority of people with myoclonus, some people have adverse reactions to these drugs.

Some studies have shown that doses of 5-hydroxytryptophan (5-HTP), a building block of serotonin, leads to improvement in people with some types of action myoclonus and PME. However, other studies indicate that 5-HTP therapy is not effective in all people with myoclonus, and, in fact, may worsen the condition in some individuals. These differences in the effect of 5-HTP on individuals with myoclonus have not yet been explained, but they may offer important clues to underlying abnormalities in serotonin receptors.

The complex origins of myoclonus may require the use of multiple drugs for effective treatment. Although some drugs have a limited effect when used individually, they may have a greater effect when used with drugs that act on different pathways or mechanisms in the brain. By combining several of these drugs, scientists hope to achieve greater control of myoclonic symptoms. Some drugs currently being studied in different combinations include clonazepam, sodium valproate, levetiracetam, and primidone. Hormonal therapy also may improve responses to antimyoclonic drugs in some people.

What Do Scientists Know about Myoclonus?

Although rare cases of myoclonus are caused by an injury to the peripheral nerves (defined as the nerves outside the brain and spinal cord or the central nervous system), most myoclonus is caused by a disturbance of the central nervous system. Studies suggest that several locations in the brain are involved in myoclonus. One such location, for example, is in the brain stem and close to structures that are responsible for the startle response, an automatic reaction to an unexpected stimulus involving rapid muscle contraction.

The specific mechanisms underlying myoclonus are not yet fully understood. Scientists believe that some types of stimulus-sensitive myoclonus may involve overexcitability of the parts of the brain that control movement. These parts are interconnected in a series of feedback loops called "motor pathways." These pathways facilitate and modulate communication between the brain and muscles. Key elements of this communication are chemicals known as "neurotransmitters," which carry messages from one nerve cell, or neuron, to another. Neurotransmitters are released by neurons and attach themselves to receptors on parts of neighboring cells. Some neurotransmitters may make the receiving cell more sensitive, while others tend to make the receiving cell less sensitive. Laboratory studies suggest that an imbalance between these chemicals may underlie myoclonus.

Some researchers speculate that abnormalities or deficiencies in the receptors for certain neurotransmitters may contribute to some forms of myoclonus. Receptors that appear to be related to myoclonus include those for two important inhibitory neurotransmitters: serotonin and gamma-aminobutyric acid (GABA). Other receptors with links to myoclonus include those for opiates and glycine, the latter an inhibitory neurotransmitter that is important for the control of motor and sensory functions in the spinal cord. More research is needed to determine how these receptor abnormalities cause or contribute to myoclonus.

What Research Is Being Done?

Within the federal government, the National Institute of Neurological Disorders and Stroke (NINDS), a component of the National Institutes of Health (NIH), has primary responsibility for research on the brain and nervous system. As part of its mission, the NINDS supports research on myoclonus at its laboratories in Bethesda, Maryland and through grants to universities and major medical institutions across the country.

Scientists are seeking to understand the underlying biochemical basis of involuntary movements and to find the most effective treatment for myoclonus and other movement disorders.

Investigators are evaluating the role of neurotransmitters and receptors in myoclonus. If abnormalities in neurotransmitters or receptors are found to play a causative role in myoclonus, future research can focus on determining the extent to which genetic alterations are responsible for these abnormalities and on identifying the nature of those alterations. Scientists also may be able to develop drug treatments that target specific changes in the receptors to reverse abnormalities, such as the loss of inhibition, and to enhance mechanisms that compensate for these abnormalities. Identifying receptor abnormalities also may help researchers develop diagnostic tests for myoclonus. NINDS-supported scientists at research institutions throughout the country are studying various aspects of PME, including the basic mechanisms and genes involved in this group of diseases.

185

Chapter 29

Potential New Treatments for Multiple Sclerosis

Partial Histocompatibility Complex Molecules May Be an Effective Multiple Sclerosis Treatment

Major histocompatibility complex (MHC) molecules are important in initiating immune responses in the body. In mice and related rodents, experimental autoimmune encephalomyelitis (EAE) is a similar illness to multiple sclerosis (MS). In a 2017 study, U.S. Department of Veterans Affairs (VA) researchers found that administering partial MHC (pMHC) molecular constructs to rodents not only reduced the severity of the disease, but also markedly reduced demyelination and damage to axons in the central nervous system. They also found that the effective dose of those constructs is sex-dependent and might be regulated by estrogen signaling.

While pMHC was already known to be an effective treatment for EAE, the study suggests the proper dosages to be used on mice and will assist in the design of future clinical trials of the construct.

Cytokines Found in Progressive Multiple Sclerosis Identified

Researchers with the VA Portland Health Care System (VAPORHCS), the Oregon Health and Science University, Yale

This chapter includes text excerpted from "Potential New Treatments for MS," U.S. Department of Veterans Affairs (VA), June 1, 2018.

187

University, and the University of California, San Francisco published a paper in 2017 in which they identified two related cytokines and associated genetic markers that may explain why some people develop MS. (Cytokines are small, specific proteins released by cells that have a specific effect on the interactions and communications between cells.)

The two cytokines, macrophage migration inhibitory factor (MIF) and D-dopachrome tautomerase (D-DT), can worsen MS by increasing inflammation within the central nervous system. The research team also identified two genetic markers that enhance the expression of both cytokines that occurred more frequently in MS patients with the progressive form of the disease, suggesting that a simple genetic test could be used to identify patients at risk of developing this form of MS. The finding may open the door to the use of precision medicine to prevent and treat the progressive form of the disease.

Lipoic Acid May Stop Brain Atrophy

Lipoic acid, also known as "alpha lipoic acid," is an antioxidant made by the body that helps turn glucose into energy. A version is sold as a dietary supplement, over the counter, at drug stores. A two-year trial by researchers at the VA Portland Health Care System and Oregon Health and Science University was completed in 2017. Researchers found that, in a double-blind study involving 51 participants, high doses of lipoic acid significantly slowed the rate of brain atrophy in patients with secondary progressive MS when compared to a placebo. In addition, the pilot study suggested improved walking times and fewer falls among study participants who took a daily dose of lipoic acid compared with those who received the placebo.

The research team is using the findings from this pilot trial to design an expanded multi-site clinical trial that has not yet begun.

Functional Electrical Stimulation Improves Walking in Multiple Sclerosis Patients

According to the National Multiple Sclerosis Society, 93 percent of patients with MS suffer gait impairment within 10 years of their diagnosis, and 13 percent report they are unable to walk twice a week. Researchers at the Advanced Platform Technology and Functional Electrical Stimulation centers at the Louis Stokes Cleveland VA Medical Center used functional electrical stimulation (FES) techniques to help a patient with MS, and another who had suffered a stroke, to effectively walk. (FES is a technique that uses low-energy electrical pulses to artificially generate body movements in individuals who have been paralyzed due to injury to the central nervous system.)

Results of the 90-day study were published in 2017, and the patient with MS who received the FES system said that at the beginning "I could barely take two steps," and "at the end, I was walking down the hallway." The research team hopes to continue their explorations in this area.

Study Promoting TREGS Underway

Regulatory T cells (TReg cells or TREGS) are a special subset of T cells in the body that prevent other immune cells from attacking the body's own tissues and other harmless environmental materials, such as food. Defects in regulatory T cells cause severe inflammatory disease.

In 2017, the VA Maryland Health Care System and the University of Maryland began a study to promote TREGS that control disease, and will explore strategies to use TREGS to control MS with a vaccine-like specificity that keeps the rest of the immune system functional. Conventional treatments for MS often compromise the immune system, leaving patients vulnerable to infection. The study is scheduled to be completed in 2021.

Evidence Lacking for Benefits of Medical Marijuana

In 2017, researchers from the VA Portland Health Care System and Oregon Health and Science University reviewed 75 publications on the effects of medical marijuana for many types of chronic pain.

They found limited evidence that marijuana use might alleviate neuropathic pain in some patients, and that it might reduce spasticity associated with multiple sclerosis. There was insufficient evidence on the benefits of marijuana for all other pain types. Between 45 and 80 percent of those who seek medical marijuana do so for pain management.

Current federal law prohibits the use or dispensing of marijuana use. As a federal agency, VA follows this prohibition and does not prescribe medical marijuana to any of its patients.

Chapter 30

Multiple Sclerosis Pain Management

Approximately two-thirds of people with multiple sclerosis (MS) experience pain at some time during the course of the disease. MS pain experts understand that MS pain is difficult to manage and is associated with depression, anxiety, and fatigue. Pain should never be ignored and should always be addressed.

Causes of Multiple Sclerosis Pain

Pain is a sensory symptom directly related to two events—the disruption of central nervous system myelin and the effects of disability. When pain is a symptom of an MS lesion or plaque, it is termed "neurogenic pain." The disability that is a result of MS causes a different type of pain originating in muscles, bones, and joints.

Neurogenic pain can be continuous and steady or spontaneous and intermittent and is reported in varying degrees of severity. Intermittent, spontaneous pain is described as shooting, stabbing, electric shock-like or searing and is often caused by sensations that normally do not cause pain.

This chapter includes text excerpted from "VA Multiple Sclerosis Centers of Excellence—A Veteran's Journey with MS," U.S. Department of Veterans Affairs (VA), 2008. Reviewed March 2019.

Tightness or band-like sensations, nagging, numbness, tingling in legs or arms, burning, aching, and throbbing pain is categorized as continuous or steady neurogenic pain. Steady pain is often worse at night, worse during temperature change, and worsened by exercise. The most common pain syndromes experienced by people with MS include headache, continuous burning pain in the extremities, back pain, and painful tonic spasms.

Treatment of Multiple Sclerosis Pain

The sensation of pain is difficult to measure, and it is what the experiencing person says it is. Pain impacts sleep, mood, and the ability to work, play, and enjoy life. Pain management is approached medically, behaviorally, physically, and, in some cases, surgically. A good pain history of the onset, location, duration, characteristics, aggravating factors, relieving factors, and treatments helps providers adequately treat pain. Keeping a pain diary helps patients explain their pain and receive the best care.

Medication

Treatment of neurogenic pain is aimed at down-regulating excitatory neurotransmitters and enhancing inhibitory transmitters of pain with topical agents, antiepileptics, antidepressants, antiarrhythmics, NMDA (N-methyl D-aspartate)-receptor antagonists, nonnarcotic, and narcotic opioids.

The use of opioids for MS neurogenic pain remains controversial. Opioids are considered when other agents become ineffective or not well tolerated. Opioids are constipating. A good bowel regimen including fiber, stool softeners, and laxatives is always considered in MS pain managed with opioids.

Antiepileptic drugs (AEDs) are commonly prescribed to manage MS pain. There is no need to discontinue these medications. Awareness of any behavior changes or depressed mood should be reported to your healthcare providers.

Behavioral

Tolerance to pain is decreased with repeated exposure to pain, stress, fatigue, anger, boredom, and sleep deprivation. Pain tolerance is increased with hypnosis, warmth, distracting activities, and strong beliefs or faith. Competing stimuli, such as distraction, socialization, and recreation, may act to increase pain tolerance. Relaxation, meditation, imagery, hypnosis, distraction, and biofeedback are strategies that increase the tolerance to pain. Getting involved in work or social activities, joining a support group or even having a good laugh are techniques that can minimize pain. Interesting to note, higher pain severity is reported by people with MS who are unemployed or homebound.

Physical

Physical agents work to enhance or limit pain transmitters and include the application of heat, cold, or pressure; physical therapy; exercise; massage; acupuncture; yoga; tai chi; and transcutaneous-electrical nerve stimulation. Use of physical agents can minimize doses of medication.

Surgical

Surgical pain management interventions are sought when medical, physical, and behavioral options fail. Procedures, such as regional nerve blocks, are reversible and safe. Neurosurgical options, rhizotomy, cordotomy, and Gamma Knife radiosurgery are known to offer relief, but carry risks.

Pain is a symptom that demands serious attention, as it has such pervasive impact on the role, mood, the capacity to work and rest, and interpersonal relationships. MS pain management is an achievable goal. The management of pain in MS is based on the mechanisms of the pain experienced. The goal of pain management is to optimize mood, sleep, and quality of life (QOL).

Chapter 31

Rehabilitation for Multiple Sclerosis

Chapter Contents

Section 31.1

How to Choose a Rehabilitation Facility

"How to Choose a Rehabilitation Facility," © 2017
Omnigraphics. Reviewed March 2019.

Stroke rehabilitation, often called "rehab," is a crucial part of recovering from a stroke. Proper rehabilitation techniques can help patients increase strength and flexibility; re-learn basic skills, such as talking, eating, and walking; regain independence; and improve their overall quality of life (QOL). Effective rehab frequently requires a team of healthcare professionals from a variety of fields, such as neurology, nursing, physical therapy, occupational therapy, psychiatry, psychology, speech therapy, nutrition, and social work. Of course, stroke patients and their families want the best rehab program available. But since each patient is different, both in terms of specific condition and individual preferences, finding the right rehab facility can be a challenging task.

Types of Rehabilitation Settings

Depending on the severity of the stroke, personal preference, insurance coverage, and other factors, rehabilitation can take place in a number of different locations, including:

- **Acute care facility.** This is often a special unit of a hospital, to which a patient is transferred after she or he is stabilized, usually a few days after the stroke. Here, for four to seven days, the patient receives ongoing medical care and testing while spending several hours per day going through progressively more complex basic tasks, such as moving limbs, sitting up, standing, bathing, and dressing.

- **Sub-acute care facility.** Sub-acute care can take place at a special hospital unit or a separate dedicated facility, such as a nursing home or skilled nursing center. This therapy is less intense than acute care, but it generally continues for a longer period of time. The patient continues to see a neurologist or other physician while receiving care by the nursing staff and undergoes a combination of physical, occupational, and speech therapy and appropriate counseling.

- **Outpatient facility.** Once stroke patients return home, they usually continue rehabilitation on an outpatient basis, which can take place at a doctor's office, a clinic, part of a hospital, or a rehab center. Here, the therapy is more intense than the patient could perform on his or her own, with the goal of regaining as much function as possible through a variety of exercises and tests.

- **Home care.** No one wants to stay in a hospital or residential facility longer than necessary, and research shows that stroke patients who are able to continue rehabilitation at home earlier generally do better. Home care is best for patients who require treatment by just one or two specialists, who can visit and supervise therapy on a regular basis. Although home care may lack the specialized equipment available at a dedicated facility, it has the advantage of allowing the patient to perform exercises and practice skills in his or her own environment.

Factors to Consider When Choosing a Rehabilitation Facility

Because of the different effects of a stroke, patient needs can vary considerably, as can the types of appropriate care facilities. But here are some factors to take into account:

- **Accreditation.** Quality standards for rehabilitation facilities are established by the Commission on Accreditation of Rehab Facilities (CARF) and the Joint Commission on Accreditation of Healthcare Organizations (JCAHO), as well as by Medicare. Ask how the facility meets these standards.

- **Specialized programs.** One of the most important factors is to be sure the facility offers programs and equipment that meet the specific needs of the patient. Ask about details of the program, such as what therapy is planned, how often it will be done, and who will be involved.

- **Trained staff.** Rehab staff must be trained and experienced in providing the particular type of therapy required by the patient. Those who require ongoing medical care, for example, will require on-site physicians and skilled nursing staff, while patients who are having difficulty walking will need a physical therapist.

- **Workload.** The number of patients served by the facility and the number seen by each medical professional or therapist

197

will have an effect on the patient's successful rehabilitation. Ask questions to ensure that staff members are not overloaded.

- **Treatment plan.** Ask about the patient's specific treatment plan, what team members were involved in developing it, and how often it will be updated.

- **Progress evaluation.** It's important to try and quantify the patient's rehabilitation to get an accurate picture of his or her progress. Ask about the facility's process for formal evaluations, how often they are done, and who is involved.

- **Additional services.** Some rehab facilities offer supplemental services, including art, music, relaxation, and pet therapy, as well as a variety of games, coordination exercises, and support groups. Some of these may appeal to certain patients and could be very beneficial to their rehabilitation.

- **Family participation.** Ask if family members are involved in developing treatment plans and participating in therapy sessions. Family support can provide important information, help improve patient morale, and also prepare family members to assist with home care at some point.

- **Transition and ongoing therapy.** Once residential therapy is completed, it's important that the facility has a process for preparing the patient for discharge with appropriate instructions for home care. In addition, some facilities are equipped to provide ongoing in-home therapy with their own trained staff.

- **Insurance.** Don't forget to ask about insurance coverage. Be sure the facility, its staff, and the anticipated therapy are covered by the patient's insurance plan before committing to a facility.

References

1. "10 Tips for Choosing a Rehab Facility," Cleveland Clinic, December 20, 2013.

2. "Choosing the Right Stroke Rehab Facility," American Stroke Association, n.d.

3. Gerber, Charlotte. "10 Questions to Ask When Choosing a Rehabilitation Facility, Verwell.com, August 12, 2016.

4. "Home Is the Best Place for Stroke Rehabilitation," Medscape. com, May 5, 2000.

5. "National Stroke Association's Guide to Choosing Stroke Rehabilitation Services," National Stroke Association, 2006.

6. "Rehab Facilities," Stroke-rehab.com, n.d.

7. "Rehabilitation," Brain Aneurysm Foundation, n.d.

Section 31.2

Rehabilitation Options for People with Multiple Sclerosis

This section contains text excerpted from the following sources:
Text in this section begins with excerpts from "Rehabilitation
Medicine," *Eunice Kennedy Shriver* National Institute of
Child Health and Human Development (NICHD), December 1, 2016;
Text under the heading "What Types of Activities Are Involved
with Rehabilitation Medicine?" is excerpted from "What Types of
Activities Are Involved with Rehabilitation Medicine?"
Eunice Kennedy Shriver National Institute of Child Health and
Human Development (NICHD), December 1, 2016.

Rehabilitation medicine includes efforts to improve function and minimize impairment related to activities that may have been hampered by illnesses or injuries. Disabling conditions, as well as musculoskeletal issues and pain, may require various levels of rehabilitation medicine.

The goal of rehabilitation medicine is two-fold:

- To maximize function, participation, independence, and quality of life (QOL) for a person with a disabling condition

- To maintain and prevent any further decline in a person's functioning

199

What Types of Activities Are Involved with Rehabilitation Medicine?

Rehabilitation medicine uses many kinds of assistance, therapies, and devices to improve function. The type of rehabilitation a person receives depends on the condition causing the impairment, the bodily function that is affected, and the severity of the impairment.

The following are some common types of rehabilitation:

- **Cognitive rehabilitation therapy** involves relearning or improving skills, such as thinking, learning, memory, planning, and decision making that may have been lost or affected by brain injury.

- **Occupational therapy** helps a person carry out daily life tasks and activities in the home, workplace, and community.

- **Pharmaco rehabilitation** involves the use of drugs to improve or restore physical or mental function.

- **Physical therapy** involves activities and exercises to improve the body's movements, sensations, strength, and balance.

- **Rehabilitative/assistive technology** refers to tools, equipment, and products that help people with disabilities move and function. This technology includes (but is not limited to):

  - Orthotics, which are devices that aim to improve movement and prevent contracture in the upper and lower limbs. For instance, pads inserted into a shoe, specially fitted shoes, or ankle or leg braces can improve a person's ability to walk. Hand splints and arm braces can help the upper limbs remain supple and unclenched after a spinal cord injury.

  - Prosthetics, which are devices designed to replace a missing body part, such as an artificial limb

  - Wheelchairs, walkers, crutches, and other mobility aids

  - Augmentative/Alternative Communication (AAC) devices, which aim to either make a person's communication more understandable or take the place of a communication method. They can include electronic devices, speech-generating devices, and picture boards.

  - Hearing aids and cochlear implants

- Retinal prostheses, which can restore useful vision in cases in which it has been lost due to certain degenerative eye conditions

- Telemedicine and telerehab technologies, which are devices or software to deliver care or monitor conditions in the home or community

- Rehabilitation robotics

- Mobile apps to assist with speech/communication, anxiety/ stress, memory, and other functions or symptoms

- **Recreational therapy** helps improve symptoms and social and emotional well-being through arts and crafts, games, relaxation training, and animal-assisted therapy.

- **Speech and language therapy** aims to improve impaired swallowing and movement of the mouth and tongue, as well as difficulties with the voice, language, and talking.

- **Surgery** includes procedures to correct a misaligned limb or to release a constricted muscle, skin grafts for burns, insertion of chips into the brain to assist with limb or prosthetic movement, and placement of skull plates or bone pins.

- **Vocational rehabilitation** aids in building skills for going to school or working at a job.

- **Music or art therapy** can specifically aid in helping people express emotion, in cognitive development, or in helping to develop social connectedness.

These services are provided by a number of different healthcare providers and specialists, including (but not limited to):

- Physiatrists (also called "rehabilitation physicians")

- Occupational therapists

- Physical therapists

- Cognitive rehabilitation therapists

- Gait and clinical movement specialist

- Rehabilitation technologists

- Speech therapists

- Audiologists

- Orthopedists/surgeons

- Neurologists

- Psychiatrists/psychologists

- Biomedical engineers

- Rehabilitation engineers

Section 31.3

Physical and Occupational Rehabilitation

This section contains text excerpted from the following sources:
Text beginning with the heading "What Is Physical Therapy?" is
excerpted from "Comparing Routine Neurorehabilitation Program
with Trunk Exercises Based on Bobath Concept in Multiple Sclerosis:
Pilot Study," Rehabilitation Research & Development Service
(RR&D), U.S. Department of Veterans Affairs (VA), November 1,
2013. Reviewed March 2019; Text beginning with the heading "What
Is Occupational Therapy?" is excerpted from "Durham VA Health
Care System—Occupational Therapy," U.S. Department of Veterans
Affairs (VA), March 1, 2019; Text under the heading "What Do
Occupational Therapists Do?" is excerpted from "VA Boston Health
Care System—Occupational Therapy," U.S. Department of Veterans
Affairs (VA), June 9, 2015. Reviewed March 2019.

What Is Physical Therapy?

Multiple sclerosis (MS) is a lifelong disease that must be supported by continuous physiotherapy to decrease adverse effects of
the symptoms. Several studies have stressed the beneficial effects of
exercises on the treatment of MS-related clinical symptoms. Therapeutic exercises can accelerate the spontaneous restoration of central
nervous system damage. Since physiotherapy and rehabilitation are
carried out over a long period of time, exercise variation is needed
according to different requirements. When studies about physiotherapy approaches for MS populations are examined, it is observed

that most routine neurorehabilitation programs concentrate on limb exercises. Therefore, in routine MS rehabilitation, most physiotherapy programs focus on the limbs. Through limb recovery, they aim to gain functions.

Loss of selective trunk control is clearly associated with limitations in balance, gait, and arm and hand function. Despite many studies indicating effects of different exercise approaches, few have concentrated on the effectiveness of trunk exercises in the MS population. Besides the fact that trunk performance is directly related to the disability, measuring the trunk is important in the examination and treatment of people with MS. In recent literature, physiotherapy based on the Bobath concept has been used to improve functions in MS patients. Bobath-based exercises have been recommended for use in MS rehabilitation. According to the Bobath concept, the trunk has a key role in functional recovery. There are many exercises focused on the trunk in the Bobath concept. The trunk can be affected at any stage of the disease, which may affect level of disability.

Studies show that exercises for trunk control are as effective as the limb exercises commonly used in MS neurorehabilitation programs. According to these studies, trunk exercises based on the Bobath concept may be another option when the physiotherapist needs to vary the exercise program in clinical practice. It was concluded from the studies that inclusion of the exercises for trunk control in physical therapy and rehabilitation would have additional benefits.

What Is Occupational Therapy?

Occupational therapy (OT) enables people of all ages to live life to its fullest by helping them promote health, prevent—or live better with—injury, illness, or disability. It is a rehabilitation profession that started in 1917 and is rooted in science. Occupational therapists and occupational therapy assistants focus on "doing," using occupations and meaningful life activities to help individuals maximize their potential. Therapeutic approaches may include strategies, modifications, or adaptations to improve function, skill building, and personal wellness to support everyday living activities.

What Do Occupational Therapists Do?

Occupational therapists (OTs) help people across the lifespan participate in the things they want and need to do through the therapeutic use of everyday activities. Common areas of treatment are:

- Activities of daily living (bathing, dressing, feeding, and grooming)
- Bathroom safety
- Kitchen safety and cooking
- Community reintegration
- Fine motor skills (difficulty using hands)
- Decreased strength or range of motion in arms
- Visual problems (legal blindness or one side neglect)
- Memory and problem solving
- Energy conservation (breathing techniques and pacing strategies)
- Joint protection for arthritic hands (how to grasp things correctly)
- Positioning (in bed, chair or wheelchair)
- Stress and/or anxiety management (relaxation techniques)
- Adaptive devices
- Assistive technology
- Wheelchair and seating
- Driver training

Section 31.4

Cognitive Rehabilitation for Multiple Sclerosis

This section includes text excerpted from "VA Multiple Sclerosis Centers of Excellence—Community Matters," U.S. Department of Veterans Affairs (VA), 2016.

Approximately 40 to 65 percent of people with multiple sclerosis (MS) experience noticeable changes in cognitive functioning related to their MS. For some, these changes are fairly minor, while for others, the cognitive changes significantly disrupt their daily lives. Declining cognitive functioning is among the top concerns for those with MS because this can affect employment, relationships, driving, health management, and other important areas of daily life. Cognition refers to a wide range of brain functions involved in thinking, including learning and memory, concentration, problem-solving, planning and organization, multitasking, language skills, and reasoning. Forgetfulness and taking a little longer to process information and respond are some of the most commonly reported cognitive complaints of people with MS. Because MS is unpredictable, it is difficult to predict in what areas, if any, a particular individual may have cognitive difficulties. For some, an assessment of cognitive functioning by a trained professional can be a helpful part of a treatment plan, allowing them to better understand their cognitive strengths and weaknesses.

Cognitive rehabilitation refers to clinical interventions to improve cognition and/or help a person develop strategies to help compensate for cognitive difficulties in daily life. While many of the activities included in cognitive rehabilitation can be practiced without the help of a clinician, some individuals may benefit from cognitive rehabilitation with a professional. Cognitive rehabilitation is often done by speech and occupational therapists, neuropsychologists, and others with appropriate training. An important part of cognitive rehabilitation is providing information about why a person with MS experiences cognitive changes and the factors that might make cognition better or worse. This can help the person feel more in control of their lives and their experience. Some examples of helpful questions that may be addressed in cognitive rehabilitation include:

- Why do I remember some things well, but not others?
- How does my energy level impact my cognitive functioning?
- Why does it take me twice as long to complete some tasks?
- How does depression impact my cognitive functioning?
- What cognitive changes can I expect in the future?

Cognitive rehabilitation can also be compensatory; that is, they help an individual compensate, or develop tools and strategies, to help cope with a cognitive problem. Examples of compensatory strategies include:

- Using a notebook to write down important information during the day

- Using an appointment calendar for scheduling, and setting alarms to prompt a reminder

- Allowing an extra 15 minutes to get to appointments

- Making "to do" lists for task completion and crossing off items when complete

- Breaking down large goals into smaller tasks, prioritizing the tasks, and scheduling the tasks into an appointment calendar

- Following a structured daily schedule

- Using imagery, grouping, or other internal memory strategies

Other approaches to cognitive rehabilitation are restorative; that is, they aim to restore lost functioning in a particular cognitive skill, and/or lead to a more general improvement in daily cognitive skills. Restorative cognitive rehabilitation is conducted in a treatment setting with a provider and usually involves a schedule of cognitive exercises administered by the clinician and or a computer.

Research Support

So far, the strongest scientific evidence for the effectiveness of cognitive rehabilitation comes from studies with individuals with traumatic brain injury (TBI) or stroke. To best understand what works and what doesn't work with people with MS, more research needs to be done with people with MS. Even though research on cognitive rehabilitation in MS is in its infancy and is far from conclusive, there are some promising findings suggesting that physical activities, such as walking, Pilates, and yoga—some of which are already frequently used by people with MS—may also help cognition. Relaxation and mindfulness exercises also show promise for improving attention, in addition to their known benefits for stress reduction.

Brain Training Computer Programing

Many people have heard about computer-based "brain training" software, some of which is available for free, but most of which costs money. While some of these training programs have shown promise for improving certain cognitive skills, it is still unclear whether they lead to lasting and generalized improvement in cognitive abilities.

The research in this area is far from conclusive. Individuals who are already mentally and physically active should not necessarily change their routines to engage in computer-based exercises; however, for some individuals who aren't as active, these activities may be a way to get them engaged in some mental stimulation.

In summary, people with MS who have memory or other cognitive difficulties may benefit from cognitive rehabilitation; however, more research is needed to better understand how and why it works. A cognitive evaluation is often the first step, to assess a person's strengths and weaknesses, in order to best guide treatment. For some, cognitive rehabilitation activities may be done in the home, while for others, office visits may be more appropriate. If you have further questions about cognition or cognitive rehabilitation, ask your healthcare provider.

Section 31.5

Music Therapy for Multiple Sclerosis

This section includes text excerpted from "Music Therapy in Multiple Sclerosis," U.S. Department of Veterans Affairs (VA), August 1, 2018.

"No wheelchair can interrupt the journeys of the mind," said cellist Jacqueline du Pre. During her struggle to maintain a brilliant career despite multiple sclerosis (MS), her musical memory was unimpaired by illness. She could easily recall the feeling of playing and used this to her advantage when teaching other aspiring cellists to achieve a high-quality musical sound. Music brought her out of depression and helped her stay active and engaged. A person does not need to be a virtuoso cellist to recognize and experience the benefits from the therapeutic effects of music. There are a variety of musical approaches that can assist people living with MS to have a better quality of life (QOL).

History of Music Therapy

The idea that music has a healing influence that can affect health and behavior has been recognized for centuries. The profession of music therapy formally began after World Wars I and II, when the therapeutic effects of music on physical and emotional traumas from the wars were recognized. From early studies in the 1800s, where psychologists used music to alter dreams for therapy, to currently using modern technology and equipment, the benefits of music therapy has become the focus of many organizations and discussions in journals worldwide.

Improving Movement and Coordination

The planning and order of movements are essential to everyday activity. Programs in which people learn to match repetitive motor actions (such as hand and foot exercises) with a computer-generated rhythmic beat can improve coordination, concentration, and physical endurance. Through these exercises, people experienced more even gait. Rhythm stimulates the impulse to move and helps people sidestep the coordination processes they cannot think through otherwise. It is almost impossible to fully lose the ability to process music because, unlike speech, it involves so many areas of the brain.

Improving Memory

Memory changes are common in people with MS. Even though some people might find it difficult to recall particular pieces of information or to remember names, words, events, etc., they can still learn to carry out new physical tasks. Studies show that the physical task of learning to play an instrument can improve cognition and memory. If long-term memories seem lost, some studies show that listening to music might actually help those memories to return. This is because hearing music is associated with the areas of the brain where long-term memories are kept. As a result, listening to music from past special events or from "the good old times" in one's life can stimulate feelings and associations with those past events and, in part, improve access to long-term memories. Familiar music can also improve attention and memory recognition.

Reducing Depression and Anxiety

Some of the hardest issues in people with MS are to cope with emotional ups and downs, such as feelings of depression and anxiety. Expressing emotions by playing or listening to music can help some people cope with their past or present feelings and also help some deal with their fears. If music therapy is done in a group, it can help establish a closer connection with others, especially since music activates areas of the brain that process social signals, language, and emotions.

Stress Management

Music can relax the mind and body and can even trigger physical reflexes, such as digestion, bladder control, and movement of the limbs. The mood may be enhanced by a particularly calming piece of music, and, as a result, some people experience less discomfort or pain.

Improved Verbal Communication

Music can also help people improve their verbal communication skills. Singing words that were otherwise difficult to recite have shown to aid in communication and verbal expression. For example, one might not be able to recite the words to "Happy Birthday," let alone speak fluently, but as soon as the words are set to music, the words can come naturally. Singing can also help with the breath support, pronunciation, and timing needed for speech.

Music therapy can help people with MS. It can help with depression, anxiety, memory, and other emotional issues. It also provides the physical benefits that come from staying active and moving. Healing through music, whether therapist-led or self-directed, can be an effective, low-risk, and low-cost endeavor. The cellist Jacqueline du Pre was able to maintain a meaningful career despite having MS. Everyone can learn from her example and from others who have used music to improve their quality of life and overall well-being.

Section 31.6

Cooling Therapy for Multiple Sclerosis

This section includes text excerpted from "Keep Cool:
Multiple Sclerosis and Heat Tolerance," U.S. Department
of Veterans Affairs (VA), August 1, 2018.

People with multiple sclerosis (MS) often have a low tolerance for changes in their body temperature caused by air temperature, activity, digestion, or metabolic changes. Small increases—as little as ½°F—in core body temperature can increase MS symptoms. Nerves that have lost their conductive coating (myelin sheath) become more sensitive to heat, and the nerve signal slows down or is blocked, resulting in an increase in symptoms. Depending on the location of the nerve damage in your body, symptoms may include increased heart rate, sweating, dizziness, muscle weakness, slowed reaction times, reduced energy, and difficulties with attention and concentration.

Causes of Increased Body Heat

Many things can cause your body temperature to rise—some we usually think of, and some that are a little harder to see. Obvious causes of increased body temperature are things such as being in a warm environment, increasing physical activity, or wearing too many clothes. All these can easily lead to increased body temperature and an increase in MS symptoms. Less obvious causes of increased body heat include having a fever, changes in metabolism, hormonal changes, or side effects of medications.

Warm environments may include things such as your kitchen during meal preparation, working hard around your home (whether cleaning the house or working outdoors), taking a hot shower, swimming in a warm pool, or being out in the sun. Your body temperature may also rise with increased physical activity, such as when walking, propelling your wheelchair, exercising, or doing other leisure activities. Wearing clothing that keeps you too warm, or being in rooms that, although they are comfortable for others, are too warm for you, may also increase your body temperature. Medical illnesses contributing to higher core body temperature may include bladder infections, colds, and/or the flu (causing a low to medium grade fever).

Keeping Cool

If heat affects you, you need to take extra precautions and use strategies to keep cool. Minimizing your symptoms will help reduce the need for additional medications and maximize your independence and safety. There are several ways you can help your body to stay cool and keep yourself healthy.

Adjust the Temperature in Your Environment

• Use an air conditioner or fan in the room you are working in or in your vehicle when traveling.

• Rest in rooms that are out of direct sunlight or have adequate shading over windows that have a western or southern exposure.

• When showering or bathing, turn the fan on in the bathroom and/or open a window if possible to help circulate the room air.

• Make sure the water temperature in your shower or bathtub is significantly lower than your body temperature and/or take a cool bath.

• Wear layered clothing that can be removed as necessary to adjust your body temperature.

• Avoid traveling to warm destinations during their hot and/or humid seasons.

When you feel hot, use a spray bottle to mist yourself with water at regular intervals during activity (or even when sitting)—as many people with MS lose the ability to perspire and release body heat.

Drink Plenty of Fluids

During periods of increased activity, your body can generate several times the amount of heat it does at rest. The body releases excess heat by sweating and evaporation. Adequate water intake is important to be able to perspire during exercise and remain hydrated. Below are some tips for better hydration.

• Place a plastic bottle of water in the freezer until frozen. Put the bottle by your bedside at night so that you have cold water available to drink without having to get out of bed.

- Drink chilled water, juices, ices, and popsicles throughout the day to help keep your body temperature down.

- Avoid drinks with caffeine (e.g., sodas, colas, coffee, tea, chocolate, and some energy drinks). Caffeinated drinks are diuretics, causing you to lose fluid by increased urination. This leaves less fluid in your body to sweat (one of our natural ways of cooling down).

Use Cooling Equipment

- Layer up with lightweight, breathable clothes. Remove the layers as necessary to keep cool. Look for clothing that is designed to have more air flow through it, making it cooler to wear.

- Use an umbrella while out in the sun.

- Wear a vented hat, sunglasses, and use sunblock while outdoors. (The sunblock will not reflect heat, but will help prevent you from skin cancer.)

- Use a cooling vest.

- Use cooling packs on your wrists, neck, and on your head (under a hat). Another strategy is to wear cloth-type hats and dip them in water, allowing the sun to evaporate the water, cooling your head.

Develop a Personal Cooling Program

Research studies show that individuals who take a cool bath or shower (not cold), sit in an air-conditioned (AC) room, or wear a cooling vest for 45 minutes a day have an overall decrease in their core body temperature. This results in an improvement in strength and less fatigue for up to 2 hours after cooling. Below are some tips.

- Take a cool bath before working around the house or in the garden.

- Avoid hot or heavy meals, especially before going outside.

- Stay inside during the midday warmer hours.

- Take a shower in a swimsuit before working outside in it. The moisture in your suit will help cool you.

- Exercise or complete home management activities in the morning, the cooler time of the day.

Cooling Vests

The above strategies work well for most people, but this does not mean that you will never have problems maintaining your body core temperature. When the "low-tech" methods (above) are not adequate, a cooling vest might meet your needs.

How Does a Cooling Vest Work?

A cooling vest is designed to keep the body's core temperature (around the heart and spinal cord) within safe levels to reduce symptoms of heat intolerance. The vest absorbs body heat, evaporates perspiration, and conducts cooler temperatures to the body through the skin. Cold packs for the neck, wrists, and head conduct cold through to the arteries, cooling the blood circulating in the body.

When Should I Wear a Cooling Vest?

The cooling vest should be worn in warm-to-hot conditions or when physical activity is planned. The vest can help keep you cool up to three hours when worn correctly, although this can depend on things, such as environmental temperature, humidity, and your level of activity.

How Do I Use the Cooling Vest?

It is beneficial to wear the cooling vest at least 30 minutes prior to physical activity. The cooling vest is more effective when worn over thin clothing and when needed when breathable fabrics are worn over the vest.

The vest usually has up to 6 Velcro closure pockets to house the cooling packs: 2 to 4 pockets on the front and 3 to 4 pockets on the back. Place each cooling pack into one of the pockets on the vest. Put the vest on, and close the front. Adjust the side straps to provide a snug, but comfortable, fit with the cold packs in place.

Are There Different Types of Cooling Vests?

An excellent summary of different cooling vests and what are recommended for MS can be found at Active MSers.

- **Active cooling:** requires an electricity source to operate the equipment that circulates air through the vest.

213

- **Passive cooling:** portable with no working components (e.g., gel inserts and ice packs, phase change—nonfreezing, cooling liquid in packs, embedded hydrogel crystals, and evaporative cooling—best in low humidity/arid environments)

How Do Traditional Cooling Pack Vests Work?

Initially, cooling packs should be put in the freezer overnight. Re-cooling them after use takes 30 to 60 minutes in the freezer. It does not harm the cooling packs to store them in the freezer.

You will need to experiment to determine which level of cooling you can tolerate and is most beneficial to you. Some cooling vests have sleeves that cover the cooling packs and provide insulation. Layering clothing can help regulate the vest temperature to your comfort.

Chapter 32

Complementary and Alternative Medicine for Multiple Sclerosis

Multiple sclerosis (MS) is a disease of the central nervous system (CNS). In MS, the body's immune system attacks myelin, which coats nerve cells. Symptoms of MS include muscle weakness (often in the hands and legs), tingling and burning sensations, numbness, chronic pain, coordination and balance problems, fatigue, vision problems, and difficulty with bladder control.

People with MS also may feel depressed and have trouble thinking clearly. MS is the most common disabling neurological disease affecting young adults. It generally strikes people between the ages of 20 and 40 and more commonly affects women. It affects some 400,000 Americans and about 2.5 million people worldwide. The most common form of the disease is called "relapsing-remitting MS (RRMS)" in which symptoms come and go.

This chapter contains text excerpted from the following sources: Text in this chapter begins with excerpts from "Multiple Sclerosis," National Center for Complementary and Integrative Health (NCCIH), October 24, 2018; Text beginning with the heading "Natural Products" is excerpted from "Multiple Sclerosis and Complementary Health Approaches: What the Science Says," National Center for Complementary and Integrative Health (NCCIH), December 2015. Reviewed March 2019.

Although MS has no cure, some conventional treatments can improve symptoms, reduce the number and severity of relapses, and delay the disease's progression. Many people with MS try some form of complementary health approach, often special diets (such as the Swank diet, which is low in saturated fats and high in polyunsaturated fatty acids, such as fish oils) and dietary supplements.

Natural Products
Cannabinoids

Orally administered cannabinoids (*cannabis* extract, synthetic tetrahydrocannabinol (THC)), mucosally delivered cannabinoids (cannabis extract oral spray, nabiximols), and smoked *cannabis* have all been studied for therapeutic effects in MS. Based on available evidence, cannabinoids may relieve spasticity and/or pain in people with MS; however, no marijuana-derived medications are approved by the U.S. Food and Drug Administration (FDA) to treat MS. Sativex (nabiximols) is licensed in the United Kingdom for use as an add-on treatment for MS-related spasticity when people have shown inadequate response to other symptomatic treatments or found their side effects intolerable. There is insufficient data to determine if smoking marijuana ameliorates symptoms of MS. Additionally, the psychoactive properties and other potential adverse effects need to be considered.

The Evidence Base

- The evidence base on the efficacy of cannabinoids consists of several small studies of short duration (6 to 15 weeks), which are the basis of the 2014 evidence-based guidelines from the American Academy of Neurology (AAN). Among the limitations of these studies was the potential for central side effects to unmask patients to treatment assignment. These factors, as stated in the guidelines, may have contributed to the discordant effects of cannabinoids on subjective and objective spasticity measures.

Efficacy

- **Oral cannabinoids.** The 2014 guidelines issued by the AAN concluded that oral cannabis extract is established as effective for reducing patient-reported spasticity symptoms and pain. This subjective benefit is possibly maintained for one year. The guidelines also concluded that tetrahydrocannabinol (THC) is probably effective for reducing patient-reported symptoms of spasticity and pain. This subjective benefit is possibly maintained for one year. However, the guidelines state that oral cannabis extract and THC are probably ineffective for reducing both objective spasticity measures and MS-related tremor symptoms. Oral cannabis extract and THC are possibly effective for reducing symptoms and objective measures of spasticity over one year.

- **Sativex oromucosal cannabinoid spray.** The 2014 AAN concluded that Sativex oromucosal cannabinoid spray is probably effective for improving subjective spasticity symptoms and is probably ineffective for reducing objective spasticity measures over 6 weeks or bladder incontinence episodes over 10 weeks. Further, the guidelines state that Sativex oromucosal spray is possibly ineffective for reducing MS-related tremor over 15 weeks. In addition, a 2010-reported meta-analysis from 666 MS patients who had spasticity that was not well controlled using existing treatments were given either nabiximols (363) or a placebo (303). Results showed nabiximols effects are typically seen within 3 weeks. Furthermore, about one-third of the MS patients given nabiximols had a 30 percent improvement from baseline. The authors noted that the treatment appeared reasonably safe.

- **Smoked cannabis.** Based on two small studies, the 2014 American Academy of Neurology (AAN) guidelines concluded that data are inadequate to determine the safety or efficacy of smoked cannabis used for spasticity/pain, balance/posture, and cognition.

Safety

- In the studies that were the basis for the 2014 AAN guidelines, cannabinoids were generally well tolerated, although some serious adverse effects were reported. Mild or moderate side effects including dizziness, somnolence, drowsiness, lightheadedness, memory disturbance, and difficulty concentrating, were more common in participants receiving cannabinoids versus the placebo. Less common effects included increased appetite, nausea, vomiting, constipation, and dry/sore mouth, myalgia, seizures, and others. The guidelines noted that because cannabinoids have known psychoactive properties, their potential for psychopathologic and neurocognitive adverse effects is a concern, especially in a patient population that may be vulnerable due to underlying disorders.

• The guidelines recommend that clinicians counsel patients about the potential for psychopathologic/cognitive and other adverse events associated with cannabinoids. Sativex oromucosal cannabinoid spray is not approved by the U.S. Food and Drug Administration (FDA) and is unavailable in the United States. Further, the guidelines suggest caution should be exercised with regard to extrapolation of results of trials of standardized oral cannabis extract (which are unavailable commercially) to other nonstandardized, nonregulated cannabis extracts (which may be commercially available in states with medical marijuana laws).

Ginkgo Biloba

There is no evidence to support the use of ginkgo biloba as an effective treatment for cognitive function in people with MS.

The Evidence Base

• The evidence base on the efficacy of ginkgo biloba for MS consists of several small randomized controlled trials, as well as a Cochrane review and evidence-based guidelines on complementary health approaches for MS issued by the AAN.

Efficacy

• The 2014 guidelines from the AAN concluded that ginkgo biloba is ineffective for improving cognitive function in people with MS, but that it is possibly effective over four weeks for reducing fatigue in MS. These conclusions are based on four small studies.

• A 2012 randomized controlled trial involving 120 participants with MS with some cognitive impairment found that ginkgo biloba twice a day for 12 weeks did not improve cognitive performance.

• A 2011 Cochrane review of four randomized controlled trials evaluated pharmacologic treatments, including ginkgo biloba, for memory disorder in MS. The reviewers concluded that based on available evidence, there is no convincing evidence to support the use of ginkgo biloba as an effective treatment for memory disorder in MS patients.

Safety

- Side effects of ginkgo may include headache, nausea, gastrointestinal upset, diarrhea, dizziness, or allergic skin reactions. More severe allergic reactions have occasionally been reported.

- There are some data from animal models to suggest that ginkgo can have an effect on the pharmacokinetics of several drugs; however, currently available clinical evidence suggests that low doses do not pose a risk for clinically relevant herb-drug interactions.

- Fresh ginkgo seeds contain large amounts of ginkgotoxin, which can cause serious adverse reactions, including seizures and death. Roasted seeds can also be toxic. Products made from standardized ginkgo leaf extracts contain little ginkgotoxin and appear to be safe when used orally and appropriately.

- National Toxicology Program (NTP) studies showed that rats and mice developed tumors after being given a specific ginkgo extract for up to two years. Further studies are needed to find out what substances in ginkgo caused the tumors and whether taking ginkgo as a dietary supplement affects the risk of cancer in people.

Omega-3 Fatty Acid Supplementation

There is insufficient data to assess any real beneficial effects of omega-3 fatty acid supplementation on MS. The 2014 guidelines from the AAN concluded that a low-fat diet with fish oil supplementation is probably ineffective for reducing MS-related relapse, disability, or magnetic resonance imaging (MRI) lesions, or for improving fatigue or quality of life.

The Evidence Base

- The evidence base on the efficacy of omega-3 supplementation for MS consists of only a few small, randomized controlled trials, as well as a Cochrane review and evidence-based guidelines on complementary health approaches for MS issued by the AAN.

Efficacy

- A 2012 Cochrane review of six randomized controlled trials examining dietary interventions, including polyunsaturated fatty acids (PUFAs) and vitamins, concluded that PUFAs seem to have no major effect on the disease progression in MS, but they may have a tendency toward reducing the frequency of relapses over two years. However, the authors noted that due to the uncertain quality of the PUFA supplementation, available data are insufficient to assess any real benefit or harm from the intervention.

Safety

- Omega-3 fatty acid supplements generally do not have adverse effects. When adverse effects do occur, they typically consist of minor gastrointestinal symptoms.

- It is unclear whether people with fish or shellfish allergies can safely consume fish oil supplements.

- People who take anticoagulants or nonsteroidal anti-inflammatory drugs (NSAIDs) should use caution when taking omega-3 supplements, because they may extend bleeding time.

Vitamin D

There is insufficient evidence to support the use of vitamin D supplementation for MS. A 2010 Cochrane review suggests clinicians may want to consider relevant guidelines on vitamin D supplementation when advising patients with MS.

The Evidence Base

- The evidence base on the efficacy of vitamin D for MS consists of a Cochrane review of a single randomized controlled trial.

Efficacy

- A 2010 Cochrane review of one randomized controlled trial concluded that the current level of evidence for the effectiveness of vitamin D supplementation in the management of people with MS does not support the use of vitamin D for MS. The reviewers noted that until more high quality evidence is available, clinicians may want to consider relevant guidelines on vitamin D supplementation when advising patients with MS.

- Results of a large, five-year randomized trial in 468 participants with MS suggest that low blood levels of vitamin D may be a risk factor for long-term disease activity and progression. However, more studies need to be conducted to determine if vitamin D supplementation affects disease course and progression.

Safety

- Limited intervention studies in MS suggest that vitamin D supplements are generally well tolerated in MS.

- High doses may cause fatigue, abdominal cramps, nausea, vomiting, renal damage, and other adverse effects.

Bee Venom

Based on a few small studies, bee venom therapy seems to have no effect on either MS symptoms or disease progression. There are serious side effects associated with bee venom, including the risk of anaphylactic reactions and death, which could limit any efficacy of bee venom therapy for the treatment of MS.

The Evidence Base

- The evidence base on the efficacy of bee venom therapy consists of only a couple of small studies.

Efficacy

- Based on a review of one small study, the 2014 guidelines from the AAN concluded that bee venom therapy is possibly ineffective for reducing MS-related relapses, disability, fatigue, total MRI lesion burden, new gadolinium-enhancing lesion volume, or health-related quality of life.

Safety

- There are serious side effects associated with bee venom, which could limit any efficacy of bee venom therapy in the treatment of MS.

Mind and Body Practices
Yoga

There is some limited evidence suggesting beneficial short-term effects of yoga on fatigue and mood in people with MS, but scientific studies overall had a high risk of bias and definitive conclusions could not be drawn.

The Evidence Base

- The evidence base on the efficacy of yoga for MS consists of a few randomized controlled trials and a systematic review and meta-analysis.

Efficacy

- A 2014 systematic review and meta analysis of 7 randomized controlled trials involving a total of 670 patients found some evidence for positive short-term effects of yoga on fatigue and mood, but not on outcomes such as mobility or cognitive function. The reviewers noted a high risk of bias in the studies included in the review, but despite the risk, yoga seems to be equally effective as exercise interventions in improving both patient-reported and clinician-rated outcomes.

- The 2014 guidelines from the AAN concluded that the data are inadequate to assess the effect of yoga on disability, spasticity, fatigue, cognition, mood, balance, or walking speed in people with MS.

Safety

- In the studies included in a 2014 systematic review and meta-analysis, yoga was not associated with serious adverse events.

- People with certain medical conditions, including MS, should modify or avoid some yoga poses.

Reflexology

There is insufficient evidence to support the use of reflexology for most symptoms of MS, including pain, health-related quality of life, disability, spasticity, fatigue, depression, and others. However, 2014 guidelines from the AAN concluded that, based on 4 studies, reflexology is possibly effective for reducing MS-associated paresthesia over 11 weeks.

The Evidence Base

- The evidence base on the efficacy of reflexology for MS consists of several small studies, four of which are the basis of a reflexology practice recommendation in 2014 evidence-based guidelines from the AAN.

Efficacy

- A 2011 update of a systematic review evaluating the evidence of 23 randomized controlled trials of reflexology in patients with any type of health condition found that 8 studies suggested that reflexology is effective for several conditions, including MS. However, the reviewers concluded that the best clinical evidence does not demonstrate convincingly that reflexology is an effective treatment for any condition.

- A 2009 double-blind, randomized, sham-controlled trial in 73 participants with MS found that reflexology was not superior to the sham control; however, significant decreases in pain, fatigue, depression, disability, spasm, and quality of life were observed in both groups.

Safety

- Reflexology is generally considered safe for most people; however, vigorous pressure applied to the feet may cause discomfort for some people.

Magnet Therapy

There is some limited, low-level evidence that suggests that magnet therapy may have modest beneficial effects on spasticity outcomes in people with MS, but the studies have been of low methodological quality. There is also some evidence, based on two studies, suggesting that magnet therapy may be useful in reducing fatigue in people with relapsing-remitting MS.

The Evidence Base

- The evidence base on the efficacy of magnet therapy for MS consists of a few randomized controlled trials, which are the basis of a 2013 Cochrane review and 2014 evidence-based guidelines from the AAN.

Efficacy

- The 2014 AAN guidelines concluded that magnet therapy is probably effective for reducing fatigue in relapsing-remitting MS, and probably ineffective for reducing depression in relapsing-remitting MS over 15 weeks. There is insufficient evidence to support the use of magnet therapy on reducing MS-related disability, bladder control problems, or spasticity, or on improving cognition, mobility, sensation, or vision.

- A 2013 Cochrane review of 9 randomized controlled trials involving a total of 301 participants concluded that there is low-level evidence for nonpharmacological interventions, including magnetic stimulation for beneficial effects on spasticity outcomes in people with MS. The studies included in the review were of low methodological quality and high risk of bias.

Safety

- Magnets may interfere with the functioning of the medical device (e.g., pacemaker, insulin pump) and may not be safe for some people. Otherwise, magnets are generally considered safe when applied to the skin.

- Reports of side effects or complications have been rare.

Hyperbaric Oxygen Therapy

Although hyperbaric oxygen therapy is often heavily marketed to people with MS, there is no consistent evidence that supports the use of hyperbaric oxygen therapy for the treatment of MS.

The Evidence Base

- The evidence base on the efficacy of hyperbaric oxygen therapy for MS consists of many studies, including reviews and a Cochrane systematic review.

Efficacy

- A 2010 meta-analysis of 12 randomized studies concluded that hyperbaric oxygen therapy does not produce any clinically significant benefits in MS.

- A 2004 Cochrane review had similar findings. The review of nine studies of hyperbaric oxygen therapy for the treatment of multiple sclerosis found no consistent evidence to confirm a beneficial effect. The reviewers also noted that based on available evidence, routine use is not justified.

Safety

- When safety guidelines are strictly adhered to, hyperbaric oxygen therapy appears to be generally safe. The predominant complication is pressure equalization problems within the middle ear. Serious complications are rare.

Chapter 33

Plasmapheresis

What Is Plasmapheresis?

Plasmapheresis, also called "plasma exchange," is a procedure in which blood is removed from the body and the liquid part, called "plasma," is separated from the red and white blood cells. The plasma is then typically discarded, and the blood cells are returned to the body, along with fresh plasma or other fluids. This procedure is a successful method of treating some autoimmune diseases, such as multiple sclerosis (MS), Guillain-Barre syndrome, Miller Fisher syndrome, chronic inflammatory demyelinating polyneuropathy, Goodpasture syndrome, and Lambert-Eaton syndrome.

An autoimmune disease causes the body's immune system to attack healthy cells or its own tissues. The immune system produces antibodies to protect the body from infections, bacteria, viruses, and other invaders, but when the antibodies, which are proteins in blood plasma, attack their own body, they became autoantibodies. Plasma exchange helps remove autoantibodies from the blood. An alternative treatment for some disorders is to use medication to suppress the immune system, but this approach can lead to serious side effects, and in some cases, the body may no longer be able to fight infection. So, plasmapheresis is often the preferred method of fighting a number of autoimmune disorders.

"Plasmapheresis," © 2017 Omnigraphics. Reviewed March 2019.

Procedure for Plasmapheresis

Anesthesia is generally not necessary for the plasmapheresis treatment itself, but it is sometimes used for the placement of the two relatively large needles that must be used. Once the needles are positioned, patients may feel some discomfort, but no pain, for the remainder of the procedure.

Before the start of plasmapheresis, the patient is asked to lie down or sit in a reclining chair. A needle or catheter tube is placed in a large vein in the crook of the arm, and another needle or tube is placed in the opposite arm or foot. In some cases, the needle or catheter is placed in the shoulder or groin area. Blood is removed through one of the tubes and passed into an apheresis machine, or cell separator. This device separates the plasma from the blood cells, either by spinning at high speed or by passing the blood through a membrane with tiny pores, which allow only the plasma to pass through, but not the blood cells.

The removed plasma is then discarded, along with the autoantibodies it contains. The replacement plasma, or a plasma substitute, is blended with the blood cells, and the mixture is returned to the body through the other tube. The amount of blood that is outside the body at any given time during the procedure is generally less than the amount a donor would contribute at a blood bank.

Plasmapheresis is usually done on an outpatient basis, and the procedure can take from 1 to 3 hours. For an average patient, treatments are repeated 6 to 10 times over span of 2 to 10 weeks. The length and number of treatments depends on the diagnosis and the general condition of the patient.

Before the Procedure

Prior to plasmapheresis, the patient will be examined by his or her physician. A thorough medical history will be taken, and all medication will be reviewed by the doctor in order to determine whether the patient will need to stop taking certain medicines for a given amount of time before and after the treatment.

A few other things to keep in mind:

- Drink plenty of fluids for several days before the procedure to stay hydrated.

- Eat a well-balanced meal prior to treatment.

- Wear comfortable clothing with sleeves that can be easily pulled above the elbows.

- Bring something to read or a portable music device with headphones to help pass the time.

After the Procedure

Following the procedure, the patient will be allowed to leave the hospital or medical center after resting for a short time. Since many people feel tired or weak after plasmapheresis, the patient will need someone to drive her or him home. After the procedure, care must be taken to follow the doctor's instructions regarding medication dosages, which may need to be adjusted, and preventing infection. The patient can show improvement within days or, at most, a few weeks, and the positive effects of the course of treatment can be expected to last for several months. But since plasmapheresis is a temporary treatment, the procedure may have to be repeated on a regular basis.

Risks and Complications

Although plasmapheresis is a safe form of treatment, and complications don't occur often, like most medical procedures, it does carry some risks. Awareness of these risks can help the patient to be better prepared.

A few of the possible risks and complications include:

- Bleeding, which can occur because of the medication given to prevent clotting during the procedure
- A drop in blood pressure, which can be helped by lowering the patient's head, raising his or her legs, and giving an intravenous fluid
- Dizziness, blurred vision, sweating, and abdominal cramps
- Allergic reaction resulting in fever, chills, or rashes
- Reactions to medication, such as tingling in the mouth or limbs or metallic taste in the mouth
- Swelling, bruises, or rashes where needles or tubes were inserted
- Infection
- Anaphylaxis, a potentially dangerous reaction to the solutions used in plasma replacement. The procedure needs to be stopped if this complication occurs.

- Severe bleeding, which can lead to irregular heartbeats or seizures; this needs immediate attention.

- Fatigue, weakness, or joint pain

- Excessive suppression of the immune system can occur during the plasma exchange; however, this generally resolves in a short time as the body produces more antibodies.

- Patients can occasionally develop an allergy to the solutions and equipment used in the procedure. If so, the medical technician or doctor would administer intravenous medication.

A doctor should be contacted immediately if any of the following serious complications develop:

- Seizures

- Signs of infection, such as chills or fever

- Severe bleeding or swelling where the needle or tube was inserted

- Persistent itching or rashes

- Severe pain

- Dizziness, shortness of breath, chest pain, or wheezing

References

1. "Plasmapheresis," Mount Sinai Hospital, 2016.

2. Heitz, David. "Plasmapheresis," Healthline, January 6, 2014.

3. Winkler, Sarah. "Plasmapheresis Procedure," How Stuff Works Health, October 10, 2011.

4. "Facts about Plasmapheresis," Muscular Dystrophy Association (MDA), July 2005.

5. "What Is Plasmapheresis?" PMWO Life Saving Organization, n.d.

Chapter 34

Stem Cell Transplant Induces Multiple Sclerosis Remission

Multiple sclerosis (MS) is an autoimmune disease in which the immune system attacks the central nervous system (CNS). It results in damage to nerve fibers, disrupting communication between the brain and the body. The disease has a wide range of symptoms that include tingling or numbness in the limbs, movement and speech difficulties, weakness, fatigue, chronic pain, vision loss, and depression.

The most common form of MS is relapsing-remitting multiple sclerosis (RRMS), which affects about 80 percent of people with the disease. It is characterized by periods of mild or no symptoms interspersed with periods of more severe symptoms, called "relapses." It can change into a progressive form where symptoms worsen over time without any symptom-free periods. RRMS can be treated with drugs that suppress the immune system and reduce inflammation. However, these drugs can cause serious side effects, are costly, and patients may become resistant to them over time.

One promising treatment for MS is high-dose immunosuppressive therapy with autologous hematopoietic cell transplant (HDIT/HCT).

This chapter contains text excerpted from the following sources: Text in this chapter begins with excerpts from "Stem Cell Transplant Induces Multiple Sclerosis Remission," National Institutes of Health (NIH), February 14, 2017; Text under the heading "Sustained Remission of Multiple Sclerosis" is excerpted from "Stem Cell Transplants May Induce Long-Term Remission of Multiple Sclerosis," National Institutes of Health (NIH), February 1, 2017.

The goal of this therapy is to "reset" a person's immune system so that it will stop attacking their central nervous system. The treatment involves first collecting a patient's hematopoietic stem cells (HSCs)—precursor cells that develop into blood cells. High-dose chemotherapy and other drugs are then used to deplete the immune system and remove disease-causing cells. Finally, the participant is infused with her or his own HSCs, which develop into red and white blood cells and re-establish their immune system.

Researchers from several sites across the country have been monitoring 24 volunteers, between the ages of 26 and 52, who underwent HDIT/HCT treatment for RRMS. The researchers found that 5 years after the procedure, 69 percent of the participants showed no signs of progression of disability, relapse of MS symptoms, or new brain lesions (viewed by magnetic resonance imaging (MRI)). Most importantly, participants did not take any MS medications after receiving HDIT/HCT. 15 of the participants—more than half—had a decrease in an index of MS disability. Side effects included infections, which are commonly associated with the toxic nature of the HDIT/HCT procedure. 3 participants had disease progression and died during the follow-up period. None of the deaths were related to the transplant procedure.

"These extended findings suggest that one-time treatment with HDIT/HCT may be substantially more effective than long-term treatment with the best available medications for people with a certain type of MS," NIAID Director Dr. Anthony S. Fauci says. "These encouraging results support the development of a large, randomized trial to directly compare HDIT/HCT to the standard of care for this often debilitating disease."

Sustained Remission of Multiple Sclerosis

New clinical trial results provide evidence that high-dose immunosuppressive therapy followed by transplantation of a person's own blood-forming stem cells can induce sustained remission of RRMS. The experimental treatment aims to suppress active disease and prevent further disability by removing disease-causing cells and resetting the immune system. During the procedure, doctors collect a participant's blood-forming stem cells, give the participant high-dose chemotherapy to deplete the immune system and return the participant's own stem cells to rebuild the immune system.

"Although further evaluation of the benefits and risks of HDIT/HCT is needed, these five-year results suggest the promise of this treatment for inducing long-term, sustained remissions of poor prognosis relapsing-remitting MS," said Richard Nash, M.D., of Colorado Blood Cancer Institute (CBCI) and Presbyterian-St. Luke's Hospital (PSLMC). Dr. Nash served as principal investigator of the HALT-MS study.

"If these findings are confirmed in larger studies, HDIT/HCT may become a potential therapeutic option for patients with active relapsing-remitting MS, particularly those who do not respond to existing therapies," said Daniel Rotrosen, M.D., director of NIAID's Division of Allergy, Immunology, and Transplantation (DAIT).

Part Four

Living with Multiple Sclerosis

Chapter 35

Resilience: Addressing the Challenges of MS

People with multiple sclerosis (MS) may find that the physical, emotional, cognitive, psychological, and spiritual challenges of living with the disease can be overwhelming. Some may feel that the challenges of living with a chronic disease are very hard to face day after day. But many people living with chronic diseases, including MS, have learned that practicing behaviors which promote resilience is the secret to not just coping with the disease, but thriving with it.

What Is Resilience?

Resilience is commonly described as the ability to bounce back from difficult circumstances—to find happiness and life satisfaction—despite challenges. These challenges can be with relationships, finances, health, or any of the myriad stressors that we face in life. It's finding hope and meaning in life, even while confronting obstacles. It's finding the motivation to take on new challenges and opportunities. It's thriving in the face of whatever life throws at you. Resilience is the ability to maintain or regain well-being and progress toward valued goals in the face of adversity. Resilience is not about acting happy all

This chapter includes text excerpted from "VA Multiple Sclerosis Centers of Excellence—Finding the Strength to Fight Back," U.S. Department of Veterans Affairs (VA), 2017.

the time or ignoring the very real difficulties in life. Resilience is not even about trying to eliminate negative thoughts or feelings. In fact, it's quite the opposite.

A significant part of being resilient involves what researchers call "positive adaptation" or "realistic optimism," which refers to remaining hopeful about the future while making plans that enable us to cope with our actual reality. It requires moving forward, despite facing difficult events and emotions. It requires courage and hope. Results of several studies suggest that people who are resilient report significantly greater satisfaction with their lives. A study in the *Journal of Health Psychology* evaluated 1,862 people with MS, muscular dystrophy, postpolio syndrome, or spinal cord injuries. The researchers used various tests to assess the participants' resilience, including levels of depression, pain, and fatigue, and overall quality of life (QOL).

The study team found that people with higher resilience scores also had lower rates of depression and a higher quality of life, even if they had high levels of pain and fatigue. Other studies suggest that when people engage in activities that boost resilience, such as stress management, social activities, or exercise, they report greater life satisfaction. Some people may be more naturally resilient than others. Researchers have found that people have a natural "set point" for resilience that is determined partly by genetics and partly by their early environmental circumstances. Together, those factors make up about half of a person's capacity to adapt positively to significant challenges. The other half of resilience comes from learning and using cognitive, behavioral, and interpersonal skills. Even if it doesn't come entirely naturally, you can learn to be more resilient.

Building Resilience

Dawn Ehde, Ph.D., a psychologist at the University of Washington, collaborated with the National Multiple Sclerosis Society and the Multiple Sclerosis Society of Canada on the program in their series, *North American Education Programs,* to create a video and workbook about resilience. The workbook describes three steps to building resilience:

1. **Understanding**—Learn as much as you can about MS and how it can change over time. Talk to others living with this chronic disease.

2. **Managing**—Use your knowledge to learn new ways to cope and live your life with MS, with physical, social, and financial adjustments. You may feel more confident and in charge.

3. **Growth**—Begin to shift your priorities, and determine what is most important in life. There are also lifestyle practices which can help people develop resilience:

    *   Maintain strong social connections—family, friends, and others who have MS

    *   Maximize physical wellness—healthy eating habits, exercise, sleep, and MS therapies

    *   Set realistic goals, and move towards them—attainable goals result in feelings of competence

    *   Practice gratitude—be mindful of positive things in life

    *   Nurture positive emotions, and savor them when they occur—hope, optimism, and humor

    *   Allow negative feelings—recognize, express, and move on

    *   Use mindfulness and relaxation approaches—develop techniques to reduce worry

    *   Practice forgiveness towards people and situations—release resentment and bitterness

    *   Plan for the future—make realistic assessments and practical adjustments

    *   Find a sense of meaning and purpose in life—relationships, activities, or other avenues

    *   Help others—volunteer

    *   Turn to faith or spirituality—seek a larger sense of belonging and meaning in life

    *   Learn to tell a different version of your story—reframe it to see both sides

    *   Nurture your sense of humor

Rather than making a chore of your resilience-building activities, focus on the ones you really enjoy. Watching a movie with your friends builds resilience. So does having a hobby and taking time to enjoy it. Taking time to meditate or engage in mindful breathing can also boost your resilience. "It's within the vast majority of humans to become more resilient—to develop the hope that leads to feeling more happy or content," says Dr. Ehde "People with MS, perhaps more than most, can benefit from building their resilience because of the ongoing, unpredictable changes they face in their health, abilities, and self-image," notes Dr. Ehde. "People who are resilient have the ability to grow from adversity. They can learn things about themselves, about what they value. They learn that they can get through tough things." To find out more about resilience, visit the National Multiple Sclerosis Society of Canada Society website and type "resilience" into the search engine window.

Chapter 36

Self-Management for Living Well

People with multiple sclerosis (MS) want to know what they can do today to feel their best and if lifestyle interventions, such as diet, stress management, and physical activity, have any benefits in reducing the impact of the disease. Over the years, the concept of health has evolved to include a dynamic sense of well-being across multiple dimensions of life and not just the absence of disease.

Wellness is attainable for everyone, even when living with a chronic illness. Achieving health and wellness is a lifelong process in which people make intentional choices, set personal priorities, and engage in health-promoting activities. Intentional choices include choosing the foods you eat, choosing whether to smoke, choosing to spend time with friends and family, choosing to engage in physical activity, devoting time to intellectual stimulation, and more.

Making Healthy Lifestyle Choices

Making healthy choices that promote satisfaction in the various dimensions of wellness can help you attain a sense of well-being and life satisfaction. Here is what we mean by the "dimensions of wellness:"

This chapter includes text excerpted from "VA Multiple Sclerosis Centers of Excellence—The Brighter Side of Life," U.S. Department of Veterans Affairs (VA), 2016.

Physical: Making positive lifestyle choices about regular physical activity/exercise (such as walking, swimming, and yoga) geared to one's abilities, healthy eating, MS care and primary care, and preventive health behaviors (including smoking cessation, limited alcohol use, and attention to personal safety).

Social: Developing positive, healthy relationships that nurture interconnectedness with family, friends, and community.

Emotional: Developing coping strategies to enhance problem-solving, manage stress, foster a positive outlook, and develop resilience in the face of unpredictable changes, while paying attention to mood changes, including depression and anxiety, that may require treatment.

Occupational: Engaging in meaningful and rewarding activities that promote a sense of purpose and accomplishment, including opportunities to contribute one's unique skills, talents, and knowledge to others at home, at work, or in the community.

Spiritual: Developing a worldview that provides a sense of peace and harmony and enables one to cope and adapt throughout life. The ultimate goal is finding meaning and purpose in the face of one's personal challenges.

Intellectual: Engaging in mentally stimulating and challenging activities that lead to personal growth, enhanced creativity, and new learning.

Selecting Medicines and Therapies

As people manage their MS, they want to understand the role of conventional medicine, including disease-modifying therapies and symptom management medications, as well as how they can integrate lifestyle interventions and complementary approaches to maximize their well-being. They may wonder about the impact of a specific diet or exercise regime on MS or about the potential benefit (or harm) of other approaches, such as vitamin supplements, probiotics, or acupuncture. Many have felt frustrated by a lack of support from healthcare professionals, who say there is not sufficient scientific evidence to provide guidance or who may not have the time or expertise to discuss it with their patients.

While many things may feel beyond one's control when living with an unpredictable and chronic disease like MS, exerting control over your personal lifestyle behaviors can help alleviate feelings of helplessness.

Tips to Incorporate Wellness Behaviors

Setting your own personal wellness objectives and discussing them with your healthcare providers are the first steps to maximizing your well-being, even in the context of MS. Some tips for incorporating wellness behaviors into everyday life include:

- Make time to relax every day, even if only for 10 to 15 minutes—listen to music, meditate, listen to guided relaxation.

- Consider making a small healthy change to your diet—replace dessert with a piece of fruit twice per week, use whole grain flour when baking.

- Explore how yoga, tai chi, or another physical activity can be modified for your level of ability and interest.

- Make a plan to enjoy time with friends or family at least once per month—watch a movie together, enjoy a meal together, take a walk together.

- Stimulate your curiosity and enhance your intellectual well-being—listen to a book on tape, attend a lecture, take an online course, visit the museum.

Chapter 37

Vaccinations and People with Multiple Sclerosis

Vaccines are important for preventing other illnesses. Preventive care is also an important part of multiple sclerosis (MS) management. You may wonder about links between MS and vaccines. Are vaccines safe to use in people with MS? Do vaccines cause MS? Are they safe for me? Should I have them? This chapter clarifies that vaccines do not cause MS and guides you in how vaccines are used safely by people with MS.

Do Vaccines Cause Multiple Sclerosis?

After mass vaccination programs for hepatitis B began, some people developed MS. This led to an investigation into a possible connection between the hepatitis B vaccine and MS. The U.S. Food and Drug Administration (FDA) reviewed the results of clinical studies used for approval of the hepatitis B vaccine and did not find any increase in MS. The World Health Organization (WHO) Global Advisory Committee on Vaccine Safety (GACVS) states that "multiple studies and review panels have concluded that there is no link between MS and hepatitis B vaccination." The Centers for Disease Control and Prevention (CDC)

This chapter includes text excerpted from "Vaccines and Multiple Sclerosis: A Practical Guide," U.S. Department of Veterans Affairs (VA), August 17, 2018.

and the National Network for Immunization Information (NNii) also support the safety of the hepatitis B vaccine.

Why Are Vaccines Important?

Vaccines are an important way to protect everyone from serious infectious diseases. Nowadays, vaccines are among the most successful and cost-effective public health tools available for preventing diseases. Thanks to vaccines, serious and often fatal diseases, such as polio, are now distant memories for most Americans. In almost all cases, getting a vaccine is much safer than getting the disease itself. Currently, vaccines to protect children and adults from at least 17 diseases are available. Travelers to foreign countries, where uncommon diseases, such as typhoid and yellow fever may be encountered, may need additional vaccines before their trips. Guidelines on vaccinations for people with MS have been established by the Multiple Sclerosis Council for Clinical Practice and by the CDC.

Several types of vaccines are available. Live, attenuated vaccines contain a version of the living microbe that has been weakened so it does not cause disease. Although live, attenuated vaccines are generally very effective, because they contain live microbes, they should not be given to people with damaged or weakened immune systems, such as those with human immunodeficiency virus (HIV). Since there may be an increased risk with live, attenuated vaccines in people taking certain MS disease-modifying medications, including natalizumab (Tysabri®), fingolimod (Gilenya®), teriflunomide (Aubagio®), and possibly dimethyl fumarate (Tecfidera®), people taking these medications should avoid live, attenuated vaccines when an alternative is available.

Vaccines that are not live are inactivated (contain microbes killed by chemicals, heat, or radiation), subunits (contain only part of the microbe), toxoids (inactivated toxins), or conjugate (a subunit linked to a toxoid) vaccines. These nonlive vaccines cannot cause disease and are, therefore, generally safe for use in people with MS. In addition to the active component of the vaccine (the part that induces disease protection), vaccines contain other substances. Anyone with a severe, life-threatening allergy to any component of a vaccine should not get that vaccine.

Nonlive Vaccines

- Influenza injectable (shot, including high dose)
- Pneumonia

- Hepatitis A
- Hepatitis B
- Tetanus
- Diphtheria
- Pertussis

Live Vaccines

- Influenza nasal spray (FluMist®)
- Chickenpox
- Shingles
- Measles, mumps, rubella (MMR)

Flu Vaccine

One of the most commonly used vaccines is the influenza (flu) vaccine. Flu vaccines are one of the most important ones we should all be sure to get because flu can be unpleasant and even fatal. There are several types of flu vaccines. The most familiar and commonly used one is the standard flu shot. The standard flu shot is an inactivated vaccine, containing only killed flu viruses. The injectable flu vaccine is recommended for everyone over 6 months of age. It has been studied extensively in people with MS and is very safe. A high-dose, injected flu vaccine is available for people over age 65. This high-dose vaccine is also an inactivated vaccine. It has not been studied in people with MS and, at present, the CDC is only recommending the high-dose vaccine over the seasonal flu vaccine for people 65 years of age or older.

Chicken Pox Vaccine (Variax)

There are some people who have never had chickenpox or the chickenpox vaccine. Because fingolimod, alemtuzumab, and ocrelizumab can increase the risk of chickenpox in people with MS, if you are going to use fingolimod and have not had chickenpox or the vaccine, the CDC recommends that you receive the varicella vaccination. The varicella vaccine is given in two doses, four weeks apart. People with MS should not start fingolimod until at least one month after the last dose of the varicella vaccine.

Shingles (Zoster) Vaccine

The shingles vaccine (Zostavax®) protects people from shingles, which is a reactivation of varicella-zoster virus if you had chickenpox earlier in life. The CDC recommends that adults 60 years of age or older should receive the shingles vaccine. The shingles vaccine is a live vaccine; however, because most people have had chickenpox earlier in their lives, and therefore, already have the virus in their bodies, the risk of getting the disease from the vaccine is much lower. If a person has had chickenpox, or tests positive for the antibodies, the shingles vaccine would generally be safe and beneficial.

Pneumonia Vaccine

The pneumonia vaccine (Pneumovax®) protects people from pneumonia caused by a bacteria called "pneumococcus." This is a nonlive, subunit vaccine. The pneumonia vaccine is recommended for people with compromised breathing or lung function, such as those who are wheelchair-dependent or bedbound, because they are more prone to pneumonia. This vaccine is generally safe for people with MS.

Other Vaccines

Both hepatitis A and hepatitis B vaccines are not live and are safe for people with MS. If you have not had these vaccines during childhood or as a condition of employment, discuss it with your healthcare provider to see if you need them. The measles, mumps, and rubella (MMR) vaccine is a live, attenuated vaccine generally given during infancy, after one year of age, and is recommended by the CDC for the general population. Tetanus vaccine, which is often given as a combined vaccination with diphtheria (Td) or with both diphtheria and pertussis (Tdap), is not a live vaccine.

Overall, vaccines are safe and effective for people with MS and are important disease prevention tools. There are no concerns for use of nonlive vaccines in people with MS. Live, attenuated vaccines should usually be avoided in people with MS when an effective, safe alternative is available. The use of live, attenuated vaccines should be avoided during and for two months after treatment with fingolimod because of the risk of infection. Additionally, vaccines should not be given during therapy with daclizumab, alemtuzumab, and ocrelizumab. If a live vaccine is required, therapy with these agents should not begin until eight weeks after the vaccination. The risk of live, attenuated vaccines for people taking natalizumab, teriflunomide, and dimethyl fumarate is uncertain; people on these medications should discuss the potential risk and benefits of live, attenuated vaccines, such as Zostavax®, with their healthcare provider. Vaccines should not be received during or within four to six weeks of an MS relapse. If you have any questions or concerns, please talk with your healthcare provider.

Chapter 38

Contraception for Women with Multiple Sclerosis

Contraception is an important consideration for women with multiple sclerosis (MS). MS is more prevalent among females, and the peak age of onset for women is during the childbearing years.

MS does not seem to significantly impair fertility, although there is emerging data on decreased ovarian reserve and higher prevalence of thyroid autoimmunity in MS patients, possibly affecting fertility.

A chronic neurologic illness may also influence pregnancy intentions. Although some patients report having completed their families prior to MS diagnosis, one study found that among women with MS who did not become pregnant after diagnosis, nearly one-third cited MS-related concerns, such as symptoms interfering with parenting, burdening their partner, and children inheriting MS.

Many women with MS use disease-modifying therapies (DMTs). DMTs are generally not recommended for women trying to become pregnant, and there are known risks to the fetus associated with some treatments; none of the DMTs are specifically approved for use in pregnancy.

If a woman is on certain DMTs, a washout period before conception is recommended. Providers are always encouraged to review

This chapter includes text excerpted from "Contraception for Women with Multiple Sclerosis: Guidance for Healthcare Providers," Centers for Disease Control and Prevention (CDC), May 2017.

up-to-date product-specific information for their practice location and scope, prior to giving advice to their patients. The optimal time for a woman with MS to conceive should be considered individually, based on the activity of her disease, her response to treatment, and the availability of resources to manage the challenges of early motherhood. As such, family planning should be an essential part of any comprehensive treatment plan for women of reproductive age with MS, including regular counseling on the use of effective contraception to optimally time desired pregnancies and prevent unintended pregnancies.

However, neurologists may not be well equipped to discuss contraception with patients. A survey of female neurologists from the United States and Canada found that most referred their patients to an obstetrician-gynecologist or internist for contraceptive counseling, and many were unsure whether their MS patients used contraception or the type of contraception used.

Many methods of contraception are available to women and couples. When choosing an appropriate contraceptive method, factors to consider include safety, availability, acceptability, and effectiveness. For women with MS, additional issues may include difficulty swallowing pills or manual dexterity needed for placing vaginal rings and barrier methods. The effectiveness of a contraceptive method depends on the inherent effectiveness of the method itself and on how consistency and correctly the method is used.

Whereas pregnancy rates during perfect use show how effective a method is in a hypothetical "perfect-use" scenario, pregnancy rates during typical use show how effective a method is during actual use, including inconsistent and/or incorrect use. The most effective reversible methods of contraception during typical use are intrauterine devices (IUDs) and implants, collectively known as "long-acting, reversible contraception" (LARC).

LARC methods are highly effective because once in place, they do not require regular user compliance. LARC methods provide pregnancy protection for 3 to 10 years, depending on the device, but can be removed at any time if the woman chooses to become pregnant (or for any other reason). Methods that are user-dependent, such as oral contraceptive pills and condoms, rely on consistent and correct use and, as a result, are less effective during typical use. When counseling women about contraceptive options, the full range, and effectiveness of methods for which they are medically eligible should be discussed.

Although several clinical reviews are available on the management of and therapeutic considerations for women with MS during the reproductive years, the focus of these reviews has largely been on issues around the time of pregnancy. Topics have included the effect of pregnancy on the MS disease course; the management of MS during pregnancy, labor, and postpartum; and safety of breastfeeding while on DMTs.

Recommendations for Women with Multiple Sclerosis

The 2016 U.S. Medical Eligibility Criteria for Contraceptive Use (U.S. MEC) includes recommendations for contraceptive use by women with MS.

Intrauterine devices (IUDs)—IUDs include the copper-containing IUD (Cu-IUD) and the levonorgestrel-releasing IUD (LNG-IUD). For both the Cu-IUD and the LNG-IUD, there are no restrictions for use by women with MS.

Progestin-only contraceptives—Progestin-only contraceptives include etonogestrel implants, DMPA, and progestin-only pills (POPs). For implants and POPs, there are no restrictions for use by women with MS. For DMPA, women with MS can generally use the method, although careful followup might be required and related to concerns about bone health. Women with MS might have compromised bone health from disease-related disability, immobility, or use of corticosteroids, and the use of DMPA has been associated with small changes in bone mineral density.

Combined hormonal contraceptives—Combined hormonal contraceptives (CHCs) include low-dose combined oral contraceptives (containing ≤35 μg ethinyl estradiol), the hormonal patch, and the vaginal ring. Classifications for CHCs for women with MS differ based on immobility status. For women with MS without prolonged immobility, there are no restrictions for use of CHCs. However, for women with MS with prolonged immobility, CHCs are usually not recommended unless other more appropriate contraceptive methods are not available or acceptable. This is because of inferred concerns about VTE risk. Although no evidence was found examining the effect of CHCs on VTE among women with MS, women with MS are at higher risk than unaffected women for VTE, and CHCs increase VTE risk.

253

Barrier methods—Barrier methods include condoms (male and female), spermicides, and diaphragm with spermicide or cervical cap. For these methods, there are no restrictions for use by women with MS.

Other methods—Other methods of contraception are included in the United States Medical Eligibility Criteria for Contraceptive Use (U.S. MEC) 2016, including fertility awareness-based methods, the lactational amenorrhea method, coitus interruptus (withdrawal), and female and male sterilization. None of these methods are restricted for women with MS.

Although a specific contraceptive method may be used with no restrictions related to safety, it does not necessarily mean that the method is the best choice for the patient. When counseling women of reproductive age with MS about contraception, providers, including neurologists, should always consider the individual social, cultural, and clinical circumstances of the patient seeking advice. For example, for a woman with MS taking potentially fetotoxic DMTs, more effective methods, such as LARC, might be the best option to avoid unintended pregnancy or to delay pregnancy until teratogenic medications are no longer needed.

Chapter 39

Multiple Sclerosis and Diet

When people are diagnosed with multiple sclerosis (MS), a common question asked is "What can I do to make myself not be affected much by MS?" It is not fully understood why MS occurs, but, increasingly, research points towards a connection between environmental factors, such as diet, exposure to sunlight, low vitamin D levels, and initial exposure to viruses, bacteria, and other microbes during childhood. Recent studies also suggest a possible connection between dietary habits and our digestive system bacteria that, in turn, can affect our immune systems and the development of autoimmune diseases, such as MS.

A report published in 2008 that surveyed people with MS from around the world, ("Atlas of Multiple Sclerosis" by the World Health Organization and Multiple Sclerosis International Federation) indicated that diet change and nutrition were the most commonly used nonconventional approaches for treating MS symptoms. Another survey done in 2008 by the Central Institute of Health at the University of Heidelberg in Germany, looked at 1,573 people with MS and found that up to 40 percent of Americans with MS use some form of diet modification after diagnosis. Based on these results, people with MS appear interested in dietary approaches for MS management.

The neurologist Dr. Roy Swank, conducted one of the pioneering studies examining the role of diet in MS in the late 1940s, an era

This chapter includes text excerpted from "VA Multiple Sclerosis Centers of Excellence—I Have MS but MS Does Not Have Me," U.S. Department of Veterans Affairs (VA), 2013. Reviewed March 2019.

when no medications for MS were available. He believed that diets rich in saturated animal fats could be bad for MS. He devised the "Swank Diet" as an MS treatment, which consists of no more than 10 to 15 grams of total saturated fat a day, fish and chicken as primary protein sources, and dairy products containing only 1 percent or less of fat. He supplemented this diet with cod liver oil, which is enriched in omega-3 fatty acids.

Dr. Swank studied the effects of this diet on survival and disability in 144 people with MS over a span of 50 years. The study included 2 groups of people with MS: 70 "good dieters" who followed a strict low-fat diet, consuming less than 20 grams of fat per day, while 74 "bad dieters" consumed more than 20 grams of fat per day. 34 years into the study, it was found that "bad dieters" had a death rate that was more than double that of the "good dieters." By 2000, 15 of the original participants in the study were alive, all of them belonging to the "good dieters" group with the majority of these participants (13 out of 15) still ambulatory. Although this study has been criticized for inadequate scientific proof, it remains a unique long-term study of an intervention showing possible benefits on survival and disability in people with MS.

Recent research involving approximately 9,000 people with MS suggests a relationship between an MS-related disability and vascular disease risk factors, such as high blood pressure, high blood fats, and heart disease. This study found that the presence of one or more of these diseases increased the risk and onset of walking disability in MS, and the risk increased with the number of each vascular condition.

In a recent two-year study, researchers studied blood fat (lipid) levels and compared them to MS-related disability and brain imaging magnetic resonance imaging (MRI) outcomes. It was found that higher low-density lipoprotein, or "bad" cholesterol, and total cholesterol levels were associated with higher MS disability, and higher high-density lipoprotein, or "good" cholesterol, was associated with lower inflammatory disease activity on the brain MRI.

Researchers at the MS Center at Oregon Health and Science University in Portland, OR are studying a very low-fat vegan diet developed by Dr. John McDougall. Within this diet, meat, fish, poultry, and animal products are eliminated, total fat is less than 20 percent of daily intake, and refined flour is restricted. This study includes 61 people with relapsing-remitting MS, and the goal of the study is to measure the effects of diet on brain MRI, MS relapse, disability, and blood-brain barrier disruption (neuroaxonal degeneration) in MS.

Upon review of the research, there appears to be a pattern supporting the idea that healthy dietary changes can be beneficial for MS and can decrease MS disability progression.

So, What a Person with Multiple Sclerosis Can Do?

First, there is no evidence that following a low-fat diet is a "cure" for MS, and it should not be used in place of appropriate use of disease-modifying therapies. Second, it is reasonable to follow a healthy, low-fat diet, such as that recommended by the American Heart Association. Third, for those who are motivated to adhere to a more stringent, well-balanced low-fat diet, following the Swank Diet or a well-balanced vegan diet, such as the McDougall Diet, is safe and may be beneficial. More research needs to be done to determine whether a low-fat diet is actually a partial treatment for MS. Until then, using common sense is prudent.

Chapter 40

Exercise Guidelines for People with Multiple Sclerosis

Chapter Contents

Section 40.1

Planning Your Activities and Designing an Exercise Program

This section includes text excerpted from "Planning Your
Activities and Designing an Exercise Program," U.S. Department
of Veterans Affairs (VA), August 1, 2018.

Learning the best way to exercise after developing a life-changing
disease, such as multiple sclerosis (MS) can be challenging.

What Is an Activity Diary?

Many people have found an activity diary to be a very useful tool.
When you keep an activity diary for three to four days in a row (and
during periods where you are doing regular activities), you start to
see patterns of what you are doing. Once you see these patterns, you
can change your activities so that during your times of energy, you do
activities that require energy, and during your low energy times, you
do things that do not take a lot of energy.

Do I Need to Change My Activities?

When you get into a habit of doing things in a certain way and then
you get a diagnosis of MS, it forces you to do some things differently.
It can be difficult to recognize that you have to change the way you
do things. It can be difficult to change life habits, and that is where
healthcare professionals fit in, as they help people through that process
of change by directing them and showing them that there are different
ways to do things. It is jarring enough to be diagnosed with MS, let
alone all of the changes that are going to have to take place in one's life.

How Do I Set Myself Up for Success?

When a person has decreased energy, setting goals and then prioritizing these goals is a very effective way of getting what is important
done. Priority setting is typically based on the list of what needs to be
done, what you would like to do, and what would be nice to do. The
activities that are ticked off on any particular day are determined by
the energy level of the day.

So How Do You Go about Identifying What a Goal Ought to Be?

It should be something realistic, something you can achieve, and it should be specific. The more specific it is, the easier it is to tell if you have achieved it. It should also be something that can be done independently. You should not have to rely on other people to achieve this goal, and you should write it down so you can review it regularly. One activity that should usually be included to help maintain function, (even if it was not a habit before) is exercise.

Why Is Exercise Important?

Exercise is important for a number of reasons. Exercise can help minimize some general health diseases, such as cardiac disease and diabetes (as well as others), that can affect people with or without MS. It is also important in helping to minimize the impact of some of the problems that MS causes, such as weakness. If you can maintain your strength and ability to move about, then you are going to minimize the impact of some of the other problems.

People with MS are at risk of becoming deconditioned. Exercising and participating in a regular exercise program can help prevent this. It is definitely one of the recommendations from the National Multiple Sclerosis Society fatigue guidelines. For it to be effective, you have to be committed to doing it and doing it regularly.

To prevent exercise from becoming boring, it should not be the same activity all the time. You should choose a variety of activities, but whatever you choose to do, you have to participate several times a week for exercise to help. To make it easier to exercise regularly, the most important thing is to schedule your exercise. By exercising regularly, you will learn more about yourself and become an expert in conserving energy, as well as become more efficient and thoughtful about how you are spending your time and energy.

What Type of Exercise Is Best?

Healthcare providers need to be aware of disease-specific issues when recommending exercise that is appropriate for people with MS. Fatigue is often a major issue when considering endurance or cardiovascular-type (aerobic) exercises, and choosing an appropriate exercise plan can be a challenge. Typical methods of exercise for people with MS (as well as others) include walking, jogging, riding an exercise (or street) bicycle, or swimming.

If people are having difficulty walking, often a safe exercise program is using an exercise bicycle. The advantage of an exercise bicycle is that when people become fatigued, they are still at home and do not have to figure out how they are going to get home.

As MS progresses, it is common to have to shift to a different mode of exercise. Some people have to make this shift early on. They might have initially been a jogger, but they no longer have the energy to keep jogging and need to explore other exercise options. Because it is easy to get into patterns and it is hard to change things on your own, it can help to have a professional evaluation.

How Often Should I Exercise?

It is generally recommended that people should exercise aerobically 3 to 5 times a week. This includes people with MS. As the goal, the duration of aerobic exercise should be 20 minutes or more of exercise each day. Unfortunately, because fatigue is a major MS symptom, starting out exercising at 20 minutes per session is usually not very realistic or possible.

Often people need to start out at three to five minutes at a time. Some will ask, "is it even worth doing if I'm only doing it three to five minutes?" The answer to this is that you have to start somewhere; so you start with what you can do, and then you build on success and slowly increase your exercise time. Most people cannot jump from 3 to 20 minutes in one exercise session. An alternate approach is trying two 10-minute sessions, which can be very beneficial.

The plan should be to start with 3 to 4 minutes, next increase from 4 to 5 minutes, and then from 5 minutes to 7 minutes etc., and go on. Remember, you can remain at those periods for as long as you need to until you are ready to go up to the next level. Exercising can help the psyche as well. Exercise endorphins, which are chemicals our bodies produce that make us feel good, are released during exercise. Therefore, there are physical and emotional benefits of exercising.

How Hard Should I Exercise?

You will hear many answers to the question "how hard should I exercise?" The "gold standard" is to monitor your heart rate, but this does not always work with people with MS. Some people find that MS causes numbness and tingling in the fingers, and it is hard to feel a heart rate. If this is an issue, it is generally recommended that you exercise to a level where a conversation can be held while still exercising. If you are having trouble carrying on a conversation, then you might be exercising a little bit too hard and need to slow down a bit. If you are able to converse without difficulty, then you probably are not exercising hard enough.

As you get stronger, you will want to increase the amount of exercise you do. One relatively painless way to get more exercise is to slowly increase the distance you park from a store (or other destination) each time you go. This will allow your body to strengthen itself while doing everyday chores. If you normally use a disabled parking pass, try parking in nondisabled spaces that are just a bit further away. You will find that you may be able to walk further as you gain strength. Of course, you can always use the disabled parking spot when you are trying to conserve your energy for the day.

This walking can be counted as exercise; although, a planned, structured exercise program is best. Keep in mind that unstructured exercise tends to wear you out, and then you are at risk for not being able to participate in an activity that might be more important to you later in the day.

Budgeting your energy is important. An example of budgeting your energy is if you have an important meeting at work, you might choose to park your car close to the entrance of the building to conserve your energy. If you need to be fully alert in the meeting, then you would want to conserve your "parking lot energy" for the energy that you will need for the business event. Walking a greater distance another day would make more sense.

People with MS need to be very careful about how they spend their energy and wisely choose their activities.

What Is Overheating When Exercising?

When people with MS exercise—in fact, when anyone exercises—we get warm. For people with MS, heat can be a big issue, because it causes more fatigue. Doing strenuous exercise can be more of a problem for people with MS because often the ability to sweat—a body cooling mechanism—does not work normally. For some people, MS can affect the ability to properly sweat and to reduce overheating while exercising.

In fact, people with MS can become overheated with little to no exercise. For example, they can experience becoming overheated when out in the sun. There are a number of things you can do to help make up for the lack of (or reduction in) sweating that we do not typically think about. One method to prevent overheating is to dress in light clothing or layers of clothing that you can peel off as you warm up during the day. Another strategy is choosing to do your exercise in a cool room or environment to help with cooling your body down. If the rooms that you are living in are not cool, you might want to try to maintain a cooler temperature at least in the room where you exercise. Some people have used circulating fans to help cool their bodies during exercise. Having a cool beverage that you can take sips of now and then will really help keep you cool as well. If you swim as part of your exercise, try to swim in a pool that maintains a cooler temperature.

Another refreshing tip is to have a water spray bottle handy to spritz yourself as needed. In addition to helping you feel more comfortable, if you are someone who does not sweat normally (or enough), the spray/misting bottle will help provide artificial sweat and help cool your body down.

Section 40.2

Tips for Exercising

This section includes text excerpted from "Six Exercise
Tips for Multiple Sclerosis," U.S. Department of Veterans
Affairs (VA), August 1, 2018.

According to the National Center on Physical Activity and Disability (NCPAD): "In addition to improving overall health, cardiovascular fitness, the range of motion, and flexibility, exercise can help one increase energy, improve balance, manage spasticity, decrease muscle atrophy, and better perform activities of daily living." Recent studies show that exercise is critical in preventing cognitive decline in those with multiple sclerosis (MS), central in lifting depression and overall mood, and may even delay the progression of the disease. Below are six exercise tips for people with MS. Consult with your doctor before starting any exercise program.

1. Stretch Daily

Flexibility exercises, such as muscle stretching and range of motion exercises, can help prevent shrinkage or shortening of muscles and can help reduce the severity of spasticity symptoms. Dedicate at least 10 to 15 minutes of stretching every day, ideally several times a day.

2. Experiment

MS affects everyone differently, so try different ways of exercising to see what works best for you. Swimming and walking are popular, as are horseback riding and biking (try a three-wheeled trike if the balance is an issue). Give a go at yoga, tai chi, or Pilates, or even an exercise class for seniors. Work out to videos at home or circuit train at the gym. Adaptive ski programs can be a great way to enjoy the cool outdoors.

3. Stay Cool

Heat, while it will not trigger an attack, can exacerbate your MS symptoms, which can range from annoying to debilitating. Go to the gym when it's cool, an exercise in the morning, seek out air conditioning, consider snow sports, and put swimming on your list. Use gear, such as cooling vests and cold packs, and don't forget to down icy drinks to keep your core temperature from rising too much.

4. Cardio Is Key

MS research continues to support the importance of cardio workouts. Not only does it improve fatigue and overall quality of life, but raising your heart rate appears to influence the progression of the disease, decreasing both damage to the brain (fewer lesions) and brain atrophy. And yes, even if you are in a wheelchair, you likely can still do seated aerobic workouts.

5. Train in Bursts

Fatigue or weakness can come on quickly, especially when doing the recommended cardio. Space out your "hard" exercise with frequent breaks if needed. High-intensity training, where you sprint for 10 to 30 seconds then rest for a few minutes, can be quite effective. Mini workouts, all combined, produce the same or even better benefits as one long one.

6. Remember, Multiple Sclerosis Is Beatable Someday

MS is beatable someday. Optimism when fighting an incurable disease is essential to good mental health. You want to be ready when that cure comes with the healthiest body and mind possible. You can do this. You can definitely do this.

Chapter 41

Sleep and Multiple Sclerosis

Sleep plays an important role in your physical health and well-being. Sleep supports healthy brain functioning, is involved in the healing and repair of your heart and blood vessels, regulates mood, reduces stress, and even helps your immune system defend your body against foreign or harmful substances. The average adult needs seven to nine hours of sleep each day to function well. Yet, many people do not get adequate amounts of sleep.

People with multiple sclerosis (MS) often say they sleep poorly at night and are fatigued in the daytime. In the general population, the three most common sleep problems reported are insomnia, sleep apnea, and restless leg syndrome (RLS). Recent research suggests that people with MS have these problems even more often.

Insomnia

Insomnia is characterized by problems getting to sleep, staying asleep, or waking up too early. Insomnia can have multiple causes and is a significant problem at some point for almost half of people with MS. Insomnia can be caused by nighttime MS symptoms that disrupt sleep, such as pain, muscle spasms, and urinary frequency. Medications, including some antidepressant (SSRIs), stimulants used to treat day-time fatigue, and corticosteroids used to treat MS exacerbations, can

This chapter includes text excerpted from "VA Multiple Sclerosis Centers of Excellence—Where There's a Will, There's a Way," U.S. Department of Veterans Affairs (VA), 2015. Reviewed March 2019.

also contribute to insomnia. Depression, which is common with MS, is also associated with insomnia. Although occasional self-medication of insomnia with over-the-counter (OTC) sleep medications containing antihistamines can help, if you use them often, they will probably stop working and will also make you sleepy or foggy during the day. Many approaches can be effective for treating insomnia, including adjusting your current medication regimen, addressing MS symptoms that are contributing to poor sleep, using nonmedication cognitive behavioral therapy (CBT) approaches, and, in resistant cases, using prescribed sleep-enhancing medications.

Sleep Apnea

Sleep apnea affects at least one in five Americans and probably an even greater proportion of people with MS. Sleep apnea is characterized by repeatedly stopping breathing during sleep. The frequent pauses in breathing can cause fragmented sleep, as well as low blood oxygen levels. Untreated, sleep apnea is associated with poor daytime functioning, mood, and memory problems and, if severe, cardiovascular disorders, such as heart disease and stroke. Sleep apnea may also lead to worsened fatigue, poor energy, and daytime tiredness common in people with MS. Treatment of sleep apnea can reduce these symptoms which may have been attributed solely to MS.

Restless Leg Syndrome

Restless leg syndrome (RLS) is characterized by an uncomfortable urge to move your legs or, more rarely, other body areas. This urge is temporarily relieved by moving your legs. RLS symptoms are generally worse in the evening or at night. RLS is three times more common in people with MS than in the general population. RLS may affect up to one-third of individuals with MS and is more common in those who are older, have had MS for longer, have primary progressive MS, and have a greater disability. The exact cause of RLS is not known, but RLS appears to be linked with iron metabolism in the brain. Checking for low iron levels with a blood test, and replacing iron when low, can improve symptoms. Decreasing the intake of caffeine, nicotine, and alcohol, massaging your legs, and taking warm baths before bedtime may decrease RLS symptoms. When these interventions fail, medications to treat RLS symptoms are available.

In summary, sleep problems, such as insomnia, sleep apnea, and RLS, are common in individuals with MS. These sleep problems may be troublesome on their own and may contribute to daytime fatigue, poorer quality of life, and may be associated with greater disability. Fortunately, treatments are available for the most common sleep problems, so if you have poor quality, unrefreshing sleep, it is important that you discuss your symptoms with your provider. Good sleep practices, such as keeping a regular bedtime and wake time, protecting your sleep time from other activities, setting up your bedroom only for sleep, and limiting caffeinated beverages, can also help. While symptoms may not completely resolve with treatment, substantial improvements in daytime functioning and an improved sense of well-being are possible.

Chapter 42

Stress and Multiple Sclerosis

Having multiple sclerosis (MS) can be incredibly stressful. Symptoms are unpredictable and can make it difficult to work, raise a family, or socialize; medications are expensive and come with a host of side effects. Many people report that stress aggravates their MS, and recent research confirms a connection between stress and worsening neurological symptoms. Thus, stress management is an essential component of a comprehensive MS treatment plan. Many of the stressful situations we experience cannot be immediately changed. If you cannot remove a specific stressor in your life, then the next best thing is to change your relationship to it, and meditation is one way to accomplish this.

What Is Meditation?

Meditation is a mental exercise. It is common for people to think that meditation is about "clearing your mind" or creating a "blank mental slate," but this is not accurate. Meditation is actually a process of getting to know your mind. There are many different types of

---

This chapter contains text excerpted from the following sources: Text in this chapter begins with excerpts from "VA Multiple Sclerosis Centers of Excellence— My 70 Years Living with MS," U.S. Department of Veterans Affairs (VA), 2015. Reviewed March 2019; Text beginning with the heading "Being Mindful of the Present Moment" is excerpted from "VA Multiple Sclerosis Centers of Excellence—A Second Generation Veteran with MS," U.S. Department of Veterans Affairs (VA), 2012. Reviewed March 2019.

meditation. Some forms encourage participants to focus their attention on the breath, other forms suggest participants focus on a word or phrase that is repeated over and over, and still other types of meditation teach that the focus should be on one's internal experience, including thoughts, feelings, and sensations.

While specific techniques may vary from one type to another, all meditative practices help cultivate self-observation, awareness, concentration, emotional regulation, and an attitude of acceptance. By practicing meditation, you can learn the patterns and habits of your mind, and then find new ways of approaching stressful life events that can lead to more satisfying and healthy experiences.

What Can Meditation Do for Me?

Regardless of the type of meditation, the general practice of focusing attention inward can induce changes in neural, immune, and endocrine function that lead to increased relaxation and improved physical and mental well-being. While research has yet to fully demonstrate how meditation effects change, studies have shown meditation can improve common MS symptoms, including fatigue, pain, sleep disturbance, depression, anxiety, and stress. More than just symptom management, meditation practice can empower participants by enhancing self-esteem, improving coping strategies, imparting a sense of control, and improving overall quality of life (QOL).

Meditation is a skill that must be practiced; the more you do it, the better the results. Like a muscle that needs exercise to become stronger, setting aside a few minutes each day to focus your attention will allow you to more readily access the physical and emotional benefits. Regular meditative practice will strengthen the neural connections associated with relaxation and emotional regulation, and with practice, you can access these connections in your day-to-day encounters with brief "meditative moments." Just a few focused breaths or a brief mindful reflection can create space between a stressful encounter and a habitual response, allowing your physiology (the way living things or any of their parts function) to shift and providing you more time for thoughtful action in a way that will help manage stress.

How Can I Get Started?

The demands of daily life are unlikely to disappear, but your response to these demands can change and that will, in turn, have a positive effect on your physiology. Commit to caring for yourself by making your stress-management plan as high a priority as taking your medications or nutritional supplements. There are many different ways to get started: The Mindful Awareness Research Center (MARC) at University of California, Los Angeles (UCLA) has a wonderful website with many resources, including free guided meditations, as well as more in-depth online courses in meditation. Check out www.headspace.com, this site provides free, daily, 10-minute guided sessions that you can listen to whenever it is convenient (they even have a free app for your smartphone). Consider reading *Full Catastrophe Living* by Jon Kabat-Zinn, Ph.D., or listen to his audiobook series entitled *Guided Mindfulness Meditation*. Find a local mindfulness-based stress reduction class, and join others as they learn how to focus attention inward. The books *Mindsight* and *The Mindful Brain* by Dan Siegel, MD, describe the neurobiological effects of meditative practice and how these effects improve health and wellbeing. There are many, many resources out there, so enjoy the exploratory process of finding a method that works for you, and start crafting your own meditative practice today.

Being Mindful of the Present Moment

Recently, classes teaching mindfulness have received a great deal of attention in healthcare. This upsurge in interest has been fueled by multiple studies showing that becoming more mindful (being more aware of what is happening in your life, thoughts, and emotions in the present moment) results in lower stress and a greater sense of well-being.

Mindfulness has been defined in the *Journal of Alternative and Complementary Medicine* as, the awareness that emerges, by way of paying attention, on purpose, in the present moment, and nonjudgmentally, to the unfolding of experience moment by moment. When this definition is examined, a lot of information can be found about how mindfulness practice reduces feelings of stress.

The first phrase, the awareness that emerges, suggests that it is indeed possible to develop a greater understanding of ourselves, others, and life circumstances and that this will occur naturally.

The second phrase, by way of paying attention, reminds us that bringing attention to our experiences helps us to grow. We begin to realize that our thoughts come and go throughout the day and that these thoughts may or may not be true. Realizing that thoughts about oneself, others, or the future are not necessarily an accurate representation of reality, can help to reduce feelings of stress. For example, the thought "I would not be able to be happy because of my MS" can be seen as an idea or thought that may or may not be true.

The third phrase, on purpose, means that it takes a conscious effort and personal motivation to help bring about a shift in perspective.

The fourth phrase, in the present moment, refers to the ability to focus on what is happening in your life at this very instant. Getting distracted by thoughts of events that occurred in the past, or carried away by worries or ideas about the future, can stand in the way of living fully in the present moment. For example, research shows that ruminating (turning things over and over in your mind) is a key factor in the relapse of depression. Learning how to let go of these cycles of rumination is an important part of mindfulness.

The fifth phrase, nonjudgmentally, refers to a noncritical, kind attitude toward experience. This nonjudgmental attitude means having an openness to all experiences, including experiences we might not choose, such as painful thoughts or feelings. This is not to be confused with being passive.

Rather, it is based on the observation that what is here, is here.

For example, if we are experiencing feelings of sadness or grief, judging yourself for having those feelings will not help the situation. Although at times, we can distract ourselves from unpleasant feelings by doing something else, in the long run, personal growth is facilitated by "staying with" a feeling and having an attitude of openness and nonjudgment. Staying with experience and having an attitude of kindness and curiosity allows us to have greater insight into our values and motivations. What makes this process easier is learning to recognize and let go of added layers of self-criticism which promotes acceptance of oneself. When a person learns to regard oneself with less judgment, this often has the effect of spilling over to others, who are then viewed with less judgment.

The sixth phrase, unfolding of experience, moment by moment, indicates that our thoughts, emotions, and life experiences are always in a state of flux. Our experiences can change gradually and change may not be so obvious, or change can be quite abrupt and very obvious. Mindfulness practice helps a person to recognize the fact that experiences are changing or "unfolding," and acceptance and recognition of change help us to adopt a realistic mindset and openness to these new experiences.

Combining the above factors helps to bring about a shift in perspective, allows an increased focus on the moment, and often reduces identification with the inner dialogue we have in our minds. The shift in perspective is one of greeting life's experience with an attitude of openness, friendliness, and with an eye toward gaining an added understanding of what is going on. This shift can lead to an enhanced quality of life, decreased stress, better coping mechanisms, improved sleep, diminished risk of depression, and possible reduced need for pain medications.

How Is Mindfulness Taught?

Mindfulness is usually taught through classes that teach mindfulness meditation. Meditation is a broad term used to describe exercises that develop skills in paying attention.

Chapter 43

Dysphagia (Swallowing Problems)

Dysphagia, which literally means "difficulty swallowing," is a condition in which people have trouble passing foods or liquids from their mouth to their digestive system. The process of swallowing involves four stages. The brain controls this process through nerves that connect to the mouth, throat, esophagus, and stomach. Dysphagia can result from problems occurring in any of the four stages.

In the oral stage, food is placed in the mouth, where it is moistened by saliva, broken down by chewing, and pushed back toward the throat by the tongue. In the pharyngeal phase, food enters the throat (pharynx). The voice box (larynx) closes briefly to prevent food from entering the airway and lungs, and then the food passes down the throat and into the esophagus. In the esophageal stage, food is pushed downward through the esophagus by wave-like muscle contractions known as "peristalsis." Finally, the food passes into the stomach through the lower esophageal sphincter, a band of muscle that relaxes to allow food to enter and tightens to prevent stomach contents from moving back upward into the esophagus.

"Dysphagia (Swallowing Problems)," © 2017 Omnigraphics. Reviewed March 2019.

Causes of Dysphagia

Swallowing difficulties have many possible causes, including the following:

- Cleft lip, cleft palate, or other problems with craniofacial development
- Dental problems
- Large tongue
- Large tonsils
- Tumors, masses, or congenital abnormalities in the throat
- Foreign objects in the esophagus
- Gastrointestinal problems that irritate or damage the esophagus, such as acid reflux
- Malformations of the digestive tract, such as esophageal atresia or tracheoesophageal fistula
- Compression of the esophagus by enlarged thyroid gland, lymph nodes, or blood vessels
- Premature birth or low birth weight
- Autism or other developmental delays
- Nervous system disorders, such as cerebral palsy
- Diseases or injuries that affect the nerves and muscles of the face and neck, such as stroke, brain injury, or muscular dystrophy
- Respiratory problems
- Tracheostomy
- Oral sensitivity or irritation of the airway from prolonged use of a ventilator
- Vocal cord paralysis
- Certain medications that decrease appetite
- Dysfunctional parent-child interaction at mealtimes

Symptoms of Dysphagia

Swallowing difficulties manifest themselves in many ways, some of which may not be obvious or may mimic other medical conditions.

Some of the more common symptoms of dysphagia include the following:

- Eating very slowly
- Chewing with difficulty
- Attempting to swallow a mouthful of food several times
- Feeling as if food becomes stuck in the throat
- Trouble coordinating breathing and swallowing
- Frequent coughing, gagging, or choking during meals
- Frequent spitting up or vomiting
- Drooling
- Stuffy nose at mealtime, or food or liquid coming out of the nose
- Hoarse, raspy, or gurgling voice during or after meals
- Chest congestion after eating, or recurring respiratory infections
- Weight loss, or less than normal weight gain and growth
- Aversion to certain textures of food
- Arching the back or stiffening while feeding
- Irritability or lack of alertness while feeding

Diagnosis of Dysphagia

The medical professional that is most often involved in diagnosing swallowing difficulties is a speech-language pathologist (SLP). The SLP may consult with a team that also includes a physician or pediatrician, a dietician or nutritionist, and a physical or occupational therapist. The team will ask about the patient's medical history, including the development of the condition, symptoms experienced, and overall health. They may also evaluate the patient's posture and behavior while eating, as well as their oral movements and the strength of muscles involved in chewing and swallowing. As needed, various tests and imaging studies may be performed to further analyze the actions of the mouth, throat, and esophagus. Some of the possible tests used to diagnose dysphagia include the following:

- **Modified Barium Swallow Study (MBSS)**—The patient consumes a small amount of a liquid containing barium, a metallic chemical that shows up well on X-rays. A series of X-rays are taken as the barium moves through the throat and esophagus, providing the SLP with valuable information about the source of swallowing difficulties.

- **Fiberoptic Endoscopic Evaluation of Swallowing (FEES)**—A small, flexible tube with a tiny camera on the end is inserted through the patient's nose to provide an internal view of the throat. The patient then consumes several varieties of solid and liquid foods while the SLP observes the function of the throat, vocal cords, and larynx.

- **Laryngoscopy**—With the patient under anesthesia, the doctor uses a small tube with a light on the end to examine the patient's throat and larynx for abnormalities or narrow areas.

- **Gastroesophageal endoscopy**—With the patient under anesthesia, the doctor inserts a small tube with a camera on the end into the patient's mouth. The tube is gently threaded through the throat and esophagus and into the stomach, and the camera captures images of the internal structures. If the doctor notices any abnormalities, the endoscope can be used to take a tissue sample.

- **Esophageal manometry**—A small tube containing a pressure gauge is inserted through the mouth and into the esophagus, where it measures the pressure. This test is used to evaluate the effectiveness of the esophagus in moving food downward to the stomach.

- **Gastrointestinal reflux testing**—Tiny probes are inserted into the patient's esophagus or stomach to measure the amount of acid present. The pH probes are used to analyze whether acid reflux may contribute to throat irritation and swallowing problems.

Treatment of Dysphagia

Based on the results of the physical examination and special tests, the medical team will recommend a course of treatment for the patient's swallowing difficulties. The treatment depends on the extent and underlying cause of the dysphagia, as well as the patient's overall health. Some of the possible forms of treatment include the following:

- Nutritional changes, including different types, tastes, textures, and temperatures of foods

- Thickening liquids to make them easier to swallow
- Medications to treat acid reflux
- Behavioral interventions
- Posture or positioning changes
- Exercises recommended by an SLP to improve chewing or sucking, strengthen muscles in the mouth, and increase tongue movement
- Referral to a dentist or craniofacial surgeon
- Surgical procedures to widen the esophagus or keep food and acid in the stomach

Prognosis

Dysphagia in children can result in dehydration, poor nutrition, and a failure to gain weight or grow properly. In addition, they may develop aversion to certain foods or liquids, embarrassment in social situations involving eating, or behavioral resistance to eating. Dysphagia can also result in aspiration of food into the trachea and lungs. Aspiration can create a choking hazard, and it also increases the risk of respiratory infections, pneumonia, and chronic lung disease. Medical treatment can help many children with dysphagia learn to swallow more effectively so that they can eat and drink with minimal difficulty. Some patients may not experience much improvement, however, especially those with health issues that affect the nerves and muscles.

References

1. "Difficulty Swallowing (Dysphagia)—Overview," WebMD, 2016.

2. "Dysphagia," Ann and Robert H. Lurie Children's Hospital of Chicago, 2016.

3. "Feeding and Swallowing Disorders (Dysphagia) in Children," American Speech-Language-Hearing Association (ASHA), 2016.

4. "Swallowing Problems (Dysphagia)," Stanford Children's Health, 2016.

Chapter 44

Speaking and Thinking Problems

Individuals with multiple sclerosis (MS) experience a wide variety of symptoms, which may impact speech or cognition. Speech-language pathologists, often called "SLPs," can evaluate and provide treatment options, should difficulties in these areas become problematic.

Speaking

Just as the muscles involved in swallowing can be impacted by MS, the muscles involved in speaking can too. Speech difficulties, called "dysarthria," are relatively common for people with MS, with about 40 to 50 percent of individuals reporting changes in their communication. Speech difficulties might include slurred-sounding speech, increased fatigue with conversation, or reduced vocal loudness. This is often mild, and may not impact overall intelligibility or successful communication, but can be of concern to the individual. Some general strategies to support effective communication include:

- Breath support and diaphragmatic or "belly" breathing

This chapter includes text excerpted from "VA Multiple Sclerosis Centers of Excellence—The Brighter Side of Life," U.S. Department of Veterans Affairs (VA), 2016.

- Increased speaking loudness

- Reduced speech rate

- Exaggerated articulation of each sound

In more severe cases of MS, speech supplementation or speech-generating devices might be necessary. When dysarthria interferes with safety, functional communication of daily needs/desires, or general quality of life (QOL), both low-tech and high-tech devices may be useful. Low-tech devices include alphabet and eye gaze boards, pictures, notebooks, or whiteboards, bells and buzzers, and simple yes/no systems. High-tech alternatives include voice amplifiers, text-to-speech devices, and applications ("apps") that can be found on smartphones and tablets. Some apps to assist with communication include Proloquo2Go, LAMP, Speak for Yourself, and SmallTalk.

If recommended, there are more complex, computer-based devices available, called "speech-generating devices." These devices have a variety of modes of access dependent upon physical abilities that may include communicating via joystick, mouse, or eye gaze technology. Tobii, Dynavox, GoTalk, and Tango might be familiar with brand names. It is important to work with a knowledgeable professional to determine the best-suited complex, computer-based device, as indicated.

Thinking

Cognition is a fancy word to refer to thinking processes, such as attention, memory, and learning, or executive functions (planning, organizing, goal setting, and time management). Some individuals with MS report changes in cognition which may include:

- Increased reliance on organizational systems, such as day planners, smartphones, or alarms

- More difficulty making decisions

- Reduced ease of remembering names, places, conversations, or recent events

- More difficulty multitasking, tuning out distractions or focusing for a long period of time

- Problems with word-finding

- Slowed information processing

Typically, these changes do not impact an individual's overall ability to function independently but may require more support and strategies, including the use of sticky notes, maps or GPS devices, day planners or smartphones, or requests for repetition or for written information. General recommendations to support cognition include:

- Focus on one task at a time.

- Reduce distractions.

- Write it down.

- Actively listen: request slower speed, repetition, and clarification as needed.

- Use calendars, day planners, computers/tablets, or smartphones to keep track of appointments and for planning/prioritization.

- Use word-finding strategies: Describe the word, think of the first letter or sound of the word, use a similar word, or use gestures.

- Keep your mind active and engaged with work, games, social activities, reading, playing music, or physical exercise.

- Eat well, get enough sleep, and practice basic healthy habits.

If an individual with MS experiences difficulty or concern about issues related to speaking, eating and drinking, or thinking, consider a visit to a speech-language pathologist who may assist you with providing more information, strategies, or possibly therapy to support cognitive, communication, and swallowing issues.

Chapter 45

Bladder Problems
Tied to Falls in
Multiple Sclerosis

Does Your Multiple Sclerosis Affect Your Bladder? Do You Fall Because of Your Multiple Sclerosis?

It's known that falls and bladder symptoms are common in people with multiple sclerosis (MS). More than 50 percent of people with MS fall in a 3- to 6-month period, and about 75 percent or more have problems with their bladder.

Recently published research by Dr. Michelle Cameron, a neurologist at U.S. Department of Veteran Affairs (VA) Portland Healthcare System, VA MS Center of Excellence-West, found that in people with MS, urinary urgency (a sudden, compelling urge to urinate) with incontinence (involuntary leakage of urine) was associated with a significantly increased risk of falling multiple times in a 3-month period. In fact, in this study, people who had both urinary urgency and incontinence had almost a 60 times greater odds of recurrent falls compared to those who did not have these bladder symptoms.

This chapter includes text excerpted from "VA Multiple Sclerosis Centers of Excellence—Finding the Strength to Fight Back," U.S. Department of Veterans Affairs (VA), 2017.

287

Interestingly, those people who only had urinary urgency or urinary frequency, but not incontinence, were not at increased risk for multiple falls. And, no bladder symptoms were associated with an increased risk of just falling once.

Participants in this study had to meet certain criteria, including a confirmed diagnosis of MS, mild-to-moderate disability due to MS, no relapse within 30 days of the study start date, and be between the ages of 18 and 50, to minimize the cause of falls being something other than MS. In addition, participants were excluded if they had balance or walking issues because of a condition other than MS, or if they could not walk at least 100 meters. In this study, a fall was defined as "an unexpected event that results in ending up on the ground, floor, or any lower surface." Of the 51 study participants, 32 people fell at least once in 3 months, and 15 people fell at least twice in 3 months.

The findings of this study are important and useful because the reasons for why people with MS fall, or how to best help prevent them from falling so much were not found. Many treatments to prevent falls in people with MS have been tried. Most of these consist of a combination of safety education and balance exercises. Although these may be helpful, they certainly don't fix the whole problem. They increase knowledge and improve people's balance, but they don't prevent all falls. Many of the reasons people with MS fall, such as weakness or numbness, cannot be fixed completely or easily. Finding out that something, such as urinary incontinence, which can often be treated easily and effectively with medications, may help prevent falls is, therefore, particularly encouraging. This study suggests that improved bladder management may be able to reduce the risk of falls in people with MS.

It is not clear why people with MS who have urinary urgency with incontinence tend to fall more. Although it is possible that they just have worse MS, this is not likely. In Dr. Cameron's study, statistical tests showed that the relationship between bladder symptoms and falls was not affected by how severe the person's MS was. So, the researchers thought that bladder problems might cause falls in people with MS because, if you have urinary urgency and incontinence, you are likely to often rush to the bathroom, not paying as much attention to your safety when walking or transferring. It is also possible that people with bladder problems avoid drinking water and become dehydrated, which can then make them dizzy when walking.

How Can Knowing That Bladder Problems and Falls Be Connected Help You?

If your MS affects your bladder, and you have frequent falls or near falls, tell your provider about it. Treatment for your bladder might not only help resolve or improve your bladder problems, but it might also help prevent you from falling.

Chapter 46

Maintaining Intimacy and Sexuality If You Have Multiple Sclerosis

Sexual arousal begins in the brain. The brain sends messages to the sexual organs along the nerve pathway in the spinal cord. Multiple sclerosis (MS)-related damage to these nerve pathways can directly or indirectly impair sexual functioning. Nerve damage can contribute to diminished sexual response and feelings. MS symptoms can get in the way of sexual initiation or satisfaction. Symptoms of fatigue can be the biggest culprit or spasms that seem to be worse at night or when lying down. Weakness contributes to exhaustion and maybe a limiting factor in initiating sexual activity.

Sexual dysfunction is a common symptom that affects more than 75 percent of people living with MS, more often than in people with other chronic diseases. Sexual dysfunction can present itself in many

This chapter contains text excerpted from the following sources: Text in this chapter begins with excerpts from "VA Multiple Sclerosis Center of Excellence— Life Is What You Make It," U.S. Department of Veterans Affairs (VA), 2018; Text under the heading "How Does Multiple Sclerosis Affect Sexuality?" is excerpted from "VA Multiple Sclerosis Center of Excellence—My Anger with MS," U.S. Department of Veterans Affairs (VA), 2008. Reviewed March 2019; Text under the heading "Sexual Dysfunction Management" is excerpted from "Sexual Dysfunction and Multiple Sclerosis," U.S. Department of Veterans Affairs (VA), August 3, 2018.

ways, as it limits your ability to be sexual with your partner, to behave as a sexual being, and to benefit from this way of expressing love and intimacy. The ability to be a sexual person is not lost because you live with MS; although, you may need to learn new ways to be sexual and accept things that are not in your control. Intimacy is a feeling of belonging to another, involves trust, and is both an emotional and physical sharing of one's most personal nature. Your MS does not need to interfere with your ability to be intimate. Recognition of sexual dysfunction can help people with MS understand the problem, find treatment, build healthier relationships, enhance self-esteem, reduce depression, and improve quality of life.

Women

For women, low desire or no desire is usually the first and foremost problem. Physical changes include lack of lubrication (dryness), genital numbness, decreased vaginal tone, and pain during intercourse. Body image is important to women, as are acceptance and personal security. Women rate affection and emotional communication as more important than orgasm. For women, a sexual partner who is tender and romantic, with touching, kissing, caressing and extended foreplay, is often ideal. Communication, honesty, warmth, and understanding are important for women.

Gentlemen

For men, sexual problems may occur with erections and ejaculation. Men often desire sexual partners who do not make demands and appreciate partners who are reassuring and supportive, without pressure regarding erections or performance. Men also want to feel secure in the relationship and share affection. The first step in managing sexual dysfunction in MS is accepting that it is a common symptom that should, and can, be addressed. Sexual dysfunction not only impacts the quality of life, but it can contribute to relationship conflict, depression, isolation, performance anxiety, and fear of intimate relationships and sexual encounters.

Talk to your provider about your symptoms and what can be done to help. Physical and occupational therapists can help with positioning, techniques and "tools," while a mental-health professional can help you address emotional issues that may be hindering intimacy. Men who experience erectile dysfunction should talk to their provider about the many medications in both pill and injectable form that can help. Before buying performance supplements, you should discuss the ingredients with your provider, so they can advise you if they are safe with your other medicines and any other medical conditions you may have. For example, yohimbine, a herbal supplement advertised to promote sexual function, may be dangerous to your liver, especially when taking some MS disease-modifying treatments.

Manage other MS symptoms that might get in the way of sexual satisfaction. If spasticity is a problem, time sexual activity between one and four hours after taking baclofen. If fatigue is a problem, take advantage of morning sex, which may be your time of peak energy. If you experience weakness, consider different positions to conserve energy and consider using supports (wedge, pillow, support chair) to reduce strain or pressure on your body. Lack of bladder or bowel control can be addressed by using the lavatory immediately before sex.

Genital stimulators can help compensate for decreased sensitivity. Know that alcohol, nicotine, some medications, and even some foods may diminish your sexual response. Intimacy and closeness are important to your life satisfaction. Intimacy can be scary, even more so with fears around performance, rejection, failing to satisfy, and fear that MS symptoms will spoil a sexual encounter. Having an open and honest conversation with your partner about your fears is a good start to fueling greater intimacy. Have realistic expectations. Focus on the process rather than the goal. Plan a date night. Enjoy intimate times, such as holding hands and making eye contact. Create romance. Light candles. Play music from your most romantic days. Touch yourself and your partner all over to discover what body mapping is all about. Engage in activities that have nothing to do with MS. You are a sexual being. Having love and intimacy is a basic human need. Sex is an important aspect of love and intimacy. Be open to making changes to improve your sexual functioning. Talk to your provider and MS team about your sexual concerns. They can refer you to resources that will help.

How Does Multiple Sclerosis Affect Sexuality?

The ways in which MS can affect sexuality and expressions of intimacy can be divided into primary, secondary, and tertiary sexual dysfunction.

Primary sexual dysfunction stems directly from MS-related changes in the brain and spinal cord that affect the sexual response or the ability to feel sexual pleasure. In both men and women, this can include a decrease or loss of sex drive, decreased or unpleasant genital sensations, and a diminished capacity for orgasm. Men may experience difficulty achieving or maintaining an erection and a decrease in or loss of ejaculatory force or frequency. Women may experience decreased vaginal lubrication, loss of vaginal muscle tone, and/or diminished clitoral engorgement.

Secondary sexual dysfunction stems from MS-related symptoms that do not directly involve nerve pathways to the genital system but nevertheless impair sexual pleasure or the sexual response. Secondary symptoms may include three bladder and bowel problems, fatigue, spasticity, muscle weakness, body or hand tremors, impairments in attention and concentration and nongenital sensory changes.

Tertiary sexual dysfunction results from disability-related psychosocial and cultural issues that can interfere with one's sexual feelings and experiences. For example, some people find it difficult to reconcile the idea of being disabled with being fully sexually expressive. Changes in self-esteem (including the way one feels about one's body), depression, demoralization, or mood swings can all interfere with intimacy and sexuality. The sexual partnership can be severely challenged by changes within a relationship, such as one person becoming the other person's caregiver. Similarly, changes in employment status or role performance within the household are often associated with emotional adjustments that can temporarily interfere with sexual expression. The strain of coping with MS challenges a couple's efforts to communicate openly about their respective experiences and their changing needs for sexual expression and fulfillment.

Communication with an MS healthcare provider on aggressive symptom management with sexual health in mind can be helpful in restoring sexual function. Although treatment of these symptoms frequently eases associated sexual complaints, it is necessary for the MS healthcare provider to know that sexual function is an ongoing concern. For example, some antidepressant medications have excellent efficacy in treating symptoms of depression, but can also cause impairments in libido and capacity for orgasm. If the person with MS and the healthcare provider have had an open dialogue about sexual function, appropriate medications and/or dosing strategies can be implemented to minimize or eliminate the sexual side effects.

In coping with sexual dysfunction, it is very important to include the sex partner in the discussion when a long-term relationship is present. This enhances intimacy by allowing both partners to learn and explore together. If partners feel inhibited about talking through these issues, counseling with a mental health professional who is knowledgeable about MS can prove to be helpful.

Sexual Dysfunction Management

The first step in the management of sexual dysfunction is to acknowledge that sexual dysfunction is a significant healthcare problem that most people with MS face at some point in their lives. It is also important to realize that sexual dysfunction is a subject that often goes underrecognized and undertreated. The second step is to talk about your sexual dysfunction concerns with your healthcare provider. Physical therapists can address positioning techniques that enhance sexual comfort. Clinical psychologists can work with individuals or couples in promoting sexually sensitive communication to enhance sexual performance. Occupational therapists can instruct people in the use of sexual devices that can enhance sexual pleasure. Additional sexual dysfunction treatments may include:

- Medical sex education materials

- Oral medications (Viagra-sildenafil, Levitra-vardenafil, Cialis-tadalafil)

- Topical hormones

- Sex therapy (body mapping other than genitals)

- Counseling

- Provision of sexual devices (vibrators, lubricants)

- Intracorporeal injection of medication into the penis

- Noninvasive physical treatments for erectile dysfunction (vacuum tumescence penis pumps)

- Surgery for erectile dysfunction (implantation of inflatable or semi-rigid rods)

Sexual dysfunction is a very prevalent problem in the MS population. It is a complex and dynamic interaction of physical, psychological, social, cognitive, and practical factors (financial). The person with MS, the healthcare team and the healthcare community must work together to reduce sexual dysfunction if we hope to improve the quality of life for all people living with MS.

Chapter 47

Driving with Multiple Sclerosis

Multiple sclerosis (MS) can affect the ability to perform activities of daily living. Driving is the most complex activity of daily living performed every day. It is important not to minimize the complexities of driving or overestimate one's abilities. Driving requires adequate vision, motor, memory, and thinking skills. MS can affect all these areas. As MS evolves, required driving skills may diminish in several domains:

- Blurred vision; poor nighttime vision; blind spots; double vision; loss of color vision; impaired visual searching, scanning, and attention

- Short-term memory loss; confusion about vehicle operation or one's location or destination; stress tolerance; impaired motor planning, multitasking, and reaction time, fatigue, and heat intolerance

- The impaired sensorimotor function may manifest as difficulty with car transfers, muscle weakness or stiffness/spasms/cramps, poor light touch and joint position sensation, pain and impaired coordination (particularly in the arms or right foot)

This chapter includes text excerpted from "VA Multiple Sclerosis Centers of Excellence—I Am Not My MS," U.S. Department of Veterans Affairs (VA), 2014. Reviewed March 2019.

297

A cardinal feature of MS is its unpredictability. Symptoms often fluctuate during the course of a day and from day to day. Most people with MS have a relapsing course, and during exacerbations (attacks, relapses, or flareups), driving may be unsafe but may return to normal upon recovery. However, with disease progression, driving can become permanently affected.

If you, your loved ones, or your healthcare provider are concerned about your driving ability, a driving evaluation performed by a driver rehabilitation specialist can help identify challenges you experience and the need for appropriate adaptive auto equipment to keep you safe on the road.

The purpose of a driving evaluation is to assess driving skills, recommend adapted auto equipment if indicated to meet specific functional needs and train the driver and family in its use, ensuring the safety of entering/exiting the vehicle, and proper storage of wheelchair, and assistive devices. It is best to consult a driver rehabilitation specialist before you buy a vehicle, as they can help you decide what vehicle best meets your needs.

Keen awareness of the fluctuating nature of MS symptoms can help you avoid the risk of unsafe driving. Here are some tips:

- Don't drive if you are having a bad day.

- Avoid driving when you have another illness because MS symptoms are often worse when the "system" is under increased stress.

- Keep trips short if you suffer from fatigue, and don't drive when fatigue is severe.

- Avoid distractions, such as cell phone calls/texting, eating, listening to the radio, and arguing with passengers.

- If you are heat intolerant, carry a cooling vest.

- Strategically plan out errands and appointments so that you can avert heavy traffic times or areas that get congested.

- Avoid driving in bad weather.

What If You Decide to Stop Driving or Are Told It Is No Longer Safe to Drive?

Just as you plan for other circumstances associated with your disease (e.g., making your home more accessible), planning for the day when driving becomes impossible can ease the transition from driver to passenger. When transitioning from driver to passenger, explore transportation options in your community.

- Ask a friend, neighbor or family member if they could give you a ride.

- Inquire about volunteer drivers at your local community center or place of worship.

- Contact your city and state public transportation agencies about transportation options.

Driving can be seen as a sign of independence, and it can be scary to think about limiting or giving up that freedom. Professional evaluation and the use of adaptive auto equipment can increase your safety on the road and promote independence for as long as it's safe for you to drive. If you feel like you can no longer safely drive, there are a variety of transportation alternatives, and your family members, friends, and healthcare professionals are here to help and support you with this transition.

Change can be hard, and if you are having difficulty accepting or adjusting to changes in your ability to drive, you might consider talking with a healthcare provider. Talking about how you feel may help you better understand and address the grief felt over these changes.

Chapter 48

Dealing with Mobility Challenges: One Step at a Time

Mobility challenges can interfere with every aspect of everyday life. This can be true for people who are just beginning to experience difficulty with balance and walking, for those using walking aids, such as canes or walkers, and for those who use wheeled mobility to get around. Strategies to improve or maintain the ability to move around are certainly important. However, there are multiple other small changes people with multiple sclerosis (MS) can put into place that can have a big impact. This is one place where thinking small and taking it one step at a time can be effective.

How Do You Budget Your Energy?

A budget approach allows you to take charge of how you spend your energy and spend it on what matters most. Think about it in the same way as budgeting money. Begin by learning how to estimate the energy cost of different activities by noticing how tired you feel during and after those things that you do regularly. Keep in mind that fatigue is not just a result of spending physical energy. There can

This chapter includes text excerpted from "Meeting Mobility Challenges One Step at a Time," U.S. Department of Veterans Affairs (VA), August 3, 2018.

be cognitive and/or emotional energy costs that are just as important to consider.

Next, evaluate how much energy you have available. Then decide where you want to spend that energy—what activities do you consider to be the most essential, have the most value to you, or have a high priority for another reason? Consider if you can reduce energy costs by doing things in a different way (e.g., shopping online). Finally, you should plan your day or week so you spend your energy on the things that matter most to you. Be proactive, and decide what you want to drop, delegate to others, ask for help with, or move to another day or time to avoid "going in the red."

In MS, the amount of energy available can vary from day to day, or even within a day, for reasons that are not always obvious or predictable. Be prepared for these unexpected fluctuations by keeping some energy on reserve in your "energy bank" and having a backup plan that focuses on your highest priority activities.

How Do You Pace Yourself?

It can be tempting to rush to finish something before you get tired or to try to do just one more thing. However, with MS, it is critical to stop and rest before you start feeling tired. This may mean taking a "micro-break," stopping to sit for a few minutes before continuing with an activity, or scheduling a regular nap or quiet time into your day. This can be hard to do when you feel like you have enough energy to keep going. However, not taking a rest before feeling tired can backfire and make you more fatigued in the long run.

What's Your Position?

You can use less energy by positioning objects and materials so they're within easy reach. Store the objects you use most often in heights between your shoulders and knees to minimize reaching and bending. Taking care in how you position yourself in relation to what you are doing can also reduce energy expenditure. Use the support of furniture (e.g., armrests) when you can, and make sure you face the task directly. This uses less energy than working from a strained or awkward position. You can also sit on a chair or stool instead of standing to do some tasks. This includes tasks that are fairly quick, such as brushing your teeth in the morning, to those that take longer, such as washing the dishes. Put chairs or stools in those locations ahead of time to make it more likely that you will use them.

What Are Activity Stations?

Set up activity stations in your home to save steps and energy by putting the objects and materials used for a task together in one place. Activity stations can be for any routine task, such as getting dressed, making sandwiches, leaving the house, or washing the car. Start with something you do often. Get help as needed to move everything you use for that task to the place where it makes sense to do the bulk of the work. Then, identify the things in that area that are not needed. Move the unneeded objects to where they will be used, and either toss or give away the things you do not use on a regular basis. This approach can reduce not just your physical energy expenditure, but also how much thinking is needed and emotional stress.

How Can You Make Life Easier?

Slide objects along countertops instead of lifting and carrying, or use a utility cart to transport objects. Save steps by using a transitional "staging area" when moving multiple items from one location to another, such as when unloading the dishwasher or setting the table. Replace heavier objects and tools with ones that are more lightweight. Use tools and devices that increase leverage, such as a long-handled jar opener, or increase friction, such as a rubber gripper. Use electrical appliances and power tools stored within easy reach for both big and small jobs.

Is There Room to Get Around?

It can be surprising how quickly clutter can accumulate. Clutter makes it more difficult to move around and can also make it more difficult to think clearly. Clearing out clutter is one way to give you enough room to get around safely. Moving furniture and electrical and phone cords out of the way is also helpful. Aim for clear, wide pathways with enough space for you and your mobility aid to move forward, change direction, and turn freely. If a narrow doorway is getting in your way, widen it by installing offset hinges. Most hardware and home supply stores carry this inexpensive solution.

How Do You Keep Things "On the Level?"

Make walking and standing surfaces safe so there is nothing to trip over, slip on, or tip over. Flooring should be level with carpet edges that are taped or tacked down. Get rid of loose rugs. If that is not an option, anchor them securely to the floor with tacks or tape. Door thresholds should be low-level with the floor is best. If needed, a mini-threshold ramp can be installed.

How Sufficient Is Your Lighting?

The goal here is sufficient lighting without glare. Aim for even lighting within and between rooms. Turn on the lights before you go into a room. If there is not a light switch within reach, move a lamp close to the entry, or use night lights to make it easier to see where you are going. It is especially important to have enough lighting in areas such as entryways, hallways, and stairs and places where you might be navigating at night, such as the bathroom.

Do You Have Something to Hold Onto?

Adequate support can reduce the risk of falls. Install stair handrails on both sides of stairs so you can hold on while going up and coming down. Use heavier furniture without caster wheels so it will stay put when you sit down or stand up, or position it against a wall to keep it in place. Transfer poles that go between the floor and ceiling are another option when there is not a place for a grab bar.

Falls in the bathroom often result in injury. This is not surprising given the hard, slippery surfaces, frequent need to move quickly, low heights, need to step over fixtures, and the possibility of overheating. A raised toilet seat can make it easier to get up and down from the toilet, or an over-the-toilet commode chair can provide additional support. Grab bars can make it safer to use the toilet and tub or shower, while nonskid mats or decals in the tub or shower can make those floors less slippery. A shower chair or a bench that goes over the edge of the tub, along with a handheld shower nozzle, can make it possible to take a shower in a seated position when standing is riskier.

Will I Need a Major Remodel?

Many of the changes described here are relatively minor in scope and can be done with a "do-it-yourself" approach. However, when faced with major remodeling and decisions about permanent changes, people with MS have found it helpful to "expect the best and prepare for the worst." This avoids having to go back and make costly changes later. Avoid person-specific solutions when possible, and use universal design principles instead. These allow you to put solutions into place that work for everyone—you, your family, and guests in your home, as well as future buyers, should you decide to move.

How Do You Get Started?

Time, energy, physical, and financial challenges can make it difficult to know where to begin. For most people, making or reviewing an energy management budget is a good first step. Then, look at the changes that give you the "biggest bang for your buck," and put those in place with the help of family, friends, and others in your support network. If you need more assistance with knowing what's best for you or how to go about making changes, a referral to an occupational therapist for additional guidance and specific suggestions may be helpful. While mobility challenges can seem overwhelming, taking one step at a time can make a difference.

Chapter 49

Features of Home Accessibility

Our home is the place where we live, and it is filled with an abundance of memories. But, what happens when your home presents challenges to your safety and independence? While moving and purchasing another home is not always an option, a home safety evaluation may help.

A home safety evaluation is a process used to identify hazards that may affect your safety in the home. It provides recommendations for eliminating these hazards through the use of assistive devices and home repairs and modifications. The benefits of a home safety evaluation include increased use of the home, as well as safety, security, and independence for you. A home safety evaluation is often helpful for those who have experienced a fall in the home, have balance issues, or have observed a decrease in their physical mobility. It is also useful for those who have noticed changes in their cognition (memory, attention, making decisions) and sensory systems (vision, hearing, taste, smell). If you have experienced any of these issues, notify your provider. Your provider will assess your concerns, request a consultation

This chapter contains text excerpted from the following sources: Text in this chapter begins with excerpts from "VA Multiple Sclerosis Centers of Excellence—A Second Generation Veteran with MS," U.S. Department of Veterans Affairs (VA), 2012. Reviewed March 2019; Text under the heading "Evaluate Yourself and Your Home" is excerpted from "VA Multiple Sclerosis Centers of Excellence—Community Matters," U.S. Department of Veterans Affairs (VA), 2016.

for an evaluation, and possibly refer you to physical therapy for an assessment of balance and gait issues.

For a home evaluation, an occupational or physical therapist will come to your home to evaluate your needs and identify the strengths and weaknesses of your home. The therapist will assess the entrance to your home, as well as the hallways, staircases, living room, kitchen, and bathrooms for various hazards. These hazards may include inadequate lighting, lack of or unstable handrails and grab bars, unsafe steps, slippery or uneven flooring, inaccessible cabinets, slippery tubs, and high or low toilet seats. Following the evaluation, the therapist will provide recommendations to improve your safety in the home.

Evaluate Yourself and Your Home

If an occupational therapist completes an evaluation in your home, they will measure rooms and doorways for wheelchair accessibility and look for safety concerns, such as tripping hazards, lighting, emergency access, etc., they will also evaluate your ability to complete activities of daily living and help determine what is limiting your independence. You can plan for this home evaluation, as well as your next clinic appointment, by gathering information.

Make a table that lists each room in your home, and write down what difficulties you are having with completing activities of daily living in that room.

Table 49.1. Room and Their Difficulties

Room	I Feel Unsafe When... I Have Difficulty With... I Need Help With...	I Am Having Difficulty Because...
Bathroom	• Getting into the tub • Getting up from the toilet • Drying off after I shower	• My wheelchair will not fit through the doorway I get too tired

If your home has more than one level, list rooms separately for each level. Remember to include entrances, steps/stairways, parking, and your yard. In each of the rooms you are having trouble, also write down why you think you are having difficulties. Is it the layout of the furniture? Are there too many things in the room? Is there good enough lighting?

Make a Plan

Once you have figured out where you are having difficulties in your home, decide what is most important to work on first. Your safety should be the most important focus, followed by things that affect your symptoms the most, such as fatigue. There are many simple changes you can make to make your home more accessible. A major remodel should be the last option.

Follow the "4 Rs" to modify your home for safety and accessibility:

- **Reduce:** Eliminate duplicates—clothing you do not use or need; extra dishes, utensils, and pans in the kitchen; and unused or expired medications in the cabinet. Overfilled storage areas require more work, energy, and time to find what you need and too many items often overflow into living spaces and walkways creating safety hazards.

- **Reorganize:** Save energy by moving heavier items to lower shelves. Create pathways for safe walker or wheelchair use. Clear areas near light switches for easier reach.

- **Relocate:** In a multilevel home, consider whether you can rearrange rooms so you spend most of your day on the most accessible level of your home. Can you convert the main floor office to a bedroom, use a dining room as a multipurpose room by putting your computer there, or move a family member or attendant bedroom to the upper level?

- **Remodel:** Make home modifications before you actually need them to reduce safety concerns and your stress level. Remodeling may include adding ramps to entries, widening doorways, changing furniture heights, adding safety equipment to your bathroom, or using technology to operate your home with handsfree or voice-activated devices.

Chapter 50

Equipment That Promotes Self-Care, Mobility, and Independence

Chapter Contents

311

Section 50.1

Assistive Technology

This section includes text excerpted from "Multiple Sclerosis and Mobility-Related Assistive Technology: Systematic Review of Literature," Rehabilitation Research & Development Service (RR&D), U.S. Department of Veterans Affairs (VA), November 3, 2010. Reviewed March 2019.

Multiple sclerosis (MS), a neurodegenerative disorder of the central nervous system, currently affects approximately 400,000 U.S. residents, with 200 newly diagnosed individuals each week. MS causes a wide variety of neurological deficits, with ambulatory impairment as the most obvious cause of disability. Within 10 to 15 years of disease onset, 80 percent of persons with MS experience gait problems due to muscle weakness or spasticity, fatigue, and balance impairments. To facilitate mobility, persons with MS frequently employ mobility assistive technology (MAT), such as canes, crutches, walkers, wheelchairs, and scooters.

Matching the most appropriate MAT to the needs of a person with MS is vital to his or her daily mobility. Mobility impairments frequently restrict participation in work, family, social, vocational, and leisure activities. Furthermore, persons with MS often experience difficulties adapting to the changing and progressive nature of mobility loss, frequently marked by exacerbations and remissions. These difficulties can compound relatively high levels of emotional distress, which can exacerbate efforts to accommodate mobility with MAT. A 2008 survey of persons with MS found that 37 percent were too embarrassed to use MAT, while 36 percent reported that they do not use their MAT as much as they should.

In addition to standard MAT, new and emerging technologies are undergoing development that could accommodate mobility needs for persons with MS. More studies are exploring the consequences and patterns of MAT use among persons with MS. However, no recent review has examined the growing scientific evidence-based literature about MAT use in MS. It's aimed to systematically review the published literature concerning MAT use among persons with MS.

Multiple Sclerosis and Risk of Falling

Persons with MS are particularly predisposed to various impairments, including fatigue and falls, due to the brain and spinal cord involvement. In an observational survey study of 1,089 persons with MS between the ages of 45 and 90, Finlayson et al. reported that 52.2 percent of participants had experienced a fall in the past 6 months. Factors associated with an increased risk of falling included being male, having a fear of falling, a deteriorating MS status, balance problems or mobility limitations, and poor concentration. In addition, another survey study found that the absence of weight-bearing activities, an unsteady gait, and the use of a cane contributed to the multifactorial nature of falls among persons with MS. The common sequelae of falls include fractures, abrasions, lacerations, compromised mobility, loss of confidence in performing tasks, and a fear of falling. Therefore, assessment of different aspects of MS-related motor impairments and the accurate determination of factors contributing to falls are necessary for disease management and therapy and for the development of fall-prevention programs.

Multiple Sclerosis and Mobility through Ambulation

Understanding the experiences of mobility loss from the perspective of persons with MS may provide insight into the development of programs, services, and advocacy efforts that support people with MS as they age. These development efforts must consider several symptoms of MS that influence ambulation, such as loss of balance, weakness, fatigue, cognitive impairment, fear of falling, spasticity, tremor, and visual impairment. In addition, resistance to using appropriate MAT must also be addressed.

A literature review conducted by Noseworthy et al. found that even though MS causes a wide variety of neurological deficits, ambulatory impairment is the most common form of resulting disability. Within 15 years of onset, 50 percent of persons with MS will require assistance with walking. Therefore, most persons with MS will require some type of mobility assistance within the course of their disease progression. A survey study conducted in 2001 with 220 participants with MS found similar results to the Noseworthy et al. study, finding that the probability of participants walking 10 to 20 meters without assistance 15 years after diagnosis was 60.3 percent, while the probability of managing to walk a few steps without using a manual wheelchair as a backup was as high as 75.0 percent.

The researchers also found that the existence of motor symptoms and advanced age at disorder onset indicated more unfavorable outcomes, but these factors were associated with the progressive course of MS. Baum and Rothschild conducted an observational study with 1,145 persons with MS and found that approximately 51 percent of participants reported they needed help with personal mobility, both indoors and outdoors. Among study participants, 4 percent reported using crutches, 12 percent walkers, and 40 percent wheelchairs at least 13 years after their original diagnosis. A survey-based study conducted with 906 persons with MS also concluded that healthcare elements, such as being seen by an occupational therapist, and the type of MS were the strongest predictors of assistive technology (AT) acquisition.

Mobility Assistive Technology

When gait difficulties do not respond to therapeutic interventions, mobility assistive technology (MAT) devices may be useful tools to enhance mobility. Most persons with MS have mobility restrictions that require MAT devices. A study with 101 persons with MS indicated that their expectancy of becoming MAT users was as follows: 22.5 percent reported that they expected to be wheelchair-dependent in the short term (2 years), 38.7 percent in the intermediate (10 years), and 54.0 percent in the long term (more than 10 years). Provision of MAT for persons with MS can potentially diminish activity limitations and participation restrictions, prevent or reduce fatigue by energy conservation, and, ultimately, improve quality of life (QOL). MAT includes any device used to maintain or improve mobility. MAT is also designed to improve functioning, enable successful living at home and in the community, and enhance independence.

Therefore, a variety of assistive devices have been used by persons with MS:

1. **Ankle-foot orthoses (AFOs)** have been an effective solution for compensating weakness, restoring energy, and helping to control unstable knee and ankle musculature. AFOs are also used for foot drop, a condition in which the individual cannot clear his or her toes in the swing-through phase of mobility, which affects normal gait. AFOs can be made from composite materials or plastics with two different mechanisms: rigid or articulated. Recently, carbon-fiber AFOs have become popular among persons with MS.

2. **Functional electrical stimulation (FES),** which has been used for the treatment of muscles deprived of nervous control, provides muscle contraction and functional movement. For persons with MS, FES has been a useful tool for foot drop,

balance, and walking training during rehabilitation treatment; advanced technology has enabled a new system unit with wireless communication. However, the decision between an AFO and/or different models of FES is ultimately clinical and needs to be made by the potential user, physical therapist, and physician together.

3. **Hip flexion assist orthosis (HFAOs)** is another option for persons with MS who do not effectively ambulate, despite the use of an AFO or FES. The HFAO is indicated for persons with unilateral lower limb weakness in the hip and knee flexors along with the ankle and dorsiflexor muscles.

4. **Canes** assist ambulation by maintaining the even distribution of weight on the hips that is characteristic of a normal gait. Canes are also beneficial when walking is only mildly unstable, reducing walking effort and risk of falls when compared with AFOs and HFAOs.

5. **Crutches** are also used to aid with ambulation by helping with balance, widening the base of support, and decreasing weight bearing on a single lower limb. Crutches provide more balance than canes during walking; they are indicated for people who need bilateral support and have good upper limb control.

6. **Walkers and/or wheeled walkers (rollators)** are indicated for persons with moderate deficits and provide increased stability as a result of the walker's larger footprint when compared with a cane or crutches. In addition, they can be purchased with wheels, brakes, and modified hand grips to aid in function and safe use. Further, to assist with fatigue, some walkers are equipped with seats for short rest periods during ambulation.

7. **Manual wheelchairs** provide a more stable wheeled option, while still providing some level of physical activity. In addition, manual wheelchairs can be used part-time or as a primary exclusive mobility option for persons who are experiencing balance difficulties and frequent falls.

8. **Power-assist push-rim activated wheelchairs (PAPAWs)** are manual wheelchairs with a force/moment-sensing push rim, which provides assistance with wheelchair propulsion while requiring less physical strain. For people with MS, PAPAWs may prove to be a good compromise between the

fatigue caused by propelling among manual wheelchair users and the lack of exercise among power wheelchair users.

9. **Scooters** are a popular mode of powered mobility among persons with MS. Some users prefer a scooter to a manual wheelchair since upper limb fatigue is not an issue. However, scooters are often less desirable than power wheelchairs because of their lack of stability during turns and limited seating system options to accommodate users with specific seating needs, as seen in progressive disorders, such as MS.

10. **Power wheelchairs** should not only be considered a mobility option for advanced stages but should also be recommended as a MAT option to address fatigue, a hallmark symptom of MS. In contrast to scooters, power wheelchairs permit power seating system upgrades that may be indicated as the client progresses, and they are configured in different types of driving base designs. Three main power wheelchair base options are available: rear-wheel, mid-wheel, and front-wheel drives.

Among the various MAT options, manual wheelchairs (60%) have been reported as the most common MAT used by persons with MS, followed by canes and crutches (44%), walkers (39%), and power wheelchairs (8%). In an observational study, Baum and Rothschild have also shown that a greater number of persons use wheelchairs (40%) than walkers/canes (12%), leg braces (6%), and crutches (4%). In a recent retrospective study, manual wheelchairs (33%) were again the most prescribed devices, followed by power wheelchairs (13%), walkers (6%), braces (6%), and canes (2%). The use of wheelchairs has been positively correlated to the duration of the disease, age, and awareness of the diagnosis.

Mobility Assistive Technology Use and Service Delivery

In advanced stages of MS, several interventions can provide assistance with independence to the individual, such as provision, education, and instruction in use of assistive devices (walking aids, power/manual wheelchairs, and car adaptations); education and instruction about compensatory strategies to accomplish an activity (safe transfers); and environmental modifications (ramps, lifts, wider doors, level-access showers, bath aids, and environmental control systems). MAT must serve as an interface between the person with a disability and the activity the person chooses to perform and must promote reintegration into community life. Services models are used as guidelines to provide a comprehensive conceptual model representing factors to be considered in the design of an AT device or the development of a service delivery program that not only meets user needs but also is in accordance with policy regulations.

New and Emerging Mobility Assistive Technologies

In a research study, Sawatzky et al. investigated the use of the Segway® Personal Transporter device (Segway Inc; Bedford, New Hampshire), another powered mobility device for persons with limited ambulatory ability, such as people with MS or lower-limb amputations. Segway® devices are described as "the first self-balancing, electric-powered transportation devices." The rider stands on a small platform that is off the ground, supported by 2 parallel wheels, and holds onto the handle-bars. A twist grip on the left bar is used to steer the device. When the rider moves forward, the Segway® moves forward; when the rider leans back, it moves back or stops. The Segway® is marketed as a revolutionary device that requires no special skills and that "virtually anyone can use." In this particular study, the authors found that the Segway® was a useful device for a wide range of disabilities (e.g., MS, spinal cord injury (SCI), amputation), and it may also increase personal mobility for some people with functional limitations.

Therefore, it would enable people with functional limitations to become more involved in meaningful activities and, hence, increase their QOL. For persons with difficulty operating a mobility device because of decreased physical strength or environmental accessibility barriers, a new concept has been developed to accommodate those issues: the Independence iBOT 3000 mobility system (Independence Technology, Johnson and Johnson; New Brunswick, New Jersey). The iBOT was recently developed with the purpose of overcoming many of the limitations of currently available mobility devices.

The iBOT has a computer system designed to provide a dynamic balance reaction and has five different operating functions:

1. Standard (similar to a traditional power wheelchair)

2. Four-wheel (four-wheel drive for outdoor mobility, including curb climbing)

3. Balance (two-wheel drive, dynamically balanced on two wheels for mobility at the elevated height of a standing person)

4. Stair-climbing (rotation of the wheel clusters to allow "stepping up" one stair at a time)

5. Remote (nonoccupied mobility device)

Even though the iBOT is a good mobility option for persons with ambulatory impairment, it is an expensive device with funding unavailable by Medicare; hence, it is no longer available on the market.

Another option in power wheelchairs designed for indoor and outdoor use and stair climbing is called the "TopChair" (HMC2 Development; Toulouse-Montrabe, France). This power wheelchair is comprised of combined wheels and a caterpillar track. The TopChair was tested in France among 25 persons with SCI, and results showed that all participants were able to successfully operate the power wheelchair indoors and outdoors. Due to its electromechanical property and caterpillar tracks, the TopChair is a little bulkier and heavier than other power wheelchairs with similar functions. However, no studies have evaluated the benefits of the TopChair among persons with MS. Even though new technologies have been developed recently to enhance mobility and community participation, a clinician must consider many factors when trying to match a person with an assistive device. Using an assistive device for mobility could vary in two ways: full-time use or part-time use, depending on the level of disability and functional characteristics. Evaluating and understanding the pros and cons of each device, either with a new design and features or with a device already on the market, are vital when MATs are prescribed. The successful use of each MAT will be based on the interaction of knowledge of the disorder stage by the rehabilitation professional and willingness of the person with MS to accept and use what is suggested.

Section 50.2

Using Power Mobility Devices

This section includes text excerpted from "Power Mobility:
Is it Time for Wheels?" U.S. Department of Veterans
Affairs (VA), August 3, 2018.

Many individuals who have multiple sclerosis (MS) begin to have difficulty with their mobility as the disease progresses. Changes in vision, decreased balance, increased spasticity, muscle weakness, changes in sensation, or a combination of these symptoms can affect mobility. When a decline in lower extremity function occurs, individuals may benefit from assistive devices, such as braces, canes, crutches, walkers, wheeled walkers, and manual wheelchairs. But, when is it time to transition to a scooter or power wheelchair?

When Do You Use Power Mobility?

There are several factors that should be considered when transitioning to power mobility. The first is your current functional status. You may be experiencing an increase in problems with your balance, near or actual falls because of muscle weakness and fatigue or other symptoms. You may also be having more difficulty completing self-care tasks and instrumental activities of daily living (home management, shopping, cooking, etc.) due to the additional effort it is taking to move around, keep your balance, and use assistive devices, such as a walker or manual wheelchair.

Generalized fatigue, impaired fine motor function, and visual changes from the fatigue effect at least two-thirds of individuals with multiple sclerosis (MS) and, also contribute to limitations in daily activities. While medications are available to combat primary fatigue in MS, many times, secondary fatigue can be effectively managed by activity modification, energy conservation, balancing work and rest, and use of adaptive equipment. The goal of using power mobility is to maximize access to your home and the community, maintain safety, and conserve energy. Power mobility is an effective tool to reduce fatigue during daily activities by limiting the need for standing, reducing walking distances, and providing a method for "mobile" rest breaks during the day.

How Do You Choose the Appropriate Power Mobility Device?

An individual assessment of mobility and function by an occupational or physical therapist will identify problem areas and lead to a stepwise intervention. The optimal outcome is a good match between your mobility needs and the power mobility device. The initial power mobility choice to be made is usually between a power scooter and a power wheelchair; selection between these two devices is based on your home environment, your functional status, and available transportation for the device.

It is very important to choose the best power mobility device to keep you as independent as possible in daily activities and assist with management of your symptoms, rather than a device that can be transported in any vehicle. With many advances in the design of power mobility devices and the large selection available, most of the time, both the goals of remaining independent and transporting your device can be met.

What Are Power Scooters?

Individuals often use a scooter for the first time at the local grocery or retail store. Scooters are three- or four-wheel power mobility devices that steer like a bicycle using the tiller and are operated with both hands (either fingers or thumbs) controlling the forward and reverse levers. Scooters are intended for part-time use during the day despite having different options for seat size and back support. The seat can be turned next to a table in a restaurant to reduce the need for transfers, and attached baskets provide storage for shopping.

Scooters range in weight from 80 pounds to over 250 pounds. Some can be disassembled and transported in a vehicle; however, frequently, a vehicle lift is more desirable to reduce the work involved in getting around for daily living and community activities. Because of their design, scooters require a large area to turn around in and, therefore, are usually not useful inside the home.

To use a scooter safely, it is important that you have good trunk control, adequate upper body strength and dexterity to operate the controls, and the ability to transfer to/from the scooter seat.

What Are Power Wheelchairs?

If MS has affected your back and arm muscles, a power wheelchair may be needed to provide adequate support to maintain good posture, reduce fatigue, and prevent deformity. A power wheelchair is operated using a single hand or other drive controls, such as head movement. Because the batteries, motors, and drive wheels are directly under the seat, a power wheelchair has a much smaller turning radius, which is helpful for in-home use and on public transportation.

There are numerous options to customize the seating system for help with transfers, reaching higher surfaces, independent pressure relief, and rest breaks. The primary disadvantage of a power wheelchair is its weight and inability to disassemble it for transport. Power wheelchairs range in weight from 200 to 500 pounds. Most private vehicles will require a vehicle lift to transport the device or an adapted van with a ramp or wheelchair lift.

Section 50.3

Medicare Coverage of Durable Medical Equipment

This section includes text excerpted from "Medicare Coverage of Durable Medical Equipment and Other Devices," Centers for Medicare & Medicaid Services (CMS), October 2017.

What Is Durable Medical Equipment?

Durable medical equipment (DME) is reusable medical equipment, such as walkers, wheelchairs, or hospital beds.

If I Have Medicare, Can I Get Durable Medical Equipment?

Anyone who has Medicare Part B (medical insurance) can get DME, as long as the equipment is medically necessary.

When Does Original Medicare Cover Durable Medical Equipment?

Original Medicare covers DME under Part B when your doctor or treating practitioner (such as a nurse practitioner, physician assistant, or clinical nurse specialist) prescribes it for you to use in your home. A hospital or nursing home that's providing you with Medicare-covered care can't qualify as your "home" in this situation. However, a long-term care facility can qualify as your home.

What If I Need Durable Medical Equipment and I'm in a Medicare Advantage Plan?

Medicare Advantage Plans (such as a Health Management Organization (HMO) or a Preferred Provider Organization (PPO)) must cover the same items and services as Original Medicare. Your costs will depend on which plan you choose. If you are in a Medicare Advantage Plan (MAP) and you need DME, call your plan to find out if the equipment is covered and how much you will have to pay.

If you are getting home care or using medical equipment and you choose to join a new MAP, you should call the new plan as soon as possible and ask for "utilization management." They can tell you if your equipment is covered and how much it will cost. If you return to Original Medicare, you should tell your supplier to bill Medicare directly after the date your coverage in the MAP ends.

If I Have Original Medicare, How Do I Get the Durable Medical Equipment I Need?

If you need DME in your home, your doctor or treating practitioner (such as a nurse practitioner, physician assistant, or clinical nurse specialist) must prescribe the type of equipment you need by filling out an order. For some equipment, Medicare may also require your doctor to provide additional information documenting your medical need for the equipment. Your supplier will work to make sure your doctor submits all required information to Medicare. If your needs and/or condition changes, your doctor must complete and submit a new, updated order.

Medicare only covers DME if you get it from a supplier enrolled in Medicare. This means that the supplier has been approved by Medicare and has a Medicare supplier number.

To find a supplier that is enrolled in Medicare, visit the Medicare website, or call 800-MEDICARE (800-633-4227). Teletypewriter (TTY) users can call 877-486-2048.

A supplier enrolled in Medicare must meet strict standards to qualify for a Medicare supplier number. If your supplier does not have a supplier number, Medicare won't pay your claim, even if your supplier is a large chain or department store that sells more than just DME.

Does Medicare Cover Power Wheelchairs and Scooters?

For Medicare to cover a power wheelchair or scooter, your doctor must state that you need it because of your medical condition. Medicare will not cover a power wheelchair or scooter that is only needed and used outside of the home. Most suppliers who work with Medicare are honest. However, there are a few who aren't. For example, some suppliers of medical equipment try to cheat Medicare by offering expensive power wheelchairs and scooters to people who do not qualify for these items.

What If My Equipment or Supplies Are Lost or Damaged in a Disaster or Emergency?

If Original Medicare already paid for DME or supplies lost or damaged due to an emergency or disaster, in certain cases, Medicare will cover the cost to repair or replace your equipment or supplies.

Generally, Medicare will also cover the cost of rentals for items (such as wheelchairs) during the time your equipment is being repaired.

If you're in a Medicare Advantage Plan (such as a HMO or PPO) or other Medicare health plan, contact your plan directly to find out how it replaces DME or supplies lost or damaged in an emergency or disaster. You can also call 800-MEDICARE to get more information about how to replace your equipment or supplies.

What's Covered, and How Much Does It Cost?

The below list shows some of the items Medicare covers and how much you have to pay for these items. This list doesn't include all covered DME. For questions about whether Medicare covers a particular item, visit Medicare.gov, or call 800-MEDICARE (800-633-4227). TTY users can call 877-486-2048. If you have a Medigap policy, it may help cover some of the costs listed.

Medicare Coverage for Durable Medical Equipment

- Air-fluidized beds and other support surfaces
- Blood sugar monitors
- Blood sugar (glucose) test strips
- Canes (however, white canes for the blind aren't covered)

- Commode chairs

- Continuous passive motion (CPM) machines

- Crutches

- Hospital beds

- Infusion pumps and supplies (when necessary to administer certain drugs)

- Manual wheelchairs and power mobility devices (power wheelchairs or scooters needed for use inside the home)

- Nebulizers and nebulizer medications

- Oxygen equipment and accessories

- Patient lifts (a medical device used to lift you from a bed or wheelchair)

- Sleep apnea and Continuous Positive Airway Pressure (CPAP) devices and accessories

- Suction pumps

- Traction equipment

- Walkers

How Much Do I Pay?

Generally, you pay 20 percent of the Medicare-approved amount after you pay your Medicare Part B deductible for the year. Medicare pays the other 80 percent. The Medicare-approved amount is the lower of the actual charge for the item or the fee Medicare sets for the item. However, the amount you pay may vary because Medicare pays for different kinds of DME in different ways. You may be able to rent or buy the equipment.

Medicare Coverage for Prosthetic and Orthotic Items

- Orthotics, as long as you go to a supplier that's enrolled in Medicare

- Orthopedic shoes only when they're a necessary part of a leg brace

- Arm, leg, back, and neck braces

- Artificial limbs and eyes

- Breast prostheses (including a surgical bra) after a mastectomy
- Ostomy bags and certain related supplies
- Urological supplies
- Cochlear implants and certain other surgically implanted prosthetic devices
- Prosthetic devices needed to replace a body part or function
- Therapeutic shoes or inserts for people with diabetes who have severe diabetic foot disease.

The doctor who treats your diabetes must certify your need for therapeutic shoes or inserts. A podiatrist or other qualified doctor must prescribe the shoes and inserts. A doctor or other qualified individual (such as a pedorthist, orthotist, or prosthetist) must fit and provide the shoes. Medicare Part B (Medical Insurance) covers the furnishing and fitting of either one pair of custom-molded shoes and inserts or one pair of extra-depth shoes each calendar year. Medicare also covers two additional pairs of inserts each calendar year for custom-molded shoes and three pairs of inserts each calendar year for extra-depth shoes. Medicare will cover shoe modifications instead of inserts.

How Much Do I Pay?

You pay 20 percent of the Medicare-approved amount after you pay your Medicare Part B deductible for the year. Medicare pays the other 80 percent. These amounts may be different if the supplier does not accept the assignment.

Medicare Coverage for Corrective Lenses

Prosthetic lenses:

- Cataract glasses (for Aphakia or absence of the lens of the eye)
- Conventional glasses and contact lenses after surgery with an intraocular lens
- Intraocular lenses

An ophthalmologist or an optometrist must prescribe these items.

Important: Only standard frames are covered. Medicare will only pay for contact lenses or eyeglasses provided by a supplier enrolled in Medicare, no matter who submits the claim (you or your supplier).

How Much Do I Pay?

You are covered for one pair of eyeglasses or contact lenses after each cataract surgery with an intraocular lens. You pay 20 percent of the Medicare-approved amount after you pay the Medicare Part B deductible for the year. Medicare pays the other 80 percent. Costs may be different if the supplier does not accept the assignment. If you want to upgrade the frames, you pay an additional cost.

What's "Assignment" in Original Medicare, and Why Is It Important?

An assignment is an agreement between you (the person with Medicare), Medicare, and doctors or other healthcare providers, and suppliers of healthcare equipment and supplies (such as DME and prosthetic or orthotic devices). Doctors, providers, and suppliers who agree to accept assignment accept the Medicare-approved amount as full payment. After you have paid the Part B deductible, you pay the doctor or supplier the coinsurance (usually 20 percent, as well as your coinsurance and any deductible) at the time you get the DME. The supplier will send the bill to Medicare for you, but you'll have to wait for Medicare to reimburse you later for its share of the charge.

Before you get DME, ask if the supplier is enrolled in Medicare. If the supplier isn't enrolled in Medicare, Medicare won't pay your claim at all. Then, ask if the supplier is a participating supplier in Medicare. A participating supplier must accept the assignment. A supplier that's enrolled in Medicare but isn't "participating" has the option of whether to accept the assignment. You will have to ask if the supplier will accept assignment for your claim.

Chapter 51

Service Animals and People with Disabilities

This chapter provides guidance on the term "service animal" and the service animal provisions in the department's revised regulations.

- Since March 15, 2011, only dogs are recognized as service animals under titles II and III of the Americans with Disabilities Act (ADA).

- A service animal is a dog that is individually trained to do work or perform tasks for a person with a disability.

- Generally, title II and title III entities must permit service animals to accompany people with disabilities in all areas where members of the public are allowed to go.

How "Service Animal" Is Defined

Service animals are defined as dogs that are individually trained to do work or perform tasks for people with disabilities. Examples of such work or tasks include guiding people who are blind, alerting people who are deaf, pulling a wheelchair, alerting and protecting a person who is having a seizure, reminding a person with mental illness to take prescribed medications, calming a person with posttraumatic

This chapter includes text excerpted from "Service Animals," ADA.gov, U.S. Department of Justice (DOJ), July 2011. Reviewed March 2019.

stress disorder (PTSD) during an anxiety attack, or performing other duties. Service animals are working animals, not pets. The work or task a dog has been trained to provide must be directly related to the person's disability. Dogs whose sole function is to provide comfort or emotional support do not qualify as service animals under the ADA.

This definition does not affect or limit the broader definition of "assistance animal" under the Fair Housing Act or the broader definition of "service animal" under the Air Carrier Access Act (ACAA). Some state and local laws also define service animal more broadly than the ADA does. Information about such laws can be obtained from that state's attorney general's office.

Where Service Animals Are Allowed

Under the ADA, state and local governments, businesses, and non-profit organizations that serve the public generally must allow service animals to accompany people with disabilities in all areas of the facility where the public is normally allowed to go. For example, in a hospital, it would be inappropriate to exclude a service animal from areas such as patient rooms, clinics, cafeterias, or examination rooms. However, it may be appropriate to exclude a service animal from operating rooms or burn units where the animal's presence may compromise a sterile environment.

Service Animals Must Be under Control

Under the ADA, service animals must be harnessed, leashed, or tethered, unless these devices interfere with the service animal's work or the individual's disability prevents from using these devices. In that case, the individual must maintain control of the animal through voice, signals, or other effective controls.

Inquiries, Exclusions, Charges, and Other Specific Rules Related to Service Animals

- When it is not obvious what service an animal provides, only limited inquiries are allowed. Staff may ask two questions:

  1. Is the dog a service animal required because of a disability?

  2. What work or task has the dog been trained to perform?

  Staff cannot ask about the person's disability, require medical documentation, require a special identification card or training documentation for the dog, or ask that the dog demonstrate its ability to perform the work or task.

- Allergies and fear of dogs are not valid reasons for denying access or refusing service to people using service animals. When a person who is allergic to dog dander and a person who uses a service animal must spend time in the same room or facility, such as, in a school classroom or at a homeless shelter, they both should be accommodated by assigning them, if possible, to different locations within the room or different rooms in the facility.

- A person with a disability cannot be asked to remove his service animal from the premises unless:

  1. The dog is out of control, and the handler does not take effective action to control it

  2. The dog is not house trained.

  When there is a legitimate reason to ask that a service animal be removed, staff must offer the person with the disability the opportunity to obtain goods or services without the animal's presence.

- Establishments that sell or prepare food must allow service animals in public areas even if state or local health codes prohibit animals on the premises.

- People with disabilities who use service animals cannot be isolated from other patrons, treated less favorably than other patrons, or charged fees that are not charged to other patrons without animals. In addition, if a business requires a deposit or fee to be paid by patrons with pets, it must waive the charge for service animals.

- If a business, such as a hotel, normally charges guests for damage that they cause, a customer with a disability may also be charged for damage caused by himself or his service animal.

- Staffs are not required to provide care or food for a service animal.

Miniature Horses

In addition to the provisions about service dogs, the department's revised ADA regulations have a new, separate provision about miniature horses that have been individually trained to do work or perform tasks for people with disabilities. (Miniature horses generally range in height from 24 to 34 inches measured to the shoulders and generally weigh between 70 and 100 pounds.) Entities covered by the ADA must modify their policies to permit miniature horses where reasonable. The regulations set out 4 assessment factors to assist entities in determining whether miniature horses can be accommodated in their facility. The assessment factors are:

1. Whether the miniature horse is house trained

2. Whether the miniature horse is under the owner's control

3. Whether the facility can accommodate the miniature horse's type, size, and weight

4. Whether the miniature horse's presence will not compromise legitimate safety requirements necessary for safe operation of the facility

Chapter 52

Developing a Support Network and Group If You Have Multiple Sclerosis

Living with a chronic illness, such as multiple sclerosis (MS), can be stressful and challenging. Uncertainty and the constant need to adapt to change can have you feeling like you are on a roller coaster ride. Many people feel they no longer have control of their life. It is common to feel you are alone, believing no one can possibly understand what you are going through. You are not alone. There are thousands of people living with MS that are struggling with many of the same issues you are. Many of these people have found that creating a supportive network of family and friends has helped them through difficult days, as well as provided the day-to-day support they may need.

What Is a Support Network?

A support network is made of family members and friends who are willing to support you. This is something you create yourself, for you. These are people that you can turn to in times of crisis, as well as for simple things, such as talking about your day, going out to lunch, or

This chapter includes text excerpted from "VA Multiple Sclerosis Centers of Excellence—MS Changed My Life," U.S. Department of Veterans Affairs (VA), 2014. Reviewed March 2019.

getting a ride to a medical appointment. These people "get it;" they understand your needs and offer help when you need it.

How Do I Set up a Support Network?

Cultivating and maintaining a network of support can take effort, and it is important you establish a support network that works best for you. Some people find that a small support network of family and friends is sufficient, while others enjoy a large, diverse support network.

Asking for or accepting help can be difficult. Try to remember that friends and family care about you and want to help. Allowing them to help gives them an opportunity to express their love for you.

MS affects everyone differently. It's up to you to let family and friends know what you need. Be specific on what you would find most helpful; no one is a mind reader. Start by making a list of everyday chores and activities. From this list, check off those things you either still enjoy doing or those things you do not feel comfortable asking others to do for you. Enlist a family member or trusted friend to "supervise" the list, and recruit members on your support team to volunteer for the remaining tasks. People will likely choose activities they enjoy or feel expertise in, assuring that they are a good fit for the task. Set realistic expectations for these tasks to avoid disappointment if things don't go exactly the way you had hoped.

If you would like to expand your social network, get involved in activities where there are people with interests similar to yours, or take some time to reconnect with old friends or colleagues. Volunteer with an organization that you find interesting, or join a cause that is important to you. Many community centers have classes you can join, as well as planned excursions that you can participate in. Having a variety of interests and activities in your life will open up opportunities to make new friends.

What Is a Support Group?

Support groups bring together people facing similar issues, allowing attendees to share experiences and advice, as well as offer emotional and moral support. While not everyone needs support beyond their family and friends, support groups may lessen feelings of isolation as attendees make connections with people experiencing similar challenges. Attendees can also gain a sense of empowerment by better understanding their disease through the eyes of others.

Support groups come in a variety of formats, including in-person, through the Internet, or over the phone. Some groups are structured moderated groups while others are more informal. If you are interested in a support group, plan to attend a few meetings to see if it is a good fit. If you're not comfortable with the group or do not find it beneficial, try a different one. It's important to find a group that works for you.

Support group options may be available through your healthcare provider. If you need help finding a support group, nonprofits, service organizations, churches, and community centers may be able to help.

Taking the time to build a network of support or participating in a support group is an investment not only in your mental well-being, but also in your overall physical health. Spending time with people you consider friends contribute to a feeling of belonging, helps ward off loneliness, and increases feelings of self-worth. Remember that the goal of building a support network is to provide support for you and to reduce your stress. Prioritize your social commitments, and watch for signs of stress and fatigue. Control your environment by choosing to surround yourself with positive people. This is not the time to keep company with people who are constantly critical or negative. Keep in mind that relationships are give and take.

Be willing to support those willing to support you. Make the effort to stay in touch with people, and be a good listener when they need you. Show appreciation to your friends and family, and do not forget to say thank you for all they do.

Chapter 53

Tips for Multiple Sclerosis Caregivers

What Is Multiple Sclerosis?

Multiple sclerosis (MS) is an unpredictable, often disabling disease of the central nervous system that interrupts the flow of information within the brain and between the brain and the body, stopping people from moving. Symptoms range from numbness and tingling to blindness and paralysis. The progress, severity, and specific symptoms of MS in any one person cannot yet be predicted.

Treatments

Treatments for MS focus on controlling the immune system and managing symptoms. It is important for people to work with their healthcare providers to find the best approach to address MS symptoms, such as extreme fatigue, bladder problems, and muscle spasms. MS symptoms, both mental and physical, can be managed with conventional medication, complementary and alternative medicine, physical therapy, mobility devices, psychotherapy, medication, and other self-care approaches.

This chapter includes text excerpted from "Caregiving Tips—Multiple Sclerosis (MS)," U.S. Department of Veterans Affairs (VA), July 12, 2017.

Physical and Mental Changes to Expect in Patients with Multiple Sclerosis

Symptoms of multiple sclerosis (MS) can vary greatly from patient to patient and from time to time in the same person. For instance, one person with MS may experience abnormal fatigue, and another person may have severe vision problems. While one person with MS may have a loss of balance, a decrease in muscle coordination, or tremors—making walking and everyday tasks difficult to perform—another person may have slurred speech and memory issues. These problems may be permanent or may come and go.

Depression is frequently experienced by MS patients and can have a significant impact on quality of life (QOL).

- **Physical changes** may include visual disturbances, difficulty in controlling strength and movements, impaired coordination and balance, numbness, tingling, sensitivity to heat and cold, bladder-control problems, urinary tract infections, mild to severe fatigue, and weakness.

- **Mental changes** may include problems with memory and concentration.

- **Emotional changes** may include mood swings, ranging from depression to euphoria.

What Does This Mean for Me?

- Caring for someone with a chronic illness, such as MS, can be deeply satisfying. Spouses and partners, family, and friends can be drawn more closely together by their shared concerns and collaborative efforts. While the primary caregiver is most often a partner or spouse, it may also be an adult, child, parent, or friend. Whoever you are, remember that paying attention to your own health and well-being is essential to being able to care for someone else.

- At times, caring for an individual with MS can be physically and emotionally exhausting, particularly for the primary caregiver. Because symptoms of MS typically fluctuate, it can make caregiving a challenge—you may find it hard to anticipate the next symptom or need of the patient you are caring for. These reactions are normal but can be challenging to deal with on your own. Remember that it's okay to ask for help and that support is available through a variety of avenues. Friends, family, support groups, and professional mental-health practitioners are all good resources.

Caregiving Tips

- Educate yourself. Understanding MS and its related physical and emotional symptoms will help you and the patient you care for cope with and manage the disease.

- Pay attention to warning signs of depression. If you begin to notice the patient is displaying signs of depression, take action. Keep contact information for a psychiatrist and/or therapist, local crisis team, and other emergency phone numbers handy. If the patient talks about suicide, take it seriously, and seek help immediately.

- Seek out emotional support. It is important that you feel comfortable discussing your concerns and fears openly.

- Plan to re-evaluate schedules and task assignments as needs and circumstances change. Make sure to schedule personal time for everyone in the household.

- If a task seems impossibly difficult or stressful, there may be an easier way to do it. Reach out to your family and friends for support or suggestions. A medical team can also provide tips, techniques, and sometimes even equipment for bathing, dressing, and safe transfers.

- Leaving the patient home alone can be a frightening proposition for both of you, especially if the patient has significant disabilities. Advance planning and making adaptations to your home can help to decrease these worries. Accessible peepholes in the front door, portable telephones with speed dial, automatic door openers, and "life-net" call systems that summon help in an emergency may provide security and peace of mind.

- Caregivers can and should make appointments with healthcare professionals to get information, advice, and training. Having a support team of committed medical experts can help you to feel at ease, determine the best treatments for the patient, and ensure that you understand medical procedures and instructions. Caring for a patient with MS can be confusing, so it is important that you surround yourself with a team that can help you navigate the caregiving system.

- It is important for your health, as well as the health of the patient, that you take some time off (or "respite") from caregiving.

Part Five

Multiple Sclerosis and Work, Financial, and Legal Issues

Chapter 54

Navigating the Workplace with Multiple Sclerosis

Chapter Contents

Section 54.1

Self-Managing the Challenges

This section includes text excerpted from "Self-Management
and Multiple Sclerosis," U.S. Department of Veterans
Affairs (VA), January 13, 2016.

The Multiple Sclerosis Center of Excellence (MSCoE) promotes a
self-management practice. This approach is traditional because the
healthcare provider stays involved with the care, diagnosis, treatment, and education to address the problems associated with multiple
sclerosis (MS). Self-management recognizes some key things. Certain
aspects, such as good treatment and education, are only beneficial if
the person can link the treatment into their everyday life. To successfully manage a disease, such as multiple sclerosis, the person needs to
receive support. This support aids them in becoming an active partner
in their healthcare.

People with multiple sclerosis are often faced with the need to manage many personal health issues all at once. These health problems
can occur during daily activities of life. For example, you may face
challenges at work, raising a family, involvement with extended family, and community concerns. For a person with multiple sclerosis, a
lot of changes can happen all at once. Self-management recognizes
that changes in behavior are not easy to make. Maintaining these
changes over a long period of time requires a good support system.
This approach also recognizes that "small changes" over time have a
large impact on a person's health.

Some ideas for self-management include choosing the most important change to work on. It may be to start an exercise program to help
manage fatigue. Self-management guidelines move this from an idea
to a specific goal. Your goal may be to walk one half mile, three times
a week, right after work. A self-management plan will also identify a
back-up plan (in case there is a problem). For example, if your goal is
to walk one half mile and it is raining, you can go to the gym or bike
indoors. A key aspect of self-management is to evaluate your level of
confidence to reach your goal. If you are not sure if the goal can be
reached, the goal may need to be changed, or additional support may
need to be provided. Planned followup is helpful to identify things that
may keep you from reaching a goal. Plan to celebrate success. You
also may need to adjust prior goals or make new ones, with the help
of your support system.

Many benefits of health practices that promote well-being or decrease chronic illness symptoms also benefit multiple sclerosis. For instance, smoking has been linked with an increased risk of developing MS. It has also been linked to a more severe course of the disease. Stopping smoking may not only improve overall health, but also improve multiple sclerosis. Smoking may also complicate other problems that people with MS face. Things such as a decreased lung capacity, fatigue, and healing of an ulcer may be worse with smoking. An exercise program has been shown to have a positive effect on multiple sclerosis, and it improves the fatigue related to MS. Exercise also can promote overall health and well-being. A healthy diet and reduced alcohol intake may improve mobility and quality of life with MS.

The Multiple Sclerosis Centers of Excellence team is able to work with you on your goals and to team up with other clinical services.

Section 54.2

Asking for Accommodations or Different Job Duties

This section includes text excerpted from "Job Applicants and the Americans with Disabilities Act," U.S. Equal Employment Opportunity Commission (EEOC), December 20, 2017.

Title I of the Americans with Disabilities Act of 1990 (ADA) makes it unlawful for an employer to discriminate against a qualified applicant or employee with a disability. The ADA applies to private employers with 15 or more employees and to state and local government employers. The U.S. Equal Employment Opportunity Commission (EEOC) enforces the employment provisions of the ADA.

The ADA defines an individual with a disability as a person who:

1. Has a physical or mental impairment that substantially limits a major life activity

2. Has a record or history of a substantially limiting impairment

3. Is regarded or perceived by an employer as having a substantially limiting impairment

An applicant with a disability, like all other applicants, must be able to meet the employer's requirements for the job, such as any education, training, employment experience, skills, or licenses. In addition, an applicant with a disability must be able to perform the "essential functions" of the job either on his or her own or with the help of "reasonable accommodation." However, an employer does not have to provide a reasonable accommodation that will cause "undue hardship," which is significant difficulty or expense.

The following section addresses common questions about how the ADA protects applicants with disabilities. This information also applies to applicants for federal employment, who are protected from discrimination by Section 501 of the Rehabilitation Act. Section 501's requirements are the same as those that apply to employers covered by the ADA. There are many other documents, some of which are listed at the end of this section, that provide more in-depth information about the employment rights of individuals with disabilities.

Reasonable Accommodation for the Application Process

1. I Have a Disability and Will Need an Accommodation for the Job Interview. Does the ADA Require an Employer to Provide Me with One?

Yes. Employers are required to provide reasonable accommodation—appropriate changes and adjustments—to enable you to be considered for a job opening. Reasonable accommodation may also be required to enable you to perform a job, gain access to the workplace, and enjoy the benefits and privileges of employment available to employees without disabilities. An employer cannot refuse to consider you because you require a reasonable accommodation to compete for or perform a job.

2. Can an Employer Refuse to Provide Me with an Accommodation Because It Is Too Difficult or Too Expensive?

An employer does not have to provide a specific accommodation, if it would cause an undue hardship, that is, if it would require significant difficulty or expense. However, an employer cannot refuse to provide an accommodation solely because it entails some costs, either financial or administrative.

If the requested accommodation causes an undue hardship, the employer still would be required to provide another accommodation that does not.

Example: A trucking company conducts job interviews in a second floor office. There is no elevator. The company calls Tanya to arrange for an interview for a secretarial position. She requests a reasonable accommodation because she uses a wheelchair. Installing an elevator would be an undue hardship, but the employer could conduct the interview in a first floor office. The employer must move the location of the interview as a reasonable accommodation.

3. What Are Some Examples of "Reasonable Accommodations" That May Be Needed during the Hiring Process?

Reasonable accommodation can take many forms. Ones that may be needed during the hiring process include (but are not limited to):

- Providing written materials in accessible formats, such as large print, braille, or audiotape
- Providing readers or sign language interpreters
- Ensuring that recruitment, interviews, tests, and other components of the application process are held in accessible locations
- Providing or modifying equipment or devices
- Adjusting or modifying application policies and procedures

Example 1: John is blind and applies for a job as a customer service representative. John could perform this job with assistive technology, such as a program that reads information on the screen. If the company wishes to have John demonstrate his ability to use the computer, it must provide appropriate assistive technology as a reasonable accommodation.

Example 2: An employer requires job applicants to line up outside its facility to apply for a job, a process that could take several hours. Tara has multiple sclerosis, and that makes her unable to tolerate prolonged exposure to temperatures in the 90s. Tara, therefore, requests that she be allowed to wait indoors, where it is air-conditioned until the human resources department is ready to take her application. The employer would need to modify its hiring procedure to accommodate Tara.

4. Because of My Learning Disability, I Need Extra Time to Complete a Written Test. Does the ADA Require an Employer to Modify the Way a Test Is given to Me?

Yes. An employer may have to provide testing materials in alternative formats or make other adjustments to tests as an accommodation for you. The format and manner in which a test is given may pose problems for persons with impaired sensory, speaking, or manual skills, as well as for those with certain learning disabilities. For example, an applicant who is blind will not be able to read a written test, but can take the test if it is provided in braille or the questions are tape recorded. A deaf person will not understand oral instructions, but these could be provided in a written format or through the use of a sign language interpreter. A 30-minute timed written test may pose a problem for a person whose learning disability requires additional time.

Thus, the ADA requires that employers give application tests in a format or manner that does not require use of your impaired skill, unless the test is designed to measure that skill.

Example 1: An employer gives a written test for a proofreading position. The employer does not have to offer this test in a different format (e.g., orally) to an applicant who has dyslexia because the job itself requires an ability to read.

Example 2: An employer gives a written test to learn about an applicant's knowledge of marketing trends. Maria is blind and requests that the test be given to her in braille. An individual's knowledge of marketing trends is critical to this job, but the employer can test Maria's knowledge by giving her the test in braille. Alternatively, the employer could explore other testing formats with Maria to determine if they would be effective, such as providing a reader or a computer version of the test.

5. When Do I Have to Tell an Employer That I Need an Accommodation for the Hiring Process?

It is best to let an employer know as soon as you realize that you will need a reasonable accommodation for some aspect of the hiring process. An employer needs advance notice to provide many accommodations, such as sign language interpreters, alternative formats for written documents, and adjusting the time allowed for taking a written test. An employer may also need advance notice to arrange an accessible location for a test or interview.

Asking for an Accommodation
6. How Do I Request a Reasonable Accommodation?

You must inform the employer that you need some sort of change or adjustment to the application/interviewing process because of your medical condition. You can make this request orally or in writing, or someone else might make a request for you (e.g., a family member, friend, health professional, or other representative, such as a job coach).

7. What Happens after I Request an Accommodation?

The employer may need to discuss your request more fully with you in order to understand your disability and why you need an accommodation. You should respond to the employer's questions as quickly as possible, and be sure to explain how a proposed accommodation would enable you to participate fully in all aspects of the application/ interviewing process. If your disability and need for accommodation are not obvious, the employer may ask you for reasonable documentation explaining the disability and why an accommodation is needed.

Example: A department store requires applicants to take a written test. Rodney has dyslexia and requests that the test be read to him as a reasonable accommodation. The human resources associate is unfamiliar with dyslexia and requests information about the condition and why the accommodation is necessary. Rodney must provide this information.

8. I Asked for a Specific Accommodation, but the Employer Offered Me a Different One Instead. Do I Have to Accept It?

An employer has to offer an accommodation that will meet your needs. If more than one accommodation meets your needs, then the employer may choose which one to provide. You cannot insist on a specific accommodation only because it is a personal preference. If the employer's proposal does not meet your needs, then you need to explain why.

Example: Charles is blind and asks that a written test be read to him as a reasonable accommodation. The employer proposes to provide Charles with a braille version of the test, but Charles explains that he cannot read braille. Thus, a braille version would not be an effective accommodation. The employer then proposes to provide Charles with an audiotape version of the test. While Charles preferred to have someone read the questions to him, the audiotape version meets his needs and thus is acceptable as a reasonable accommodation.

Discussing Disability with the Potential Employer

The ADA prohibits employers from asking questions that are likely to reveal the existence of a disability before making a job offer (i.e., the preoffer period). This prohibition covers written questionnaires and inquiries made during interviews, as well as medical examinations. However, such questions and medical examinations are permitted after extending a job offer but before the individual begins work (i.e., the postoffer period).

9. What Are Examples of Questions That an Employer Cannot Ask on an Application or during an Interview?

Examples of prohibited questions during the preoffer period include:

- Do you have a heart condition? Do you have asthma or any other difficulties breathing?
- Do you have a disability which would interfere with your ability to perform the job?
- How many days were you sick last year?
- Have you ever filed for workers' compensation? Have you ever been injured on the job?
- Have you ever been treated for mental-health problems?
- What prescription drugs are you currently taking?

10. May the Employer Ask Me These Questions after Making a Job Offer?

Yes. An employer can ask all of the questions listed in question nine, and others that are likely to reveal the existence of a disability, after they extend a job offer, as long as they ask the same questions of other applicants offered the same type of job. In other words, an employer cannot ask such questions only of those who have obvious disabilities. Similarly, an employer may require a medical examination after making a job offer, as long as it requires the same medical examination of other applicants offered the same type of job.

11. May an Employer Ask Me Whether I Will Need a Reasonable Accommodation for the Hiring Process?

Yes. An employer may tell all applicants what the hiring process involves (for example, an interview, timed written test, or job demonstration), and then ask whether they will need a reasonable accommodation for this process. (See question 16 for a discussion about employers asking about an applicant's need for reasonable accommodation for the job.)

12. I Have an Obvious Disability. Can an Employer Ask Me Medical Questions during an Interview?

No. Except as explained in question 15 below, an employer cannot ask questions about an applicant's disability either because it is visible or because the applicant has voluntarily disclosed a hidden disability.

13. After I Got a Job Offer, the Employer Had Me Take a Medical Examination in Which I Revealed I Have Epilepsy. Can the Employer Withdraw My Job Offer?

While the employer had the right to require a postoffer medical examination, they cannot withdraw the job offer solely because you revealed you have a disability. Instead, the employer can withdraw the job offer only if it can show that you are unable to perform the essential functions of the job (with or without reasonable accommodation), or that you pose a significant risk of causing substantial harm to yourself or others.

Example: Darla receives a job offer to be a cook at a hotel resort, and, during the medical examination, she discloses that she has epilepsy. The hotel doctor expresses concern about Darla working around stoves and using sharp utensils. Darla tells the doctor that her seizures are controlled with medication and offers to bring information from her neurologist to answer the doctor's concerns. Darla also points out that she has worked as a cook for seven years without any incidents. The hotel will violate the ADA if it withdraws Darla's job offer based on her epilepsy.

14. During the Hiring Process, I Gave the Employer Medical Information That I Do Not Want Anyone Else to Know About. Must the Employer Keep This Information Confidential?

Yes. The ADA contains strict confidentiality requirements. Medical information revealed during the hiring process (pre- or post-offer) must be kept confidential, with certain exceptions. The confidentiality requirements protect both information voluntarily revealed as well as information revealed in response to an employer's written or oral questions or during a medical examination.

An employer may share medical information with other decision-makers involved in the hiring process who need it, so they can make employment decisions consistent with the ADA. The ADA also permits an employer to share medical information with the following individuals:

- Supervisors and managers may be told about necessary restrictions on the work or duties of an employee and about reasonable accommodations

- First aid and safety personnel may be told if the disability might require emergency treatment

- Government officials investigating compliance with the ADA

- State workers' compensation offices, state second injury funds, or workers' compensation insurance carriers

An employer also may use the information for insurance purposes.

Discussing Accommodation to Perform the Job
15. May an Employer Ask Applicants on an Application Form or during an Interview Whether They Will Need Reasonable Accommodation to Perform the Job?

Generally, no. An employer cannot ask all applicants whether they would need reasonable accommodation to perform a job because the answer to this question is likely to reveal whether an applicant has a disability.

However, if the employer knows that an applicant has a disability, and it is reasonable to question whether the disability might pose difficulties for the individual in performing a specific job task, then the employer may ask whether she would need reasonable accommodation to perform that task. An employer might know that an applicant has a disability because it is obvious, or she has voluntarily revealed the existence of one. If the applicant indicates that accommodation will be necessary, then the employer may ask what accommodation is needed.

Example 1: Carl has a severe limp and uses a cane because of his prosthetic leg. He applies for an assembly line job which does not require employees to move around, but does require that they stand for long periods of time. The employer asks Carl about his ability to stand and whether he will need reasonable accommodation to perform the job. Carl replies that he will need accommodation. The employer asks Carl for examples of accommodations, and Carl suggests two possibilities: a tall stool so that he can sit down but still reach the conveyor belt or, alternatively, a "sit-stand" chair which will provide support and enable him to do the job.

Also, if the employer believes an applicant with an obvious disability will need a reasonable accommodation to do the job, it may ask the applicant to describe or demonstrate how she would perform the job with or without reasonable accommodation.

Example 2: Alberto uses a wheelchair and applies for a job that involves the retrieval of files that would seem to be beyond his reach. The employer can show him the files and ask him to explain or demonstrate how he would perform this task.

16. Do I Have to Tell the Employer during the Application Process That I Might Need an Accommodation to Perform the Job?

No. The ADA does not require that an applicant inform an employer about the need for a reasonable accommodation at any particular time, so this information need not be volunteered on an application form or in an interview.

Determining the best moment to tell a prospective employer about the need for reasonable accommodation on the job is a personal decision. Sometimes, applicants are not aware they may need a reasonable accommodation until they have more information about the job, its requirements, and the work environment. Some applicants choose to inform an employer during the application process after they better understand the job and its requirements. Others choose to wait until they have a job offer.

Being "Qualified" for the Job

17. What If My Disability Prevents Me from Performing Some Job Duties?

An employer does not have to hire you if you are unable to perform all of the essential functions of the job, even with reasonable accommodation. However, an employer cannot reject you only because the disability prevents you from performing minor duties that are not essential to the job.

Example: Wei is deaf and applies for a file clerk position. The essential functions for this job are to file and retrieve written materials. While the job description states that the clerk must also answer the phone, in practice, the clerk rarely does this because other employees have responsibility for this duty. The employer cannot reject Wei solely because she is unable to answer the phone since that is not an essential part of performing this job.

18. Can an Employer Refuse to Hire Me Because They Believe That My Disability Makes It Unsafe for Me to Perform a Job?

An employer can refuse to hire you only if your disability poses a significant risk of substantial harm to you or others. If an employer has such concerns, they must seek appropriate information to assess the level of risk and the nature of the harm. This can include asking questions about prior work experience and requesting specific information from your doctor related to health and safety.

An employer cannot refuse to hire you based on a slightly increased risk, speculation about future risk, or generalizations about your disability. The employer must also consider whether a risk can be eliminated or reduced to an acceptable level with a reasonable accommodation.

Example: An employer learns, during a postoffer medical examination, that Simone has major depression. She has been offered a high-level managerial position, but the employer is concerned that the job will be too stressful, causing Simone's illness to worsen. But, Simone's depression is well-controlled with medication, and she has been working for two years in a similar position with no effect on her depression or her performance. Based on this information, Simone's disability would not pose a high level of risk of harm, and therefore, the employer could not refuse to hire her based on fears that she will experience an increased number of depressive episodes or that she would be unable to perform the job.

Section 54.3

Employment Support and Opportunities for People with Disabilities

This section includes text excerpted from "Employment Support for Persons with Disabilities," Bureau of Alcohol, Tobacco, Firearms, and Explosives (ATF), U.S. Department of Justice (DOJ), October 17, 2018.

Through the Americans with Disabilities Act Amendment Acts (ADAAA) 2009, the Bureau of Alcohol, Tobacco, Firearms and Explosives (ATF) can hire through traditional competitive hiring processes or by means of a noncompetitive, or special appointing, authority. In addition, ATF is committed to providing reasonable accommodation throughout the hiring process and employment.

Eligibility Requirements

To be considered as an individual with a disability, you must meet one of the following criteria:

Definition of Disability

Not everyone with a medical condition is protected by the law. In order to be protected, a person must be qualified for the job and have a disability as defined by the law.

A person can show that she or he has a disability in one of three ways:

- A person may be disabled if she or he has a physical or mental condition that substantially limits a major life activity (such as walking, talking, seeing, hearing, or learning).

- A person may be disabled if she or he has a history of a disability (such as cancer that is in remission).

- A person may be disabled if she or he is believed to have a physical or mental impairment that is not transitory (lasting or expected to last six months or less) and minor (even if she or he does not have such an impairment).

Reasonable Accommodation

Bureau of Alcohol, Tobacco, Firearms, and Explosives (ATF) provides reasonable accommodation to applicants with disabilities. If you need a reasonable accommodation for any part of the job application and hiring process, and you meet the eligibility requirements listed above, please notify the human resources specialist, or contact the ATF's Office of Equal Employment Opportunity at 202-648-8760. The decision to grant a reasonable accommodation is decided on a case-by-case basis.

Personal Assistant Services

Federal agencies are required to provide personal assistant services (PAS) during working hours to qualified persons with disabilities who need assistance with performing activities of daily living that an individual would typically perform if she or he did not have a disability, and that is not otherwise required as an accommodation. These services include, for example, assistance with removing and putting on clothing, eating, and using the restroom. Individuals may use the U.S. Department of Justice (DOJ) reasonable accommodation process to request PAS.

Special Appointing Authorities

The Office of Personnel Management (OPM) has established special appointing authorities for people with disabilities. The DOJ has the authority to use a special appointing authority to hire a qualified person with a disability for vacant positions. These special appointing authorities include:

- **5 CFR 213.3102(ll)** for hiring readers, interpreters, and personal assistants. This excepted authority is used to appoint readers, interpreters, and personal assistants for employees with severe disabilities.

- **5 CFR 213.3102(t)** for hiring people with intellectual disabilities. This excepted authority is used to appoint persons with intellectual disabilities who have demonstrated satisfactory performance through a temporary appointment, or have been certified as likely to succeed in performing the duties of the job. They may qualify for conversion to permanent status after two years of satisfactory service.

- **5 CFR 213.3102(u)** for hiring people with severe physical disabilities. This excepted authority is used to appoint persons with severe physical disabilities who have demonstrated satisfactory performance through a temporary appointment, or have been certified as likely to succeed in performing the duties of the job. After two years of satisfactory service, they may qualify for conversion to permanent status.

- **5 CFR 213.3102(gg)** — Positions filled by persons with psychiatric disabilities who have demonstrated their ability to perform satisfactorily under a temporary appointment [such as one authorized in 213.3102(i)(3)] or who are certified as likely to be able to perform the essential functions of the job, with or without reasonable accommodations, by a state vocational rehabilitation counselor, a U.S. Department of Veterans Affairs (VA) Veterans Benefits Administration psychologist, vocational rehabilitation counselor, or psychiatrist. Upon completion of two years of satisfactory service under this authority, the employee can be converted, at the discretion of the agency, to competitive status under the provisions of Executive Order 12125 as amended by Executive Order 13124.

Chapter 55

Financial Planning: Security for the Years Ahead

Disability is something most people do not like to think about. But the chances that you'll become disabled are probably greater than you realize. Studies show that a 20-year-old worker has a 1 in 4 chance of becoming disabled before reaching full retirement age. This chapter provides basic information on Social Security disability benefits, but it is not meant to answer all questions. For specific information about your situation, you should speak with a Social Security representative. The disability benefits are provided through two programs: the Social Security disability insurance (SSDI) program and the Supplemental Security Income (SSI) program. This chapter is about the Social Security disability program.

Who Can Get Social Security Disability Benefits?

Social Security pays benefits to people who can't work because they have a medical condition that's expected to last for at least one year or result in death. Federal law requires this very strict definition of disability. While some programs give money to people with partial disability or short-term disability, Social Security does not. Certain family members of disabled workers can also receive money from Social Security.

This chapter includes text excerpted from "Disability Benefits," U.S. Social Security Administration (SSA), August 2018.

How Do I Meet the Earnings Requirement for Disability Benefits?

In general, to get disability benefits, you must meet two different earnings tests:

1. A recent work test, based on your age at the time you became disabled

2. A duration of work test to show that you worked long enough under Social Security

Certain blind workers have to only meet the duration of work test.

The following table shows the rules for how much work you need for the recent work test, based on your age when your disability began. The rules are based in this table on the calendar quarter in which you turned or will turn a certain age.

The calendar quarters are:

First Quarter: January 1 through March 31

Second Quarter: April 1 through June 30

Third Quarter: July 1 through September 30

Fourth Quarter: October 1 through December 31

Table 55.1. Work Requirement for Disability Benefits

If You Become Disabled...	Then You Generally Need:
In or before the quarter you turn age 24	1.5 years of work during the 3-year period ending with the quarter your disability began.
In the quarter after you turn age 24 but before the quarter you turn age 31	Work during half the time for the period, beginning with the quarter after you turned 21 and ending with the quarter you became disabled. Example: If you become disabled in the quarter you turned age 27, then you would need 3 years of work out of the 6-year period ending with the quarter you became disabled.
In the quarter you turn age 31 or later	Work during 5 years out of the 10-year period ending with the quarter your disability began.

You must have a minimum of 6 quarters of coverage to meet the duration requirement. This minimum requirement for 6 quarters of coverage is also applicable for those who have not yet attained age 22 and may apply for disability based on their own earnings.

Table 55.2. Disability Benefits Requirement

If You Become Disabled...	Then You Generally Need:
Before age 28	1.5 years of work
Age 30	2 years
Age 34	3 years
Age 38	4 years
Age 42	5 years
Age 44	5.5 years
Age 46	6 years
Age 48	6.5 years
Age 50	7 years
Age 52	7.5 years
Age 54	8 years
Age 56	8.5 years
Age 58	9 years
Age 60	9.5 years

This table is an estimate only and does not cover all situations.

How Do I Apply for Disability Benefits?

There are two ways that you can apply for disability benefits. You can:

1.   Apply online at www.socialsecurity.gov.

2.   Call the U.S. Social Security Administration's (SSA) toll-free number, 800-772-1213, to make an appointment to file a disability claim at your local Social Security office or to set up an appointment for someone to take your claim over the telephone. The disability claims interview lasts about one hour. If you are deaf or hard of hearing, you may call SSA's toll-free TTY number, 800-325-0778, between 7 a.m. and 7 p.m. on business days. If you schedule an appointment, the SSA send you a "Disability Starter Kit" to help you get ready for your disability claims interview. The Disability Starter Kit also is available online, through the SSA's website. You have the right to representation by an attorney or other qualified person of your choice when you do business with Social Security.

When Should I Apply and What Information Do I Need?

You should apply for disability benefits as soon as you become disabled. Processing an application for disability benefits can take three to five months. To apply for disability benefits, you'll need to complete an application for Social Security benefits. You can apply online on the SSA's website. They may be able to process your application faster if you provide all needed information.

The information needed includes:

- Your Social Security number

- Your birth or baptismal certificate

- Names, addresses, and phone numbers of the doctors, caseworkers, hospitals, and clinics that took care of you, and the dates of your visits

- Names and dosage of all the medicine you take

- Medical records from your doctors, therapists, hospitals, clinics, and caseworkers that you already have in your possession

- Laboratory and test results

- A summary of where you worked and the kind of work you did

- A copy of your most recent W-2 Form (Wage and Tax Statement) or, if you are self-employed, your federal tax returns for the past year

In addition to the basic application for disability benefits, you'll also need to fill out other forms. One form collects information about your medical condition and how it affects your ability to work. Other forms give doctors, hospitals, and other healthcare professionals who have treated you permission to send in information about your medical condition. Do not delay applying for benefits if you can't get all of this information together quickly; the SSA can help you get it.

Who Decides If I Am Disabled?

Social Security will review your application to make sure you meet some basic requirements for disability benefits. They'll check whether you worked enough years to qualify and evaluate any current work activities. If you meet these requirements, the SSA will process your application and forward your case to the Disability Determination Services office in your state.

This state agency completes the initial disability determination decision for the SSA. Doctors and disability specialists in the state agency ask your doctors for information about your condition. They'll consider all the facts in your case. They will use the medical evidence from your doctors, hospitals, clinics, or institutions where you have been treated and all other information. They'll ask your doctors about:

- Your medical condition(s)

- When your medical condition(s) began

- How your medical condition(s) limit your activities

- Medical tests results

- The treatment(s) you have received

They'll also ask the doctors for information about your ability to do work-related activities, such as walking, sitting, lifting, carrying, and remembering instructions. Your doctors do not decide if you are disabled. The state agency staff may need more medical information before they can decide if you are disabled. If your medical sources can't provide needed information, the state agency may ask you to go for a special examination. Social Security prefers this examination to be conducted by your own doctor, but, sometimes, the exam may have to be done by someone else. Social Security will pay for the exam and for some of the related travel costs.

How Social Security Makes the Decision

Social Security uses a five-step evaluation process, in a set order, to decide if you are disabled.

1. Are You Working?

If you are working, and your earnings average more than a certain amount each month, the SSA generally won't consider you to be disabled. The amount (referred to as "substantial gainful activity") changes each year.

If you are not working, or your monthly earnings average to the current amount or less, the state agency then looks at your medical condition at step two.

361

2. Is Your Medical Condition "Severe"?

For you to be considered to have a disability by Social Security's definition, your medical condition must significantly limit your ability to do basic work activities—such as lifting, standing, walking, sitting, and remembering—for at least 12 months. If your medical condition isn't severe, the SSA won't consider you to be disabled. If your condition is severe, Social Security proceeds to step three.

3. Does Your Medical Condition Meet or Medically Equal a Listing?

Social Security has a listing of impairments (the listings) that describes medical conditions that are considered severe enough to prevent a person from doing any gainful activity, regardless of their age, education, or work experience. Within each listing, the SSA specifies the objective medical and other findings needed to satisfy the criteria of that listing. If your medical condition meets, or medically equals (meaning it is at least equal in severity and duration to), the criteria of a listing, the state agency will decide that you have a qualifying disability. If your medical condition doesn't meet or medically equal the criteria of a listing, the state agency goes on to step four.

4. Can You Do the Work You Did Before?

At this step, Social Security decides if your medical condition(s) prevents you from performing any of your past work. If it doesn't, the SSA will decide that you do not have a qualifying disability. If it does, they'll proceed to step five.

5. Can You Do Any Other Type of Work?

If you can't do the work you did in the past, SSA looks to see if there's other work you can do despite your medical condition(s). They consider your age, education, past work experience, and any skills you may have that could be used to do other work. If you can't do other work, the SSA will decide that you are disabled. If you can do other work, they'll decide that you do not have a qualifying disability.

Special Rules for Blind People

There are special rules for people who are blind. For more information, you can visit the SSA's website and navigate to "If You Are Blind Or Have Low Vision—How We Can Help."

Social Security Will Tell You Their Decision

When the state agency makes a determination on your case, the SSA will send a letter to you. If your application is approved, the letter will show the amount of your benefit, and when your payments start. If your application isn't approved, the letter will explain why and tell you how to appeal the determination if you do not agree with it.

What If I Disagree

If you disagree with a decision made on your claim, you can appeal it. The steps you can take are explained in The Appeals Process, which is available from Social Security.

How Social Security Will Contact You

Generally, the SSA will mail a letter or call you when they want to contact you about your benefits, but sometimes, a Social Security representative may come to your home. The representative will show you identification before talking about your benefits. Calling the Social Security office to ask if someone was sent to see you is a good idea. If you are blind or have low vision, you can choose to receive notices from the SSA in one of the following ways:

- Standard print notice by first-class mail

- Standard print notice by certified mail

- Standard print notice by first-class mail and a follow-up telephone call

- Braille notice and a standard print notice by first-class mail

- Microsoft Word file on a data compact disc (CD) and a standard print notice by first-class mail

- Audio CD and a standard print notice by first-class mail or

- Large print (18-point size) notice and a standard print notice by first-class mail

For more information, visit the notices page on the Social Security website, or call them toll-free at 800-772-1213. If you are deaf or hard of hearing, you may call their TTY number at 800-325-0778.

What Happens When My Claim Is Approved

Social Security will send a letter to you telling you that your application is approved, the amount of your monthly benefit, and the effective date. Your monthly disability benefit is based on your average lifetime earnings. Your first Social Security disability benefits will be paid for the sixth full month after the date your disability began.

Here is an example: If the state agency decides your disability began on January 15, your first disability benefit will be paid for the month of July. Social Security benefits are paid in the month following the month for which they are due, so you'll receive your July benefit in August.

You'll also receive a booklet titled "What You Need To Know When You Get Disability Benefits," which gives you important information about your benefits and tells you what changes you must report to the SSA.

Can My Family Get Benefits?

Certain members of your family may qualify for benefits based on your work. They include:

- Your spouse, if she or he is 62 years of age or older

- Your spouse at any age, if she or he is caring for a child of yours who is younger than the age of 16 or disabled

- Your unmarried child, including an adopted child, or, in some cases, a stepchild or grandchild. The child must be younger than the age of 18 (or younger than 19 years of age if still in high school).

- Your unmarried child, 18 years of age or older, if she or he has a disability that started before the age of 22. The child's disability must also meet the definition of disability for adults.

NOTE: In some situations, a divorced spouse may qualify for benefits based on your earnings, if she or he was married to you for at least 10 years, is not currently married, and is at least 62 years of age. The money paid to a divorced spouse doesn't reduce your benefit or any benefits due to your current spouse or children.

How Do Other Payments Affect My Benefits?

If you are getting other government benefits (including those from a foreign country), the amount of your Social Security disability benefits may be affected. For more information, you should see the following publications, all available on the SSA's website:

- "How Workers' Compensation And Other Disability Payments May Affect Your Benefits"
- "Windfall Elimination Provision"
- "Government Pension Offset"

What Do I Need to Tell Social Security?
If You Have an Outstanding Warrant for Your Arrest

You must tell Social Security if you have an outstanding arrest warrant for any of the following felony offenses:

- Flight to avoid prosecution or confinement
- Escape from custody
- Flight-escape

You can't receive regular disability benefits, or any underpayments you may be due, for any month in which there is an outstanding arrest warrant for any of these felony offenses.

If You Are Convicted of a Crime

Tell Social Security right away if you are convicted of a crime. Regular disability benefits, or any underpayments that may be due, aren't paid for the months a person is confined for a crime, but any family members who are eligible for benefits based on that person's work may continue to receive benefits.

Monthly benefits, or any underpayments that may be due, are usually not paid to someone who commits a crime and is confined to an institution by court order and at public expense. This applies if the person has been found:

- Not guilty by reason of insanity or similar factors (such as mental disease, mental defect, or mental incompetence)
- Incompetent to stand trial

If you violate a condition of parole or probation, you must tell the SSA if you are violating a condition of your probation or parole, as imposed under federal or state law. You can't receive regular disability benefits or any underpayment that may be due for any month in which you violate a condition of your probation or parole.

When Do I Get Medicare?

You'll get Medicare coverage automatically after you've received disability benefits for two years. You can find more information about the Medicare program, in the Medicare section of the SSA's website.

What Do I Need to Know about Working?

After you start receiving Social Security disability benefits, you may want to try working again. Social Security has special rules, called "work incentives," that allow you to test your ability to work and still receive monthly Social Security disability benefits. You can also get help with education, rehabilitation, and training you may need to work.

If you do take a job or become self-employed, tell the SSA about it right away. They need to know when you start or stop work, and if there are any changes in your job duties, hours of work, or rate of pay. You can call them toll-free at 800-772-1213. If you are deaf or hard of hearing, you may call their TTY number, 800-325-0778.

For more information about helping you return to work, ask for the "Working While Disabled—How We Can Help" booklet. A guide to all of Social Security's employment supports can be found in SSA's "Red Book," which is a summary guide to employment support for individuals with disabilities under the Social Security disability insurance and supplemental security income programs.

The Ticket to Work Program

Under the Ticket to Work program, Social Security and Supplemental Security Income disability beneficiaries can get help with training and other services they need to go to work at no cost to them. Most disability beneficiaries are eligible to participate in the Ticket to Work program and can select an approved provider of their choice who can offer the kind of services they need.

Contacting Social Security

There are several ways to contact Social Security, including online, by phone, and in person. They are here to answer your questions and to serve you. For more than 80 years, Social Security has helped secure today and tomorrow by providing benefits and financial protection for millions of people throughout their life's journey.

Visit Their Website

The most convenient way to conduct Social Security business from anywhere at any time, is to visit www.socialsecurity.gov. There, you can:

- Create a my Social Security account to review your Social Security Statement, verify your earnings, print a benefit verification letter, change your direct deposit information, request a replacement Medicare card, get a replacement SSA-1099/1042S, and more.

- Apply for Extra Help with Medicare Prescription Drug Plan Costs.

- Apply for retirement, disability, and Medicare benefits.

Call

If you do not have access to the Internet, the SSA offers many automated services by telephone, 24 hours a day, 7 days a week. Call toll-free at 800-772-1213 or at the TTY number, 800-325-0778, if you are deaf or hard of hearing. If you need to speak to a person, Social Security can answer your calls from 7 a.m. to 7 p.m., Monday through Friday.

Chapter 56

Healthcare Options: Home Care, Assisted Living, Skilled Nursing Care

At some point, support from family, friends, and local programs may not be enough. People who require help full-time might move to a residential facility that provides many, or all, of the long-term care services they need. Facility-based long-term care services include board and care homes, assisted living facilities, nursing homes, and continuing care retirement communities (CCRCs).

Some facilities have only housing and housekeeping, but many also provide personal care and medical services. Many facilities offer special programs for people with Alzheimer disease (AD) and other types of dementia.

Board and Care Homes

Board and care homes, also called "residential care facilities" or "group homes," are small private facilities, usually with 20 or fewer residents. Rooms may be private or shared. Residents receive personal

---

This chapter includes text excerpted from "Residential Facilities, Assisted Living, and Nursing Homes," National Institute on Aging (NIA), National Institutes of Health (NIH), May 1, 2017.

care and meals, and have staff available around the clock. Nursing and medical care are usually not provided on site.

Assisted Living

Assisted living is for people who need help with daily care, but not as much help as a nursing home provides. Assisted living facilities range in size from as few as 25 residents to 120 or more. Typically, a few "levels of care" are offered, with residents paying more for higher levels of care.

Assisted living residents usually live in their own apartments or rooms, and share common areas. They have access to many services, including up to three meals a day; assistance with personal care; help with medications, housekeeping, and laundry; 24-hour supervision, security, and on-site staff; and social and recreational activities. Exact arrangements vary from state to state.

Nursing Homes

Nursing homes, also called "skilled nursing facilities," provide a wide range of health and personal care services. Their services focus on medical care more than most assisted living facilities. These services typically include nursing care, 24-hour supervision, three meals a day, and assistance with everyday activities. Rehabilitation services, such as physical, occupational, and speech therapy, are also available.

Some people stay at a nursing home for a short time after being in the hospital. After they recover, they go home. However, most nursing home residents live there permanently because they have ongoing physical or mental conditions that require constant care and supervision.

Continuing Care Retirement Communities

Continuing care retirement communities, also called "life care communities," offer different levels of service in one location. Many of them offer independent housing (houses or apartments), assisted living, and skilled nursing care all on one campus. Healthcare services and recreation programs are also provided.

In a CCRC, where you live depends on the level of service you need. People who can no longer live independently move to the assisted living facility or sometimes receive home care in their independent living unit. If necessary, they can enter the CCRC's nursing home.

There are many sources of information about facility-based long-term care. A good place to start is the Eldercare Locator at 800-677-1116 or eldercare.acl.gov. You can also call your local Area Agency on Aging (AOA), Aging and Disability Resource Center (ADRC), department of human services or aging, or a social service agency.

Chapter 57

A Guide to Disability Rights Laws

Americans with Disabilities Act

The Americans with Disabilities Act (ADA) prohibits discrimination on the basis of disability in employment, state and local government, public accommodations, commercial facilities, transportation, and tele-communications. It also applies to the United States Congress.

To be protected by the ADA, one must have a disability or have a relationship or association with an individual with a disability. An individual with a disability is defined by the ADA as "a person who has a physical or mental impairment that substantially limits one or more major life activities, a person who has a history or record of such an impairment, or a person who is perceived by others as having such an impairment." The ADA does not specifically name all of the impairments that are covered.

ADA Title I: Employment

Title I requires employers with 15 or more employees to provide qualified individuals with disabilities an equal opportunity to benefit from the full range of employment-related opportunities available

This chapter includes text excerpted from "A Guide to Disability Rights Laws," ADA.gov, U.S. Department of Justice (DOJ), July 2009. Reviewed March 2019.

to others. For example, it prohibits discrimination in recruitment, hiring, promotions, training, pay, social activities, and other privileges of employment. It restricts questions that can be asked about an applicant's disability before a job offer is made, and it requires that employers make reasonable accommodation to the known physical or mental limitations of otherwise qualified individuals with disabilities, unless it results in undue hardship. Religious entities with 15 or more employees are covered under title I.

Title I complaints must be filed with the U. S. Equal Employment Opportunity Commission (EEOC) within 180 days of the date of discrimination or within 300 days, if the charge is filed with a designated state or local fair employment practice agency. Individuals may file a lawsuit in federal court only after they receive a "right-to-sue" letter from the EEOC.

Charges of employment discrimination on the basis of disability may be filed at any EEOC field office. Field offices are located in 50 cities throughout the United States and are listed in most telephone directories under "U.S. government."

ADA Title II: State and Local Government Activities

Title II covers all activities of state and local governments regardless of the government entity's size or receipt of federal funding. Title II requires that state and local governments give people with disabilities an equal opportunity to benefit from all of their programs, services, and activities (e.g., public education, employment, transportation, recreation, healthcare, social services, courts, voting, and town meetings).

State and local governments are required to follow specific architectural standards in the new construction and alteration of their buildings. They also must relocate programs or otherwise provide access in inaccessible older buildings, and communicate effectively with people who have hearing, vision, or speech disabilities. Public entities are not required to take actions that would result in undue financial and administrative burdens. They are required to make reasonable modifications to policies, practices, and procedures where necessary to avoid discrimination, unless they can demonstrate that doing so would fundamentally alter the nature of the service, program, or activity being provided.

Complaints of title II violations may be filed with the U.S. Department of Justice (DOJ) within 180 days of the date of discrimination. In certain situations, cases may be referred to a mediation program sponsored by the DOJ. The DOJ may bring a lawsuit where it has investigated a matter and has been unable to resolve violations.

Title II may also be enforced through private lawsuits in federal court. It is not necessary to file a complaint with the DOJ or any other federal agency, or to receive a "right-to-sue" letter, before going to court.

ADA Title II: Public Transportation

The transportation provisions of title II cover public transportation services, such as city buses and public rail transit (e.g., subways, commuter rails, Amtrak). Public transportation authorities may not discriminate against people with disabilities in the provision of their services. They must comply with requirements for accessibility in newly purchased vehicles, make good faith efforts to purchase or lease accessible used buses, remanufacture buses in an accessible manner, and, unless it would result in an undue burden, provide paratransit where they operate fixed-route bus or rail systems. Paratransit is a service where individuals who are unable to use the regular transit system independently (because of a physical or mental impairment) are picked up and dropped off at their destinations.

ADA Title III: Public Accommodations

Title III covers businesses and nonprofit service providers that are public accommodations, privately operated entities offering certain types of courses and examinations, privately operated transportation, and commercial facilities. Public accommodations are private entities who own, lease, lease to, or operate facilities such as restaurants, retail stores, hotels, movie theaters, private schools, convention centers, doctors' offices, homeless shelters, transportation depots, zoos, funeral homes, day care centers, and recreation facilities including sports stadiums and fitness clubs. Transportation services provided by private entities are also covered by title III.

Public accommodations must comply with basic nondiscrimination requirements that prohibit exclusion, segregation, and unequal treatment. They also must comply with specific requirements related to architectural standards for new and altered buildings; reasonable modifications to policies, practices, and procedures; effective communication with people with hearing, vision, or speech disabilities; and other access requirements. Additionally, public accommodations must remove barriers in existing buildings where it is easy to do so without much difficulty or expense, given the public accommodation's resources.

Courses and examinations related to professional, educational, or trade-related applications, licensing, certifications, or credentialing must be provided in a place and manner accessible to people with disabilities, or alternative accessible arrangements must be offered.

Commercial facilities, such as factories and warehouses, must comply with the ADA's architectural standards for new construction and alterations.

Complaints of title III violations may be filed with the DOJ. In certain situations, cases may be referred to a mediation program sponsored by the DOJ. The DOJ is authorized to bring a lawsuit where there is a pattern or practice of discrimination in violation of title III, or where an act of discrimination raises an issue of general public importance. Title III may also be enforced through private lawsuits.

ADA Title IV: Telecommunications Relay Services

Title IV addresses telephone and television access for people with hearing and speech disabilities. It requires common carriers (telephone companies) to establish interstate and intrastate telecommunications relay services (TRS) 24 hours a day, 7 days a week. TRS enables callers with hearing and speech disabilities who use TTYs (also known as "TDDs"), and callers who use voice telephones to communicate with each other through a third party communications assistant. The Federal Communications Commission (FCC) has set minimum standards for TRS services. Title IV also requires closed captioning of federally funded public service announcements.

Telecommunications Act

Section 255 and Section 251(a)(2) of the Communications Act of 1934, as amended by the Telecommunications Act of 1996, require manufacturers of telecommunications equipment and providers of telecommunications services to ensure that such equipment and services are accessible to and usable by persons with disabilities, if readily achievable. These amendments ensure that people with disabilities will have access to a broad range of products and services, such as telephones, cell phones, pagers, call-waiting, and operator services, that were often inaccessible to many users with disabilities.

Fair Housing Act

The Fair Housing Act, as amended in 1988, prohibits housing discrimination on the basis of race, color, religion, sex, disability, familial status, and national origin. Its coverage includes private housing, housing that receives federal financial assistance, and state and local government housing. It is unlawful to discriminate in any aspect of selling or renting housing or to deny a dwelling to a buyer or renter because of the disability of that individual, an individual associated with the buyer or renter, or an individual who intends to live in the residence. Other covered activities include, for example, financing, zoning practices, new construction design, and advertising.

The Fair Housing Act requires owners of housing facilities to make reasonable exceptions in their policies and operations to afford people with disabilities equal housing opportunities. For example, a landlord with a "no pets" policy may be required to grant an exception to this rule and allow an individual who is blind to keep a guide dog in the residence. The Fair Housing Act also requires landlords to allow tenants with disabilities to make reasonable access-related modifications to their private living space, as well as to common use spaces. (The landlord is not required to pay for the changes.) The act further requires that new multifamily housing with four or more units be designed and built to allow access for persons with disabilities. This includes accessible common use areas, doors that are wide enough for wheelchairs, kitchens, and bathrooms that allow a person using a wheelchair to maneuver, and other adaptable features within the units.

Additionally, the DOJ can file cases involving a pattern or practice of discrimination. The Fair Housing Act may also be enforced through private lawsuits.

Air Carrier Access Act

The Air Carrier Access Act (ACAA) prohibits discrimination in air transportation by domestic and foreign air carriers against qualified individuals with physical or mental impairments. It applies only to air carriers that provide regularly scheduled services for hire to the public. Requirements address a wide range of issues including boarding assistance and certain accessibility features in newly built aircraft and new or altered airport facilities. People may enforce rights under the Air Carrier Access Act by filing a complaint with the U.S. Department of Transportation (DOT), or by bringing a lawsuit in federal court.

Voting Accessibility for the Elderly and Handicapped Act

The Voting Accessibility for the Elderly and Handicapped Act (VAEHA) of 1984 generally requires polling places across the United States to be physically accessible to people with disabilities for federal elections. Where no accessible location is available to serve as a polling place, a political subdivision must provide an alternate means of casting a ballot on the day of the election. This law also requires states to make available registration and voting aids for disabled and elderly voters, including information by TTYs or similar devices.

National Voter Registration Act

The National Voter Registration Act (NVRA) of 1993, also known as the "Motor Voter Act," makes it easier for all Americans to exercise their fundamental right to vote. One of the basic purposes of the act is to increase the historically low registration rates of minorities and persons with disabilities that have resulted from discrimination. The Motor Voter Act requires all offices of state-funded programs that are primarily engaged in providing services to persons with disabilities to provide all program applicants with voter registration forms, to assist them in completing the forms, and to transmit completed forms to the appropriate state official.

Civil Rights of Institutionalized Persons Act

The Civil Rights of Institutionalized Persons Act (CRIPA) authorizes the U.S. attorney general to investigate conditions of confinement at state and local government institutions, such as prisons, jails, pretrial detention centers, juvenile correctional facilities, publicly operated nursing homes, and institutions for people with psychiatric or developmental disabilities. Its purpose is to allow the attorney general to uncover and correct widespread deficiencies that seriously jeopardize the health and safety of residents of institutions. The attorney general does not have authority under CRIPA to investigate isolated incidents or to represent individual institutionalized persons.

The attorney general may initiate civil lawsuits where there is reasonable cause to believe that conditions are "egregious or flagrant," that they are subjecting residents to "grievous harm," and that they are part of a "pattern or practice" of resistance to residents' full enjoyment of constitutional or federal rights, including title II of the ADA and section 504 of the Rehabilitation Act.

Individuals with Disabilities Education Act

The Individuals with Disabilities Education Act (IDEA) (formerly called "P.L. 94-142" or the "Education for all Handicapped Children Act of 1975") requires public schools to ensure that all eligible children with disabilities receive a free, appropriate public education in the least restrictive environment appropriate to their individual needs.

IDEA requires public school systems to develop appropriate Individualized Education Programs (IEP's) for each child. The specific special education and related services outlined in each IEP reflect the individualized needs of each student.

IDEA also mandates that particular procedures be followed in the development of the IEP. Each student's IEP must be developed by a team of knowledgeable persons and must be at least reviewed annually. The team includes the child's teacher; the parents, subject to certain limited exceptions; the child, if determined appropriate; an agency representative who is qualified to provide or supervise the provision of special education; and other individuals at the parents' or agency's discretion.

If parents disagree with the proposed IEP, they can request a due process hearing and a review from the state educational agency if applicable in that state. They also can appeal the state agency's decision to state or federal court.

Rehabilitation Act

The Rehabilitation Act prohibits discrimination on the basis of disability in programs conducted by federal agencies, in programs receiving federal financial assistance, in federal employment, and in the employment practices of federal contractors. The standards for determining employment discrimination under the Rehabilitation Act are the same as those used in title I of the ADA.

Section 501

Section 501 requires affirmative action and nondiscrimination in employment by federal agencies of the executive branch. To obtain more information or to file a complaint, employees should contact their agency's U.S. Equal Employment Opportunity Office (EEOC).

Section 503

Section 503 requires affirmative action and prohibits employment discrimination by federal government contractors and subcontractors with contracts of more than $10,000.

Section 504

Section 504 states that "no qualified individual with a disability in the United States shall be excluded from, denied the benefits of, or be subjected to discrimination under" any program or activity that either receives federal financial assistance or is conducted by any Executive agency or the United States Postal Service (USPS).

Each federal agency has its own set of Section 504 regulations that apply to its own programs. Agencies that provide federal financial assistance also have Section 504 regulations covering entities that receive federal aid. Requirements common to these regulations include reasonable accommodation for employees with disabilities; program accessibility; effective communication with people who have hearing or vision disabilities; and accessible new construction and alterations. Each agency is responsible for enforcing its own regulations. Section 504 may also be enforced through private lawsuits. It is not necessary to file a complaint with a federal agency or to receive a "right-to-sue" letter before going to court.

Section 508

Section 508 establishes requirements for electronic and information technology developed, maintained, procured, or used by the federal government. Section 508 requires federal electronic and information technology to be accessible to people with disabilities, including employees and members of the public.

An accessible information technology system is one that can be operated in a variety of ways and does not rely on a single sense or ability of the user. For example, a system that provides output only in visual format may not be accessible to people with visual impairments, and a system that provides output only in audio format may not be accessible to people who are deaf or hard of hearing. Some individuals with disabilities may need accessibility-related software or peripheral devices in order to use systems that comply with Section 508.

Architectural Barriers Act

The Architectural Barriers Act (ABA) requires that buildings and facilities that are designed, constructed, or altered with federal funds, or leased by a federal agency, comply with federal standards for physical accessibility. ABA requirements are limited to architectural standards in new and altered buildings and in newly leased facilities. They do not address the activities conducted in those buildings and facilities. Facilities of the USPS are covered by the ABA.

Chapter 58

Put It in Writing: Advance Directives

Avoid Confusion: Let Others Know What You Want

Advance directives explain how you want medical decisions to be made when you are too ill to speak for yourself. These legal documents tell your family, friends, and healthcare professionals:

- What kind of healthcare you want

- Who you want to make decisions for you

Types of Advance Directives

A healthcare proxy is a document that names someone you trust to make health decisions if you can not. This is also called a "durable power of attorney."

This chapter contains text excerpted from the following sources: Text beginning with the heading "Avoid Confusion: Let Others Know What You Want" is excerpted from "Advance Directives and Long-Term Care," Centers for Medicare & Medicaid Services (CMS), February 20, 2018; Text beginning with the heading "Decisions That Could Come Up" is excerpted from "Advance Care Planning: Healthcare Directives," National Institute on Aging (NIA), National Institutes of Health (NIH), January 15, 2018.

A living will tell which treatment you want if your life is threatened, including:

- Dialysis and breathing machines

- Resuscitation if you stop breathing or if your heart stops

- Tube feeding

- Organ or tissue donation after you die

How to Get Advance Directives

Get an advance directive from any of these:

- Your healthcare provider

- Your attorney

- Your local Area Agency on Aging

- Your state health department

What to Do with Your Advance Directives

1. Keep the original copies of your advance directives where you can easily find them.

2. Give a copy to your healthcare proxy, healthcare providers, hospital, nursing home, family, and friends.

3. Carry a card in your wallet that says you have an advance directive.

4. Review your advance directives each year.

Decisions That Could Come Up

Sometimes, decisions must be made about the use of emergency treatments to keep you alive. Doctors can use several artificial or mechanical ways to try to do this. Decisions that might come up at this time relate to:

- Cardiopulmonary resuscitation (CPR)

- Ventilator use

- Artificial nutrition (tube feeding) and artificial hydration (IV, or intravenous fluids)

- Comfort care

Cardiopulmonary resuscitation (CPR). CPR might restore your heartbeat if your heart stops or is in a life-threatening abnormal rhythm. It involves repeatedly pushing on the chest with force, while putting air into the lungs. This force has to be quite strong, and sometimes ribs are broken or a lung collapses. Electric shocks, known as "defibrillation," and medicines might also be used as part of the process. The heart of a young, otherwise healthy person might resume beating normally after CPR. Often, CPR does not succeed in older adults who have multiple chronic illnesses or who are already frail.

Ventilator use. Ventilators are machines that help you breathe. A tube connected to the ventilator is put through the throat into the trachea (windpipe), so the machine can force air into the lungs. Putting the tube down the throat is called "intubation." Because the tube is uncomfortable, medicines are often used to keep you sedated while on a ventilator. If you are expected to remain on a ventilator for a long time, a doctor may perform a tracheotomy or "trach" (rhymes with "make"). During this bedside surgery, the tube is inserted directly into the trachea through a hole in the neck. For long-term help with breathing, a trach is more comfortable, and sedation is not needed. People using such a breathing tube are not able to speak without special help, because exhaled air does not go past their vocal cords.

Artificial nutrition and hydration. If you are not able to eat, you may be fed through a feeding tube that is threaded through the nose and down to your stomach. If tube feeding is needed for an extended period, a feeding tube may be surgically inserted directly into your stomach. Hand feeding (sometimes called "assisted-oral feeding") is an alternative to tube feeding. This approach may have fewer risks, especially for people with dementia.

If you are not able to drink, you may be provided with IV fluids. These are delivered through a thin plastic tube inserted into a vein.

Artificial nutrition and hydration can be helpful if you are recovering from an illness. However, studies have shown that artificial nutrition toward the end of life does not meaningfully prolong life. Artificial nutrition and hydration may also be harmful if the dying body cannot use the nutrition properly.

Comfort care. Comfort care is anything that can be done to soothe you and relieve suffering, while staying in line with your wishes. Comfort care includes managing shortness of breath; limiting medical testing; providing spiritual and emotional counseling; and giving medication for pain, anxiety, nausea, or constipation.

Getting Started

Start by thinking about what kind of treatment you do or do not want in a medical emergency. It might help to talk with your doctor about how your current health conditions might influence your health in the future. For example, what decisions would you or your family face if your high blood pressure leads to a stroke? You can ask your doctor to help you understand and think through your choices before you put them in writing. Medicare or private health insurance may cover advance-care planning discussions with your doctor.

If you do not have any medical issues now, your family medical history might be a clue to help you think about the future. Talk with your doctor about decisions that might come up if you develop health problems similar to those of other family members.

In considering treatment decisions, your personal values are key. Is your main desire to have the most days of life? Or, would your focus be on the quality of life (QOL), as you see it? What if an illness leaves you paralyzed or in a permanent coma, and you need to be on a ventilator? Would you want that?

What makes life meaningful to you? If your heart stops, or you have trouble breathing, would you want to undergo life-saving measures if it meant that, in the future, you could be well enough to spend time with your family? Would you be content if the emergency leaves you simply able to spend your days listening to books on tape or gazing out the window?

But, there are many other scenarios. Here are a few. What would you decide?

- If a stroke leaves you unable to move and then your heart stops, would you want CPR? What if you were also mentally impaired by a stroke—does your decision change?

- What if you are in pain at the end of life? Do you want medication to treat the pain, even if it will make you more drowsy and lethargic?

- What if you are permanently unconscious and then develop pneumonia? Would you want antibiotics and to be placed on a ventilator?

For some people, staying alive as long as medically possible, or long enough to see an important event, such as a grandchild's wedding, is the most important thing. An advance directive can help make that possible. Others have a clear idea about when they would no longer want to prolong their life. An advance directive can help with that too.

Your decisions about how to handle any of these situations could be different at 40 years of age than at 85 years of age. Or, they could be different if you have an incurable condition as opposed to being generally healthy. An advance directive allows you to provide instructions for these types of situations and then change the instructions as you get older or if your viewpoint changes.

Making Your Wishes Known

There are two main elements in an advance directive—a living will and a durable power of attorney for healthcare. There are also other documents that can supplement your advance directive. You can choose which documents to create, depending on how you want decisions to be made. These documents include:

- A living will
- A durable power of attorney for healthcare
- Other advance-care planning documents

Living will. A living will is a written document that helps you tell doctors how you want to be treated if you are dying or permanently unconscious and cannot make your own decisions about emergency treatment. In a living will, you can choose which the procedures described in the "Decisions That Could Come Up" section, you would want, which ones you would not want, and under which conditions each of your choices apply.

Durable power of attorney for healthcare. A durable power of attorney for healthcare is a legal document naming a healthcare proxy, someone to make medical decisions for you at times when you are unable to do so. Your proxy, also known as a "representative," "surrogate," or "agent," should be familiar with your values and wishes. This means that she or he will be able to decide as you would when treatment decisions need to be made. A proxy can be chosen in addition to or instead of a living will. Having a healthcare proxy helps you plan for situations that cannot be foreseen, such as a serious auto accident.

Some people are reluctant to put specific health decisions in writing. For them, naming a healthcare agent might be a good approach, especially if there is someone they feel comfortable talking with about their values and preferences. A named proxy can evaluate each situation or treatment option independently.

Other advance-care planning documents. You might also want to prepare documents to express your wishes about a single medical issue or something not already covered in your advance directive. A living will usually covers only the specific life-sustaining treatments discussed earlier. You might want to give your healthcare proxy specific instructions about other issues, such as blood transfusion or kidney dialysis. This is especially important if your doctor suggests that, given your health condition, such treatments might be needed in the future.

Medical issues that might arise at the end of life include:

- Do not resuscitate (DNR) orders

- Organ and tissue donation

- POLST (Physician Orders for Life-Sustaining Treatment) and MOLST (Medical Orders for Life-Sustaining Treatment) forms

A DNR order tells medical staff in a hospital or nursing facility that you do not want them to try to return your heart to a normal rhythm, by using CPR or other life-support measures, if it stops or is beating unsustainably. Sometimes this document is referred to as a "DNAR" (do not attempt resuscitation) or an "AND" (allow natural death) order. Even though a living will might say CPR is not wanted, it is helpful to have a DNR order as part of your medical file if you go to a hospital. Posting a DNR next to your bed might avoid confusion in an emergency situation. Without a DNR order, medical staff will make every effort to restore your breathing and the normal rhythm of your heart.

A similar document, called a "DNI" (do not intubate) order, tells medical staff in a hospital or nursing facility that you do not want to be put on a breathing machine.

A nonhospital DNR order will alert emergency medical personnel to your wishes regarding measures to restore your heartbeat or breathing if you are not in the hospital.

Organ and tissue donation allows organs or body parts from a generally healthy person who has died to be transplanted into people who need them. Commonly, the heart, lungs, pancreas, kidneys, corneas, liver, and skin are donated. There is no age limit for organ and tissue donation. You can carry a donation card in your wallet. Some states allow you to add this decision to your driver's license. Some people also include organ donation in their advance-care planning documents.

At the time of death, family members may be asked about organ donation. If those close to you, especially your proxy, know how you feel about organ donation, they will be ready to respond. There is no cost to the donor's family for this gift of life. If the person has requested a DNR order but wants to donate organs, she or he might have to indicate that the desire to donate supersedes the DNR. That is because it might be necessary to use machines to keep the heart beating until the medical staff is ready to remove the donated organs.

POLST and MOLST forms provide guidance about your medical care preferences in the form of a doctor's orders. Typically you create a POLST or MOLST when you are near the end of life or critically ill and know the specific decisions that might need to be made on your behalf. These forms serve as a medical order in addition to your advance directive. They make it possible for you to provide guidance that healthcare professionals can act on immediately in an emergency.

A number of states use POLST and MOLST forms, which are filled out by your doctor or, sometimes, by a nurse practitioner or physician's assistant. The doctor fills out a POLST or MOLST after discussing your wishes with you and your family. Once signed by your doctor, this form has the same authority as any other medical order. Check with your state department of health to find out if these forms are available where you live.

Selecting Your Healthcare Proxy

If you decide to choose a proxy, think about people you know who share your views and values about life and medical decisions. Your proxy might be a family member, a friend, your lawyer, or someone in your social or spiritual community. It is a good idea to also name an alternate proxy. It is especially important to have a detailed living will if you choose not to name a proxy.

You can decide how much authority your proxy has over your medical care—whether she or he is entitled to make a wide range of decisions or only a few specific ones. Try not to include guidelines that make it impossible for the proxy to fulfill his or her duties. For example, it is probably not unusual for someone to say in conversation, "I do not want to go to a nursing home," but think carefully about whether you want a restriction like that in your advance directive. Sometimes, for financial or medical reasons, that may be the best choice for you.

Of course, check with those you choose as your healthcare proxy and alternate before you name them officially. Make sure they are comfortable with this responsibility.

Making It Official

Once you have talked with your doctor and have an idea of the types of decisions that could come up in the future and whom you would like as a proxy, if you want one at all, the next step is to fill out the legal forms detailing your wishes. A lawyer can help, but it is not required. If you decide to use a lawyer, do not depend on her or him to help you understand different medical treatments. Start the planning process by talking with your doctor.

Many states have their own advance directive forms. Your local Area Agency on Aging can help you locate the right forms.

Some states require your advance directive to be witnessed; a few require your signature to be notarized. A notary is a person licensed by the state to witness signatures. You might find a notary at your bank, post office, or local library, or you can call your insurance agent. Some notaries charge a fee.

Some states have registries that can store your advance directive for quick access by healthcare providers, your proxy, and anyone else to whom you have given permission. Private firms also will store your advance directive. There may be a fee for storing your form in a registry. If you store your advance directive in a registry and later make changes, you must replace the original with the updated version in the registry.

Some people spend a lot of time in more than one state—for example, visiting children and grandchildren. If that's your situation, consider preparing an advance directive using forms for each state—and keep a copy in each place too.

After You Set up Your Advance Directive

Give copies of your advance directive to your healthcare proxy and alternate proxy. Give your doctor a copy of your medical records. Tell close family members and friends where you keep a copy. If you have to go to the hospital, give the staff there a copy to include in your records. Because you might change your advance directive in the future, it is a good idea to keep track of who receives a copy.

Review your advance-care planning decisions from time to time—for example, every 10 years, if not more often. You might want to revise your preferences for care if your situation or your health changes. Or, you might want to make adjustments if you receive a serious diagnosis; if you get married, separated, or divorced; if your spouse dies; or if something happens to your proxy or alternate. If your preferences change, you will want to make sure your doctor, proxy, and family know about them.

Be Prepared

What happens if you have no advance directive or have made no plans and you become unable to speak for yourself? In such cases, the state where you live will assign someone to make medical decisions on your behalf. This will probably be your spouse, your parents if they are available, or your children if they are adults. If you have no family members, the state will choose someone to represent your best interests.

Always remember: an advance directive is only used if you are in danger of dying and need certain emergency or special measures to keep you alive, but you are not able to make those decisions on your own. An advance directive allows you to make your wishes about medical treatment known.

It is difficult to predict the future with certainty. You may never face a medical situation where you are unable to speak for yourself and make your wishes known. But having an advance directive may give you and those close to you some peace of mind.

Chapter 59

Guardianship for People with Disability

According to the National Guardianship Association (NGA), Inc., "Guardianship, also referred to as 'conservatorship,' is a legal process, utilized when a person can no longer make or communicate safe or sound decisions about his/her person and/or property or has become susceptible to fraud or undue influence. Because establishing a guardianship may remove considerable rights from an individual, it should only be considered after alternatives to guardianship have proven ineffective or are unavailable."

Before evaluating guardianship or making recommendations for how to improve it, it is important to define and ensure a basic understanding of what guardianship is. Although the previous quote may seem like a reasonable definition, it contains value judgments—which are worthy of consideration—such as what constitutes "safe or sound decisions," who gets to make that determination for an individual, and how an individual's safety should balance against his or her right to experience the dignity of risk.

Despite the oft-cited proposition that all people have certain inalienable rights, once someone is declared incapacitated and is appointed

This chapter includes text excerpted from "Beyond Guardianship: Toward Alternatives That Promote Greater Self-Determination," National Council on Disability (NCD), March 22, 2018.

a guardian, many of their rights are taken away, and their ability to make decisions in a wide variety of areas is given to another person.

Therefore, although guardianship is largely a creature of state law, it nonetheless raises fundamental questions concerning federal civil rights and constitutional due process. An adult usually becomes subject to guardianship when the court finds that:

- The individual is incapable of making all or some of their own financial or personal decisions.

- It is necessary to appoint a guardian to make those choices on their behalf.

Rights at Risk in Guardianships

Guardianships are typically separated into two categories, guardianships of the person and guardianships of the property (also sometimes referred to as "conservatorship"). When the guardian controls decisions regarding both person and property, the guardianship is called "plenary." However, there are really three types of rights that are at issue in guardianships:

- Rights that can be taken from an individual but not given to another individual

- Rights that can be taken from a person and exercised by someone else on their behalf

- Rights that a guardian needs a court order to exercise on the individual's behalf

A person who is determined incapacitated generally can have the following rights removed, but these rights cannot be exercised by someone else. These include the right to:

- Marry

- Vote

- Drive

- Seek or retain employment

Still, other rights can be removed and transferred to a guardian who can exercise these rights on behalf of the individual, such as the right to:

- Contract

- Sue and defend lawsuits
- Apply for government benefits
- Manage money or property
- Decide where to live
- Consent to medical treatment
- Decide with whom to associate or be friends

In many states, there are also some rights that a guardian can exercise on behalf of the individual subject to guardianship, but only after the court has issued a specific order allowing the action, such as:

- Committing the person to a facility or institution
- Consenting to biomedical or behavioral experiments
- Filing for divorce
- Consenting to the termination of parental rights
- Consenting to sterilization or abortion

A Word on Language

When a petition is filed with the court that alleges that the individual is incapacitated, the individual is often referred to as the "alleged incapacitated person," or AIP for short. If the court finds that the person does lack capacity and appoints a guardian to manage some or all of their affairs, the individual is often referred to as the "ward."

In this report, the term AIP will be used, but because the term "ward" is viewed by many as stigmatizing and inappropriate, whenever possible, consistent with National Council on Disability's (NCD) longstanding commitment of avoiding stigmatizing language, individuals for whom a guardian has been appointed as an individual subject to guardianship will be referred to. This is also consistent with the Uniform Guardianship, Conservatorship and Other Protective Arrangements Act (UGCOPAA), which is the latest iteration of the uniform guardianship statute that has been approved by the Uniform Law Commission (ULC). However, it should be noted that the term "ward" will appear when it appears in a direct quote.

Process of Obtaining Guardianship

Guardianship petitions may be filed in a wide variety of situations, such as by parents when a child with an intellectual disability reaches 18 years of age, by a son or daughter when a parent begins to show signs of dementia severe enough that there is concern for their safety, for a person with a severe disability due to sudden trauma, or when there is concern that a bad actor is exercising undue influence over a person with a disability in order to exploit the individual in some way. There are also times when guardianship is filed for less altruistic reasons, such as to gain access to the person's assets or public benefits or to exploit the individual. Whether the guardianship is over person, property, or both, or whether it is limited or plenary may be determined, at least in part, by the circumstances that give rise to the perceived need for guardianship. Due to our federalist system of government, guardianship is a creature of state, rather than federal law, and all 50 states and the District of Columbia have revised their statutes regarding guardianship numerous times.

However, it is not clear that, in statute or in practice, guardianship law has been able to keep pace with the nation's changing understanding of disability, autonomy, and due process. Although the process is different in every state, making it difficult to provide a singular description of the guardianship process, there are certain generalities that are helpful to discuss before examination of whether or not guardianship is working for people with disabilities, their families, and communities. The following steps are generalities that may or may not align with the laws in a given state, so it is important for interested individuals to consult their state's laws for more accurate, detailed information.

General Steps to Guardianship

1. Filing the petitions

2. Notice that a guardianship petition has been filed

3. Appointment of an attorney to represent the alleged incapacitated person

4. Capacity evaluation

5. Hearing

6. Letters of guardianship

7. Guardianship plan and initial reports

Guardianship as a Disability Policy Issue

Guardianship is often overlooked, and, when it becomes part of the national policy conversation, it is often viewed as an issue impacting older Americans and not thought of as an important disability issue. However, guardianship must be understood as a disability policy issue worthy of examination, reflection, and reform. After all, an adult becomes subject to guardianship only if a court has determined that she or he cannot manage property or meet essential requirements for health and safety.

Additionally, at least 11 states have laws that provide for alternate, and generally less rigorous, procedures when the individual who allegedly needs a guardian is an adult with intellectual and/or developmental disabilities. Regardless of whether one is a young adult with a congenital developmental disability subject to guardianship because the court determined she or he lacked the ability to make decisions her or himself, or whether one is in his or her 80s and the court believes that Alzheimer disease (AD) has advanced to the point where she or he can no longer make decisions for his or herself, the reason to impose guardianship is disability in both instances. In order to fully understand guardianship as a disability issue, we need to come from a common understanding of it within the context of the evolution of disability policy, particularly as it relates to issues of liberty, autonomy, and self-determination.

Part Six

Clinical Trials on Multiple Sclerosis

Chapter 60

Understanding Clinical Trials

Clinical trials are medical studies that involve people like you. They help find new ways to prevent, detect, or treat diseases that are safe and effective.

Clinical trials are an important part of the research spectrum. The idea for a clinical trial often starts in the lab. After researchers test new treatments or procedures in the lab and in animals, the most promising treatments are moved into clinical trials. As studies about new treatments move through a series of steps called "phases," researchers learn more information about the treatment, its risks, and its effectiveness.

Each clinical trial has criteria describing who can join. Children, as well as adults, healthy volunteers and patients and people of a diverse range of ethnic and racial backgrounds can and are encouraged to participate in clinical trials.

Clinical trials follow a plan, called a "protocol," that describes what you will be doing and what you can expect from the research team. It is important to understand the risks and benefits of participation before joining. You also have rights and protections as a participant in clinical trials.

Types of Clinical Trials

The institutes and centers within the National Institutes of Health (NIH) support many types of clinical trials that contribute to medical

This chapter includes text excerpted from "Clinical Trials," National Heart, Lung, and Blood Institute (NHLBI), September 27, 2018.

knowledge and practice. Clinical trials can be described in a number of different ways, including by their purpose or by the phase.

Purpose of Clinical Trials

Clinical trials have different purposes. The purpose then helps define the type of trial it is.

- Behavioral trials evaluate or compare ways to promote behavioral changes designed to improve health.

- Diagnostic trials study or compare tests or procedures for diagnosing a particular disease or condition.

- Prevention trials look for better ways to prevent a disease in people who have never had the disease or to prevent the disease from returning. Approaches may include medicines, vaccines, or lifestyle changes.

- Quality of life (QOL) trials, or supportive care trials, explore and measure ways to improve the comfort and quality of life for people with conditions or illnesses.

- Screening trials test new ways for detecting diseases or health conditions.

- Treatment trials test new treatments, new combinations of medicines, or new approaches to surgery or radiation therapy.

Clinical Trial Phases

Researchers conduct clinical trials in phases. Each phase has a different purpose and helps researchers answer different questions.

- **Phase I trials.** Researchers test a medicine or other treatment in a small group of people for the first time. The purpose is to learn about the best dose, if it is a medicine, as well as its safety and side effects.

- **Phase II trials.** Researchers study the new medicine or treatment in a larger group of people to determine its effectiveness and to further study its safety.

- **Phase III trials.** Researchers give the new medicine or treatment to an even larger group of participants to confirm its effectiveness, monitor side effects, compare it with standard or similar treatments or a placebo, and collect information that will allow the new medicine or treatment to be used safely.

- **Phase IV trials.** After the U.S. Food and Drug Administration (FDA) approves a medicine and it is made available to the public, researchers track its safety in the general population, seeking more information about a medicine or treatment benefits and optimal use.

What to Expect

As a participant in a clinical trial, you may work with a healthcare team, and you may need to go to a hospital or other location. Everything that happens throughout your experience follows a plan called a "clinical trial protocol." Governing bodies called "Institutional Review Boards (IRBs)" approve protocols and are responsible for ensuring your safety. The research team will also operate by other national and international standards that protect you and help produce reliable study results. Before you join a clinical trial, you will be told all about the study, what procedures you will be undergoing, how much time you will be spending on aspects of the study, and any other information you need to know. Once your questions have been answered and you are comfortable, you will be asked to give your consent to participate.

Clinical Trial Experience

During a clinical trial, you may see doctors, nurses, social workers, and other healthcare providers who will monitor your health closely. You may have more tests and medical exams than you would if you were not taking part in a clinical trial. You may also be asked to do other tasks, such as keeping a log about your health or filling out forms about how you feel.

You may need to travel or stay in a hospital to take part in clinical trials. For example, the NIH Clinical Center in Bethesda, Maryland, runs clinical trials. It is the largest research hospital in the world. Many other clinical trials take place in medical centers and doctors' offices around the country. If you decide that a trial is not for you, it is important to remember that you can withdraw at any time. Whether you participate or not will not affect your regular medical care.

Clinical Trial Protocols

The protocol is carefully designed to balance the potential benefits of a trial with the risks to participants. It also answers specific research questions. A protocol describes the following:

- Goals of the study

- Eligibility requirements

- Protections against risks to participants

- Details about tests, procedures, and treatments

- Expected duration, or how long the study will last

- Information to be gathered

A clinical trial team is led by a principal investigator (PI). Members of the research team regularly monitor the participants' health to determine the study's safety and effectiveness.

Clinical Trial Designs

There are different types of clinical trials and different trial designs. However, many clinical trials include standard design elements.

Randomization is the process by which participants are randomly assigned a treatment instead of being selected for one. This is done to avoid bias when making assignments. The effects of each treatment are compared at specific points during a trial. If one treatment is found superior, the study is stopped so that all the volunteers receive the more beneficial treatment.

Blinded or masked studies are designed to prevent members of the research team and study participants from influencing the results. Blinding allows the collection of scientifically accurate data.

- In single-blind (single-masked) studies, you are not told what is being given, but the research team knows.

- In a double-blind study, neither you nor the research team are told what you are given; only the pharmacist knows. Members of the research team are not told which participants are receiving which treatment, in order to reduce bias. If medically necessary, however, it is always possible to find out which treatment you are receiving.

When the Study Is Finished

After a clinical trial is completed, the researchers carefully examine information collected during the study before making decisions about the meaning of the findings and about the need for further testing. After a phase I or II trial, the researchers decide whether to move on to the next phase or to stop testing the treatment or procedure because it was unsafe or not effective. When a phase III trial is completed, the researchers examine the information and decide whether the results have medical importance.

Results from clinical trials are often published in scientific journals in articles that have gone through peer review. Results that are particularly important may be featured in the news, and discussed at scientific meetings and by patient advocacy groups. Once a new approach has been proven safe and effective in a clinical trial, it may become a new standard of medical practice. In many cases, if you participated in a blinded or masked study, you will get information about the treatment you received.

Who Can Participate?

Many different types of people take part in clinical trials. Some studies include healthy volunteers, while other studies include patient volunteers. Some studies include both healthy and patient volunteers. This includes studies specific to children's needs. Eligibility criteria determine who can participate in a clinical trial.

How much of your time is needed, discomfort you may feel, or risk involved depends on the clinical trial. While some studies require minimal amounts of time and effort, other studies may require a major commitment of your time and effort and may involve some discomfort. The clinical trial may also carry some risk. The informed consent process for volunteers includes a detailed discussion of what you will be asked to do as part of the study and any possible risks.

Healthy Volunteers

Clinical trials with healthy volunteers are designed to develop new knowledge, not to provide direct benefit to those taking part. Researchers take measurements and make observations. Researchers may use the data to compare patient volunteers and healthy volunteers.

Patient Volunteers

Research with patient volunteers also helps develop new knowledge. Depending on the stage of knowledge about the disease or condition, these procedures may or may not benefit the patient volunteer. Patients may volunteer for studies similar to those in which healthy volunteers take part.

Diverse Volunteers

In the past, clinical trial volunteers often were white men. Researchers assumed that study results were valid for other populations as well. Nowadays, researchers realize that women and people from different racial and ethnic groups sometimes respond differently to the same medical approach.

Children

Children need clinical trials that focus on them, as medical treatments and approaches often differ for children. For example, children may need lower doses of certain medicines or smaller medical devices. A child's stage of development also can affect how safe a treatment is or how well it works.

Eligibility Criteria

A clinical trial's protocol describes who is eligible to take part in the research. Each study must include only people who meet the requirements for that study. These are the study's eligibility criteria.

Eligibility criteria are different for each trial. They include whether you are a healthy or patient volunteer. They also include factors such as your age and sex, the type and stage of disease, and whether you have had certain treatments or have other health problems.

The criteria ensure that new approaches are tested on similar groups of people. This makes it clear to whom a clinical trial's results apply. Eligibility criteria are not used to reject people personally. Instead, the criteria are used to identify appropriate participants and keep them safe, and to help ensure that researchers can find the new information they need.

Benefits and Risks

Clinical trials offer hope for many people, while giving researchers a chance to find treatments that could benefit patients in the future. Healthy volunteers say they take part to help others and contribute to moving science forward. People with an illness or disease may take part to help others, but also to have a chance to receive the newest treatment and get added care and attention from the clinical trial staff. Clinical trials may involve risk, as can routine medical care and the activities of daily living. When weighing the risks of clinical trials, consider the possible harms that could result from taking part in the study, the level of harm, and the chance of any harm occurring.

Possible Benefits

• Well-designed and well-performed clinical trials provide benefits to you, while allowing you to help others by contributing to knowledge about new treatments or procedures.

• You gain access to new research treatments before they are widely available.

• You receive regular and careful medical attention from a research team that includes doctors and other healthcare professionals.

Possible Risks

Clinical trials do come with some risks.

• Most clinical trials pose the risk of minor discomfort, which often lasts only a short time. However, some study participants experience complications that require medical attention. Rarely, participants have experienced serious or life-threatening complications resulting from their participation in trials of experimental treatments.

• The study may require more time and attention than standard treatment would, including visits to the study site, more blood tests, more procedures, hospital stays, or complex dosage schedules.

In clinical trials that compare a new product or therapy with another that already exists, researchers try to determine if the new one is as good, or better than, the existing one. In some studies, you may receive a placebo. Comparing a new product with a placebo can be the fastest and most reliable way to show the new product's effectiveness. However, placebos are not used if you would be put at risk—particularly in the study of treatments for serious illnesses—by not having effective therapy. You will be told if placebos are used in the study before entering a trial.

You can learn about the risks and benefits of any clinical trial and how your rights are protected before you agree to take part in the trial. A member of the research team will explain the study and answer any questions about the study. A member of the research team will also ask you to consider and sign an informed consent document, which will describe in detail the specific risks associated with a research protocol. Before deciding to participate, carefully consider risks and possible benefits. You can also talk with your doctor about specific clinical trials you are interested in.

Protecting Your Safety

Protecting the safety of people who take part in clinical trials is a high priority. You also have rights to help protect your safety.

Scientific Oversight

Each study has scientific oversight, including the following:

- **Institutional Review Board (IRB).** An IRB approves and monitors most, but not all, clinical trials in the United States to ensure that the risks are minimal when compared with potential benefits. An IRB is an independent committee that consists of physicians, statisticians, and members of the community who ensure that clinical trials are ethical and that the rights of participants are protected. You should ask the research coordinator if an IRB reviewed the research in which you are considering participating.

- **Office for Human Research Protections.** The U.S. Department of Health and Human Services' (HHS) Office for Human Research Protections (OHRP) external link oversees all research done or supported by HHS. The OHRP helps protect the rights, welfare, and well-being of healthy volunteers and patient participants. The OHRP provides guidance and oversight to the IRBs, develops educational programs and materials, and offers advice on research-related issues.

- **Data and Safety Monitoring Board.** Many clinical trials supported or conducted by the NIH are required to have a Data and Safety Monitoring Board (DSMB). This board consists of a group of research and study topic experts. A DSMB's role is to review data from a clinical trial for safety problems or differences in results among different groups. The DSMB also reviews research results from other relevant studies. Scientific oversight informs decisions about a study while it is underway. For example, researchers stop some studies early if benefits from a strategy or treatment are obvious to make wider access to the new strategy available sooner. Researchers also may stop a study, or part of a study, early if the intervention or treatment is having harmful effects.

- **U.S. Food and Drug Administration (FDA).** In the United States, the FDA provides oversight for clinical trials that are testing new medicines or medical devices. The FDA reviews applications for new medicines and devices before studies begin with human volunteers. They check to make sure that the proposed studies have followed proper informed consent and protection procedures. The FDA also provides oversight and guidance at various stages throughout the studies. For example, before phase III trials begin, the FDA provides input on how these studies should be done.

Patient Rights

As a participant in a clinical trial, you have rights that help protect your safety. These rights include:

- **Informed consent.** Informed consent is the process of learning the key facts about a clinical trial before deciding whether to participate. The process of providing information to participants continues throughout the study. To help you decide whether to take part, members of the research team explain the study. The research team provides an informed consent document, which includes details about the study, such as its purpose, duration, required procedures, and who to contact for various purposes. The informed consent document also explains risks and potential benefits. If you decide to enroll in the trial, you will need to sign the informed consent document. You can withdraw from the study at any time.

- **Rights and protection for children.** Children under the age of 18 get special protection as research participants. Almost always, a parent must give legal consent for his or her child to take part in a clinical trial. Sometimes, both parents must give permission for their child to enroll. Also, children 7 years of age and older often must agree to take part in clinical trials.

Chapter 61

Nutritional Approaches in Multiple Sclerosis

Study Description
Brief Summary

Multiple sclerosis (MS) is a chronic inflammatory disease affecting the central nervous system (CNS) and is characterized by damage (lesions) on the brain and spinal cord. These lesions are associated with the destruction of the covering (the myelin sheath) that protects the body's nerves and promotes the efficient transmission of nerve impulses.

The aim of this project is to characterize the influence of a ketogenic diet and intermittent therapeutical fasting on the course of the disease, as measured by T2-hyperintense cerebral lesions with magnetic resonance tomography (MRT) in patients with relapse-remitting multiple sclerosis (RRMS). The investigators expect in both intervention groups fewer cerebral T2 lesions occurring after 18 months in comparison to the control group and as detectable by MRT. According to current recommendations of the German Society of Nutrition (DGE), the control group receives a vegetarian-focused, anti-inflammatory diet.

This chapter includes text excerpted from "Nutritional Approaches in Multiple Sclerosis," ClinicalTrials.gov, National Institutes of Health (NIH), November 29, 2018.

411

Eligibility Criteria

Ages Eligible for Study: 18 to 65 Years (Adult, Older Adult)
Sexes Eligible for Study: All
Accepts Healthy Volunteers: No

Inclusion Criteria

- Existing health insurance, so that in case of random findings these can also be clarified

- Patients with relapse-remitting multiple sclerosis (RRMS) according to the multiple sclerosis (MS) diagnostic criteria according to McDonald 2010

- Age 18 to 65

- Consent ability and written consent

- Body mass index (BMI) between 19 and 45 kg/m2

- Expanded Disability Status Scale (EDSS) < 4.5

- Stable immunomodulatory therapy or no immunomodulatory therapy > 6 months before confinement

- In the last 2 years ≥ 1 relapse or within the last 2 years, ≥ 1 new T2 lesions, or ≥ 1 contrast-sensitive lesion in MRT

- Consent that possible random findings are reported

Exclusion Criteria

- Initiation or modification of immunomodulatory therapy during the study

- Cortisone treatment in the last 30 days before enrollment

- Relapse in the last 30 days before enrollment

- Insulin-dependent diabetes mellitus (type I)

- Intake of omega-3 fatty acids (docosahexaenoic acid (DHA), eicosapentaenoic acid (EPA))—more than 1 g/day

- Significant cognitive impairment, clinically relevant or progressive disease (e.g., liver, kidney, cardiovascular system (CVS), and conditions involving the respiratory tract, vascular system, brain, metabolism, or thyroid) that could affect the course of the study

- Malignant disease

- Simultaneous participation in an interventional study or participation in an interventional study in the last two months before study inclusion

- Clinically relevant addiction or substance-abuse disorder (defined as alcohol, drug, and drug abuse)

- Nicotine consumption of > 5 cigarettes per day and no willingness to stop consumption during therapeutic fasting

- Insufficient mental possibility of cooperation

- Eating disorder

- Kidney stones

- Known metabolic disorders (e.g., fatty acid oxidation disorders, ketolysis / ketogenesis or glucogenesis disorder, hyperinsulinism (e.g., nesidioblastoma), pyruvate carboxylase (PC) deficiency)

- Therapy with oral anticoagulants (e.g., Marcumar)

- Pregnancy and breastfeeding period

- Suspected lack of compliance

Chapter 62

Physical Telerehabilitation in Multiple Sclerosis

Study Description
Brief Summary

The study aims to evaluate the efficacy of the Multiple Sclerosis Home Automated Telemanagement System (MS HAT) as an adjunct to the current standard of medical care for patients with multiple sclerosis (PwMS). The individual patient with multiple sclerosis (MS) will be the unit of analysis. For each participant, the investigators will assess the effect of Home Automated Telemanagement (HAT) on functional outcomes; levels of disablement, including impairment, activity and participation, socio-behavioral parameters; and satisfaction with medical care as described below.

Detailed Description

People with multiple sclerosis may develop severe disability over the time. Physical therapy including regular exercise helps patients with severe disability to maintain muscle strength, reduce disease symptoms, and improve quality of life (QOL). However, physical therapy programs at clinical settings require constant travel, which may

This chapter includes text excerpted from "Physical Telerehabilitation in Multiple Sclerosis," ClinicalTrials.gov, National Institutes of Health (NIH), July 27, 2017.

limit access of patients with mobility disability to these services on a continuous basis. Technology can allow patients with mobility disability exercise at home under the supervision of their rehabilitation team. Currently, it is unclear how effective this approach is. The study aims to demonstrate that the patients who were helped by the new technology to exercise at home will have better fitness, less symptoms, and better quality of life. If so, other patients with significant mobility disability will be able to take advantage of this technology. This approach can be extended to people with different diseases causing mobility impairment, and it can be used not only for physical therapy, but also for cognitive and occupational rehabilitation.

Eligibility Criteria

Ages Eligible for Study: 22 Years and older (Adult, Older Adult)
Sexes Eligible for Study: All
Accepts Healthy Volunteers: No

Inclusion Criteria

- Age > 21

- Confirmed diagnosis of multiple sclerosis based on McDonald criteria

- Expanded Disability Status Scale (EDSS) range 5.0 to 8.0

- Mini-Mental State Examination (MMSE) > 22 or presence of a caregiver to assist in a daily exercise regimen

Exclusion Criteria

- Coronary artery disease (CAD)

- Congestive heart failure (CHF)

- Uncontrolled hypertension

- Epilepsy

- Pacemaker or implanted defibrillator

- Unstable fractures or other musculoskeletal diagnoses

Chapter 63

Spinal Cord Analysis in Multiple Sclerosis

Study Description
Brief Summary

Research project in which patients with multiple sclerosis (MS) are examined clinically and with magnetic resonance imaging (MRI). To evaluate spinal cord (SC) grey and white matter changes (including lesions) using fast, high-resolution MRI sequences with high contrast between the SC and cerebrospinal fluid (CSF), as well as high contrast within the SC (grey-white matter contrast).

Detailed Description

The Swiss Multiple Sclerosis Cohort (SMSC-Study) aims to better evaluate specific multiple sclerosis (MS) phenotypes through the systematic and standardized documentation and acquisition of clinical course and paraclinical tests, such as magnetic resonance imaging (MRI), and blood and cerebrospinal fluid (CSF) specimens.

Determination of the relative contribution of SC metrics (cervical cord volume, cervical grey matter (GM) cord volume, cervical white matter (WM) cord volume, SC lesion load) to disability in MS.

This chapter includes text excerpted from "Spinal Cord Analysis in Multiple Sclerosis," ClinicalTrials.gov, National Institutes of Health (NIH), February 15, 2019.

Eligibility Criteria

Ages Eligible for Study: 18 to 60 Years (Adult)
Sexes Eligible for Study: All
Accepts Healthy Volunteers: Yes
Sampling Method: Probability Sample

Study Population

The recruitment of MS patients will take place within the ongoing SMSC study at the MS Clinic of the Department of Neurology (Neurologische Klinik und Poliklinik), and at the University Hospital Basel (Universitätsspital Basel). Healthy subjects will be recruited by public announcements on the university hospital's and the university's notice board.

Inclusion Criteria

• Diagnosis of multiple sclerosis

• Steroid-free period: > 4 weeks

• Healthy controls without any history of severe neurological, internistic, or psychiatric disease

Exclusion Criteria

• History of severe (other) neurological, internistic, or psychiatric disease

• MRI-related exclusion criteria:

  1. Paramagnetic and/or superparamagnetic foreign objects in the body

  2. Pacemaker

  3. Claustrophobia

  4. Pregnancy, lactation

Chapter 64

Early Exercise Efforts in Multiple Sclerosis

Study Description
Brief Summary

This study seeks to investigate whether early exercise efforts can expand the use of exercise in multiple sclerosis (MS), from symptom treatment only to early supplementary disease-modifying treatment (DMT).

The study will be conducted in a randomized and controlled manner, with single blinding. Participants will be allocated to either a systematic aerobic exercise intervention or an educational programme on exercise and physical activity. Both interventions will last one year and involve a one year follow-up period.

It is hypothesized that early exercise efforts can modify disease activity and disability progression.

Detailed Description

Multiple sclerosis (MS) is an autoimmune and neurodegenerative disease in the central nervous system (CNS), characterized by complex pathogenesis and heterogeneous symptoms. The histopathological hallmark of the disease is sclerotic lesions. These inflammatory

This chapter includes text excerpted from "Early Exercise Efforts in Multiple Sclerosis," ClinicalTrials.gov, National Institutes of Health (NIH), April 17, 2018.

lesions manifest as disabling relapses, and the number of relapses in the first few years after disease onset is associated with progression of disability, with a higher number of relapses leading to a more rapid progression. In addition, diffuse neurodegeneration seems to occur early in the disease, and even though it is not always clinically evident it is associated with disease progression. A reduction in relapse rate and neurodegeneration early in the MS disease course may slow the progression of disabilities and can possibly reduce the overall disease burden. For the individual person with MS (PwMS), a reduction in overall disease burden will often improve quality of life (QOL), and since MS is a lifelong disease this is of great interest. Preventing disability in PwMS is also highly relevant in a societal perspective, as it lowers the large costs associated with increased disability. As a consequence, the importance of early treatment have been emphasized.

Treatment of MS has seen great advances in recent years, resulting in an increasing number of available disease-modifying treatments (DMT). Despite the fact that the current DMTs alter a number of clinical outcomes and the course of the disease, it is still a serious and deteriorating condition with significant disease activity, impaired neurological functions, and, thus, the progression of disabilities. New and supplemental treatment strategies are, therefore, still warranted, and exercise has gained attention as a safe and tolerable rehabilitation strategy. Recently, exercise has gained substantial attention, as the first indications of neuroprotective and disease-modifying effects of exercise has been published. However, despite the focus on early treatment in medical DMTs, no studies have investigated the effects of exercise as a supplemental treatment strategy early in the disease course of MS.

Consequently, the purpose of this study is to investigate the effects of early exercise efforts on disease activity and disability progression. In a subgroup, the effects will furthermore be investigated on brain volume, specific brain regions, and inflammation.

It is hypothesized that early exercise efforts can modify the disease activity and disability progression, by reducing the relapse rate, the progression of multiple sclerosis functional composite (MSFC) and Expanded Disability Status Scale (EDSS) scores. The rate of brain atrophy and the lesion load, obtained by MRI scans, is also hypothesized to be reduced. This is expected to be due to an exercise-induced reduction in inflammation.

The study will be a randomized and controlled study with randomization to either a systematic aerobic exercise intervention or an educational programme on exercise and physical activity. Both interventions are in addition to standard treatment and will last one year. The exercise intervention will consist of two supervised exercise sessions per week in the complete duration of the study, while the standard treatment plus exercise education program will consist of four educational sessions on the health benefits associated with exercise and physical activity held every third month throughout the intervention period. The training in the exercise group will be aerobic exercise (running, cycling, rowing, or on a cross-trainer) and is planned by exercise physiologists and performed in a progressive manner. To allow handling of a large number of participants, who are also geographically spread, the exercise intervention will be locally anchored, but at the same time supervised by student employees from Section for Sports Science and controlled by Internet and telephonic communication. In addition to the two intervention groups, data from the Danish MS registry will serve as population-based standard treatment control data. All groups will be followed up to one year after cessation of the interventions.

To set the estimated number of participants, a two-sample two-sided power calculation has been conducted. The basis for this calculation is an report from Tallner et al. who have shown a difference in relapse rate during a two-year period (equal to 1 year intervention, and 1 year follow-up) of 0.65 relapses between physically active and physically inactive MS patients (active: 0.95 +/- 0.97 relapses in 2 years; inactive: 1.60 +/- 1.64 relapses in 2 years). 83 patients with MS should be enrolled in each intervention group (a 20% drop-out rate has been included). Newly published data on the brain atrophy in the percentage of total brain volume after 24 weeks of resistance training have been the basis for a similar calculation of the number of participants in the subgroup, from whom magnetic resonance imaging (MRI) scans and blood samples will be obtained. 41 participants from each intervention group should form this subgroup.

MS is a complex disease with heterogeneous symptoms, and by combining the disciplines of exercise physiology, neurology, and radiology, this study can be the first long-term and large-scale exercise study to investigate the possible neuroprotective and disease-modifying effects of exercise when initiated early in the disease course of MS. Consequently, this project has the potential to change present clinical practice and generate further attention to exercise, not only as a symptom treatment but also as a supplemental disease-modifying treatment strategy early in the course of MS.

Eligibility Criteria

Ages Eligible for Study: 18 to 60 Years (Adult)
Sexes Eligible for Study: All
Accepts Healthy Volunteers: No

Inclusion Criteria

• Signed consent

• Definite diagnosis with relapsing-remitting multiple sclerosis
  (RRMS)

• No more than two years since diagnosis

• Expectedly able to carry out high-intensity aerobic training

• Able to transport themselves to and from training sessions

Exclusion Criteria

• Pregnancy

• Dementia, alcohol abuse, or pacemaker

• Metallic implants, hindering MRI scans

• Comorbidities hindering participation in high-intensity aerobic
  training

Chapter 65

Tele-Exercise and Multiple Sclerosis

Study Description
Brief Summary

The purpose of this study is to compare the effects of two delivery models of an evidence-based complementary alternative medicine (CAM) program that combines neurorehabilitative (functional) exercise, yoga, and Pilates for adults age 18 to 70 with multiple sclerosis (MS). CAM will be delivered as a 12-week program through two different delivery forms: on-site at a clinic (DirectCAM) and telerehabilitation (TeleCAM). Participants will be randomly assigned to one of these two groups.

Detailed Description

There are few primary care and multiple sclerosis (MS) clinics that provide full exercise and rehabilitation services for patients with MS, especially in mostly rural, low-income areas, such as Alabama, Mississippi, and Tennessee. Telerehabilitation, or the delivery of rehabilitation services over the telephone and/or the Internet, can help fill service gaps for underserved MS patient populations in this region.

This chapter includes text excerpted from "Tele-Exercise and Multiple Sclerosis (TEAMS)," ClinicalTrials.gov, National Institutes of Health (NIH), October 15, 2018.

The proposed study will determine if our evidence-based rehabilitation and exercise program produces similar health outcomes when delivered in clinic or at home, using preloaded tablets and Interactive Voice Response (IVR) system technology among 820 participants with MS from 38 clinics across Alabama, Mississippi, and Tennessee.

Outcomes to be achieved through the proposed rehabilitation and exercise program, referred to as "complementary alternative medicine," are improved physical activity, decreased pain and fatigue, and an improved quality of life. Improvement in attitudes and behaviors related to physical activity, such as outcome expectations for physical activity, social support from family and friends for physical activity, self-efficacy (i.e., confidence in one's ability to be active), and self-regulation (i.e., setting exercise goals) will happen. The variation in outcomes by patient characteristics, such as age and severity of disability, will be examined to determine for whom the intervention is effective.

This project is important to patients with MS because it seeks to reduce their barriers to receiving exercise treatment and increase the convenience and appeal of such programs through technology. Furthermore, findings and resources from this study will be quickly provided to MS patients and clinicians across the United States (e.g., via training webinars through the National Center on Health, Physical Activity, and Disability [NCHPAD]) and thereby improve the quality and reach of exercise treatment for patients with MS.

The patient and stakeholder partners include MS patients, caretakers, and clinicians, who have been actively guiding the development of this project. In stakeholder meetings, members have provided insight into exercise treatment needs and preferences (e.g., individually tailored approaches that account for varying levels of mobility), outcomes of interest to the patient population (e.g., pain, fatigue, quality of life), and strategies for engaging/motivating participants with MS who may be discouraged and experiencing fatigue and pain (e.g., IVR calls and feedback). Moreover, their ongoing program satisfaction feedback will be important to the recruitment and retention success. Finally, the stakeholders will help make this project successful by continuing to emphasize the importance of long-term gains in health outcomes and promote (through NCHPAD) the sustainability of the program.

Eligibility Criteria

Ages Eligible for Study: 18 to 70 Years (Adult, Older Adult)
Sexes Eligible for Study: All
Accepts Healthy Volunteers: No

Inclusion Criteria

- Physician permission to participate in the study
- Mild to moderate disability (i.e., ambulate with/without assistive device, Patient-Determined Disease Steps [PDDS] 0 to 7)
- Able to use arms/legs for exercise

Exclusion Criteria

- Significant visual acuity that prevents seeing a tablet screen to follow home exercise program
- Cardiovascular disease event within the last six months, several pulmonary disease, and/or renal failure
- Active pressure ulcers
- Currently pregnant
- Within 30 days of receiving a rehabilitation program
- Already meeting physical activity guidelines (GLTEQ > 24)

Chapter 66

Dual-Task Performance in Patients with Multiple Sclerosis

Study Description
Brief Summary

Multiple sclerosis (MS) is a chronic inflammatory disease affecting the central nervous system (CNS). It is reported that 85 percent of patients with multiple sclerosis have gait disturbance, 88 percent have balance difficulties, and 35 to 90 percent experience fatigue. In addition, 65 percent of patients reported that their cognitive functions have regressed.

It is important to increase the independence of the MS patients in activities of daily living (ADL). Almost all of ADL requires many activities at the same time. For example, toothbrushing involves both the standing balance and the motor activity of the upper limb at the same time. It also requires cognitive tasks, such as attention and focusing. Many activities that seem to be the only task are actually multitasking.

This chapter includes text excerpted from "Dual-Task Performance in Patients with Multiple Sclerosis," ClinicalTrials.gov, National Institutes of Health (NIH), January 30, 2019.

The aim of this study is to investigate the effects of motor and cognitive task on top of balance, mobility, and upper limb performances in MS patients and to determine the factors associated with dual-task performance.

Detailed Description

Patients with MS between 0 to 5.5 score, according to the Extended Disability Status Scale (EDSS), and healthy individuals of similar age and sex to patients will be included in the study. The balance, mobility, upper extremity performance, cognitive function, fatigue, physical activity level, mood, sleep quality, quality of life (QOL) will be evaluated once.

The descriptive statistics and t-tests will be used to compare demographic characteristics between groups and for the categorical variables chi-square. Effect of the group (MS patients or healthy controls), condition (Single task and dual-task conditions), and group × condition interaction will be compared using two-way repeated measures analysis of variance (ANOVA). The correlations between fatigue severity, physical activity level, mood, sleep quality, quality of life will be examined using Pearson bivariate correlations. The significance level is set at $p < 0.05$.

Eligibility Criteria

Ages Eligible for Study: 18 to 65 Years (Adult, Older Adult)
Sexes Eligible for Study: All
Accepts Healthy Volunteers: Yes
Sampling Method: Probability Sample

Study Population

MS patients who apply to the Neurological Rehabilitation Unit of Gazi University Faculty of Health Sciences will be invited to this study.

Inclusion Criteria

• Participants who are 18 to 65 years of age

• MS patients who are ambulatory (Expanded Disability Status Scale (EDSS) score ≤ 5.5), in a stable phase of the disease, and without relapses in the last three months

Exclusion Criteria

- Participants who have orthopedic, vision, hearing, or perception problems

Chapter 67

Speed of Processing Training to Improve Cognition in Multiple Sclerosis

Study Description
Brief Summary

Multiple sclerosis (MS) affects myelin that wraps around nerve fibers. Researchers have learned that MS also damages the nerve cell bodies, which are found in the brain's gray matter, as well as the axons themselves in the brain, spinal cord, and optic nerve. As the disease progresses, the brain's cortex shrinks.

The purpose of this research study is to investigate the effectiveness of a computerized technique designed to improve processing speed (i.e., the amount of time it takes for a person's brain to process information) in an MS population. The study is designed to study how well this technique can help people with MS increase their processing speed and their ability to function better in everyday life. This treatment protocol has been studied extensively with older adults, showing improvements

This chapter includes text excerpted from "Speed of Processing Training to Improve Cognition in Multiple Sclerosis," ClinicalTrials.gov, National Institutes of Health (NIH), August 7, 2018.

on standard laboratory measures of processing speed and performance of activities of daily living.

Detailed Description

This study is a double-blind, placebo-control randomized clinical trial examining the efficacy of Speed of Processing Training (SPT) for improving processing speed (PS) deficits in persons with multiple sclerosis (MS). Slowed PS is one of the most common deficits in individuals with MS, and such deficits have been shown to exert significant negative impact on multiple aspects of everyday life, including occupational and social functioning. Despite these findings, few studies have attempted to remediate PS deficits in order to improve the everyday functioning of individuals with MS.

This study is designed to apply a treatment protocol for PS impairments well-validated in an aging population to individuals with MS with objectively observable deficits in PS and document its efficacy on standard neuropsychological outcome measures. In addition, the investigators will assess the effectiveness of the intervention utilizing global measures of everyday life, including an objective measure (the Timed Activities of Daily Living (TIADL)), as well as additional questionnaires to be completed by both the participant and a significant other. This study is also designed to examine the influence of degree of PS impairment on treatment efficacy using neuropsychological tests, evaluating the long-term effects of the treatment protocol and examining the utility of booster sessions to facilitate long-term treatment effects.

Eligibility Criteria

Ages Eligible for Study: 18 to 59 Years (Adult)
Sexes Eligible for Study: All
Accepts Healthy Volunteers: No

Inclusion Criteria

* English as a primary language

* Diagnosis of multiple sclerosis

* Processing speed impairment (based on evaluation)

Exclusion Criteria

- Most recent exacerbation within one month

- Currently taking steroids or benzodiazepines

- History of significant psychiatric illness (bipolar disorder, schizophrenia, or psychosis), or a current diagnosis of major depressive disorder

- Significant alcohol or drug abuse history

Chapter 68

E-Support Groups in Multiple Sclerosis

Study Description
Brief Summary
Primary Objectives

- To determine the feasibility of the program (80% retained with 75% overall attendance, and completed immediate follow-up questionnaires from 75% of participants)

- To determine the efficacy of the program (evaluated by decreased loneliness, operationalized as decreased total score on the University of California, Los Angeles (UCLA) Loneliness Scale from pre to post intervention)

Secondary Objective

- To determine whether the program will affect depression and quality of life (QOL)

This chapter includes text excerpted from "E-Support Groups in Multiple Sclerosis (eSupport)," ClinicalTrials.gov, National Institutes of Health (NIH), July 18, 2018.

Detailed Description

This study involves prospective data collection from an intervention to investigate the impact of participation by MS patients in a 12-week guided online social support group. All outcomes will be compared to active control group. At the completion of a 12-week interval, all participants (placebo and treatment) will complete follow-up questionnaires. Three months after completing, participants will be sent follow-up questionnaires that will be evaluated as a 6-month follow-up, to assess retention of benefits.

Social support has been linked to better health outcomes in many clinical populations. An unpredictable disease of the central nervous system, multiple sclerosis (MS) can range from relatively benign to somewhat disabling to devastating, as communication between the brain and other parts of the body is disrupted. MS affects over 400,000 people in the United States, involves physical and cognitive disability that can have negative consequences on social integration. This can lead to social isolation, which may be dynamically related to depression, fatigue, and disease progression. The aim of the present study is to investigate the impact of support group involvement on persons with MS. Outcomes of interest include mood, loneliness, and quality of life (QOL).

Many people with MS feel isolated and are unable to participate in support groups that meet in locations that may be far from home, difficult to travel to (due to physical disability or lack of resources), or may not be convenient for their schedules. Another hindrance is the apprehension that MS patients sometimes experience when they encounter patients with severe physical disability or worse impairment than their own. For these reasons, the study is introducing remote support groups to be conducted via the Internet, "e-Support." Attending a remote, Internet-based support group may be more appealing to patients with MS as it obviates the need to travel, thereby reducing cost, time, and energy.

Eligibility Criteria

Ages Eligible for Study: 18 Years and older (Adult, Older Adult)
Sexes Eligible for Study: All
Accepts Healthy Volunteers: No

Inclusion Criteria

- Diagnosis of MS (any disease type)
- Age 18 or over
- Willingness to sign informed consent document

Exclusion Criteria

- Unable to obtain access to the Internet

Chapter 69

Intermittent Fasting in Multiple Sclerosis

Study Description
Brief Summary

This is a randomized controlled trial that will test the effects of intermittent fasting (IF) in subjects with relapsing-remitting multiple sclerosis (RRMS). The goal of this clinical trial is to acquire objective evidence regarding whether an intermittent fasting (IF) diet has beneficial effects in multiple sclerosis (MS) patients. Two dietary regimens, IF and western diet, will be compared in a randomized, controlled, single-blinded 12-week trial in RRMS patients. This is a single-center study.

Detailed Description

RRMS patients will be enrolled in a randomized, controlled, single-blinded 12-week trial in which IF will be compared to a standard western diet. Patients will be recruited at the John L. Trotter MS Center and randomly assigned to either a standard western diet or an IF diet (1:1). Enrolled subjects will complete a clinical and laboratory assessment before starting the diet (baseline), at week 6, and at the

This chapter includes text excerpted from "Intermittent Fasting in Multiple Sclerosis (IFMS)," ClinicalTrials.gov, National Institutes of Health (NIH), May 28, 2018.

end of the study (week 12). The primary outcome will be leptin at week 12, as measured in the peripheral blood. Secondary outcomes will be:

1. Peripheral blood metabolic profiling

2. Anthropometric (body mass index (BMI) and waist circumference) and total body fat measures

3. Gut microbiota richness and composition

Eligibility Criteria

Ages Eligible for Study: 18 Years and older (Adult, Older Adult)
Sexes Eligible for Study: All
Accepts Healthy Volunteers: No

Inclusion Criteria

- Diagnosis of RRMS (2010 Mc Donald criteria)

- Expanded Disability Status Scale (EDSS) < 6.0 and disease duration ≤ 15 years

- On an injectable therapy for MS, glatiramer acetate (GA) or beta interferon (beta IFN) for at least 3 months prior to the study and with no anticipated changes of the medication for the 12-week study duration

- Age ≥ 18 years

- BMI > 22 and < 35 kg/m², with stable weight in the 3 months prior to screening

Exclusion Criteria

- History of any chronic disease process (excluding MS) that could interfere with the interpretation of results

- Diagnosis in the past of an eating disorder (anorexia, bulimia, or binge eating)

- Relapsing at the time of enrollment

- On corticosteroid treatment (oral or intravenous) in the past month. Nasal corticosteroid treatments are allowed.

- Diagnosis of diabetes or at time of oral glucose tolerance test (OGTT) (fasting glucose > 126 mg/dl or > 200 mg/dl at 2 hours with a load of 75 g of glucose

- History of food allergies or food intolerance that would interfere with the study

- History of antibiotic treatment within the past 3 months prior to enrollment

- Use of anticoagulant drugs (such as Warfarin or Coumadin) that need to monitor their intake of vegetables containing high levels of vitamin K

- Currently on a special diet and not willing to stop at least one month prior to enrollment

- Currently taking omega 3/fish oil supplements and not willing to stop administration one month prior to enrollment

- Currently pregnant or plan to become pregnant within 6 months

- Current tobacco or e-cigarette smoker

Part Seven

Additional Help and Information

Chapter 70

Glossary of Terms Related to Multiple Sclerosis

absorption: The process of taking in. For a person or an animal, absorption is the process of a substance getting into the body through the eyes, skin, stomach, intestines, or lungs.

addiction: A chronic, relapsing disease characterized by compulsive drug seeking and use despite serious adverse consequences, and by long-lasting changes in the brain.

adverse effect: An unexpected medical problem that happens during treatment with a drug or other therapy. Adverse effects may be mild, moderate, or severe, and may be caused by something other than the drug or therapy being given. Also called adverse event.

affinity: In chemistry and biology, the strength of the attraction between two substances, such as two chemicals, or an antigen and an antibody.

alcohol: A chemical substance found in drinks such as beer, wine, and liquor. It is also found in some medicines, mouthwashes, household products, and essential oils (scented liquid taken from certain plants). It is made by a chemical process called fermentation that uses sugars and yeast.

This glossary contains terms excerpted from documents produced by several sources deemed reliable.

alcoholism: A chronic disease in which a person craves drinks that contain alcohol and is unable to control his or her drinking.

amenorrhea: The abnormal absence of menstrual periods. Early amenorrhea caused by overtraining can cause bones to become brittle and break.

amino acid: One of several molecules that join together to form proteins. There are 20 common amino acids found in proteins.

amphetamine: A stimulant drug that acts on the central nervous system (CNS). Amphetamines are medications prescribed to treat attention deficit hyperactivity disorder (such as Adderall®) and narcolepsy.

anemia: A condition in which the number of red blood cells is below normal.

anesthetic: A drug that causes insensitivity to pain and is used for surgeries and other medical procedures.

antibiotic: A drug used to treat infections caused by bacteria and other microorganisms.

antibody: A protein made by plasma cells (a type of white blood cell) in response to an antigen (a substance that causes the body to make a specific immune response). Each antibody can bind to only one specific antigen.

antigen: Any substance that causes the body to make an immune response against that substance. Antigens include toxins, chemicals, bacteria, viruses, or other substances that come from outside the body.

anxiety: Feelings of fear, dread, and uneasiness that may occur as a reaction to stress. A person with anxiety may sweat, feel restless and tense, and have a rapid heart beat.

aspiration: The removal of fluid or tissue through a needle. Also, the accidental breathing in of food or fluid into the lungs.

assessment: The process of gathering evidence and documentation of a student's learning.

assistive devices: Tools that enable individuals with disabilities to perform essential job functions (e.g., telephone headsets, adapted computer keyboards, and enhanced computer monitors).

asthma: A chronic disease in which the bronchial airways in the lungs become narrowed and swollen, making it difficult to breathe. Symptoms include wheezing, coughing, tightness in the chest, shortness of breath, and rapid breathing.

autoimmune disease: A condition in which the body recognizes its own tissues as foreign and directs an immune response against them.

axon: A nerve fiber in the peripheral nervous system that conducts impulses away from the cell body.

baclofen: A drug that is used to treat certain types of muscle spasms. Baclofen relaxes muscles by blocking certain nerve receptors in the spinal cord. It is a type of antispasmodic.

bacteria: A large group of single-cell microorganisms. Some cause infections and disease in animals and humans.

bladder: The organ in the human body that stores urine. It is found in the lower part of the abdomen.

blood: A tissue with red blood cells (RBCs), white blood cells (WBCs), platelets, and other substances suspended in fluid called plasma. Blood takes oxygen and nutrients to the tissues, and carries away wastes.

body mass index (BMI): A measure of body fat based on a person's height and weight. BMI can be used to screen for weight categories that may lead to health problems but it is not diagnostic of the body fatness or health of an individual. A high BMI can be an indicator of high body fatness.

bone: A living, growing tissue made mostly of collagen.

breast cancer: Cancer that forms in tissues of the breast. The most common type of breast cancer is ductal carcinoma, which begins in the lining of the milk ducts (thin tubes that carry milk from the lobules of the breast to the nipple).

calcium: A mineral that is an essential nutrient for bone health. It is also needed for the heart, muscles, and nerves to function properly and for blood to clot.

cannabis: The dried leaves and flowering tops of the *Cannabis sativa* or *Cannabis indica plant*. *Cannabis* contains active chemicals called cannabinoids that cause drug-like effects all through the body, including the central nervous system and the immune system.

cancer: A term for diseases in which abnormal cells in the body divide without control. Cancer cells can invade nearby tissues and can spread to other parts of the body through the blood and lymphatic system, which is a network of tissues that clears infections and keeps body fluids in balance.

cervix: The lower, narrow part of the uterus (womb). The cervix forms a canal that opens into the vagina, which leads to the outside of the body.

chemotherapy: Treatment with anticancer drugs.

childbearing age: Range of ages during which a woman may become pregnant. For example: Can be defined as 16 to 49 years of age.

chromosome: An organized package of deoxyribonucleic acid (DNA) found in the nucleus of the cell. Different organisms have different numbers of chromosomes. Humans have 23 pairs of chromosomes—22 pairs of numbered chromosomes, called autosomes, and one pair of sex chromosomes, X and Y.

chronic disease: A disease that has one or more of the following characteristics: is permanent; leaves residual disability; is caused by nonreversible pathological alteration; requires special training of the patient for rehabilitation; or may be expected to require a long period of supervision, observation, or care.

chronic pain: Pain that can range from mild to severe, and persists or progresses over a long period of time.

cigarette: A tube-shaped tobacco product that is made of finely cut, cured tobacco leaves wrapped in thin paper. It may also have other ingredients, including substances to add different flavors.

computed tomography (CT): A procedure for taking X-ray images from many different angles and then assembling them into a cross-section of the body. This technique is generally used to visualize bone.

constipation: A decrease in frequency of stools or bowel movements with hardening of the stool. Some forms of osteogenesis imperfecta are associated with increased risk for constipation caused by increased perspiration, growth impairment, pelvic malformation, and diminished physical activity.

corticosteroids: Steroid-type hormones that have antitumor activity in lymphomas and lymphoid leukemias. In addition, corticosteroids may be used for hormone replacement and for the management of some of the complications of cancer and its treatment.

diabetes: A disease in which blood glucose (blood sugar) levels are above normal. There are two main types of diabetes. Type 1 diabetes is caused by a problem with the body's defense system, called the immune system.

diet: What a person eats and drinks. Any type of eating plan.

e-cigarette: A device that has the shape of a cigarette, cigar, or pen and does not contain tobacco. It uses a battery and contains a solution of nicotine, flavorings, and other chemicals, some of which may be harmful.

enzyme: A protein that speeds up chemical reactions in the body.

estrogen: A group of female hormones that are responsible for the development of breasts and other secondary sex characteristics in women. Estrogen is produced by the ovaries and other body tissues. Estrogen, along with progesterone, is important in preparing a woman's body for pregnancy.

exercise: A type of physical activity that involves planned, structured, and repetitive bodily movement done to maintain or improve one or more components of physical fitness.

exposure: Swallowing, breathing, or touching a substance through the skin or eyes. Exposure duration may be immediate, short term (14 days or less), intermediate, or long term (more than 1 year).

fetus: A developing unborn offspring in the uterus (womb). This stage of pregnancy begins 8 weeks after conception and lasts until birth.

fracture: Broken bone. People with osteoporosis, osteogenesis imperfecta, and Paget disease are at greater risk for bone fracture.

gynecologist: A doctor who diagnoses and treats conditions of the female reproductive system and associated disorders.

hepatitis B: A viral disease transmitted by infected blood or blood products, or through unprotected sex with someone who is infected.

hormone: Substance produced by one tissue and conveyed by the bloodstream to another to affect a function of the body, such as growth or metabolism.

human immunodeficiency virus (HIV): A virus that infects and destroys the body's immune cells and causes a disease called AIDS, or acquired immunodeficiency syndrome.

hypertension: Also called high blood pressure, it is having blood pressure greater than 140 over 90 mmHg (millimeters of mercury). Long-term high blood pressure can damage blood vessels and organs, including the heart, kidneys, eyes, and brain.

immune system: A complex system of cellular and molecular components having the primary function of distinguishing self from not self and defense against foreign organisms or substances.

inflammatory bowel disease (IBD): Diseases, including ulcerative colitis (UC) and Crohn disease, that cause swelling in the intestine and/or digestive tract, which may result in diarrhea, abdominal pain, fever, and weight loss. People with IBD are at an increased risk for osteoporosis.

intestines: Also known as the bowels, or the long, tube-like organ in the human body that completes digestion or the breaking down of food. They consist of the small intestine and the large intestine.

lesion: An area of abnormal tissue. A lesion may be benign (not cancer) or malignant (cancer).

lupus: A chronic inflammatory disease that occurs when the body's immune system attacks its own tissues and organs. Also, called systemic lupus erythematosus (SLE). Inflammation caused by lupus can affect many different body systems including joints, skin, kidneys, blood cells, heart, and lungs. People with lupus are at increased risk for osteoporosis.

magnetic resonance imaging (MRI): A noninvasive procedure that uses magnetic fields and radio waves to produce three-dimensional computerized images of areas inside the body.

marijuana: The dried leaves and flowering tops of the *Cannabis sativa* or *Cannabis indica plant.* Marijuana contains active chemicals called cannabinoids that cause drug-like effects all through the body, including the central nervous system and the immune system.

menopause: The cessation of menstruation in women. Bone health in women often deteriorates after menopause due to a decrease in the female hormone estrogen.

metabolism: The chemical changes that take place in a cell or an organism. These changes make energy and the materials cells and organisms need to grow, reproduce, and stay healthy. Metabolism also helps get rid of toxic substances.

migraine: A medical condition that usually involves a very painful headache, usually felt on one side of the head. Besides intense pain, migraine also can cause nausea and vomiting and sensitivity to light and sound. Some people also may see spots or flashing lights or have a temporary loss of vision.

multiple sclerosis (MS): A disorder of the brain and spinal cord that causes decreased nerve function associated with the formation of scars on the covering of nerve cells. Symptoms range from numbness to paralysis and blindness. A person with MS slowly loses control over his or her body.

neuroimaging: The process of determining the structure or function of the brain through various imaging techniques.

neurotransmitter: A chemical produced by neurons that carry messages from one nerve cell to another.

nicotine: Chemical in tobacco that causes and maintains the powerful addicting effects of tobacco products.

nutrition: The taking in and use of food and other nourishing material by the body. Nutrition is a 3-part process. First, food or drink is consumed. Second, the body breaks down the food or drink into nutrients.

organ: A part of the body that performs a specific function. For example, the heart is an organ.

osteoporosis: Literally means "porous bone." This disease is characterized by too little bone formation, excessive bone loss, or a combination of both, leading to bone fragility and an increased risk of fractures of the hip, spine, and wrist.

over-the-counter (OTC): Diseases, including ulcerative colitis (UC) and Crohn disease, that cause swelling in the intestine and/or digestive tract, which may result in diarrhea, abdominal pain, fever, and weight loss. People with IBD are at an increased risk for osteoporosis.

panic: Sudden extreme anxiety or fear that may cause irrational thoughts or actions. Panic may include rapid heart rate, flushing (a hot, red face), sweating, and trouble breathing.

penis: An external male reproductive organ. It contains a tube called the urethra, which carries semen and urine to the outside of the body.

physical activity: Any bodily movement that is produced by the contraction of skeletal muscle and that substantially increases energy expenditure.

placenta: During pregnancy, a temporary organ joining the mother and fetus. The placenta transfers oxygen and nutrients from the mother to the fetus, and permits the release of carbon dioxide and waste products from the fetus.

pregnancy: The condition between conception (fertilization of an egg by a sperm) and birth, during which the fertilized egg develops in the uterus. In humans, pregnancy lasts about 288 days.

prevention: Actions that reduce exposure or other risks, keep people from getting sick, or keep disease from getting worse.

prognosis: The likely outcome or course of a disease; the chance of recovery or recurrence.

prostate: A gland in the male reproductive system. The prostate surrounds the part of the urethra (the tube that empties the bladder) just below the bladder, and produces a fluid that forms part of the semen.

prostate cancer: A disease in which abnormal tumor cells develop in the prostate gland. Men who receive hormone deprivation therapy for prostate cancer have an increased risk of developing osteoporosis and broken bones.

protein: A molecule made up of amino acids. Proteins are needed for the body to function properly. They are the basis of body structures, such as skin and hair, and of other substances such as enzymes, cytokines, and antibodies.

psychosis: A mental disorder characterized by delusional or disordered thinking detached from reality; symptoms often include hallucinations.

puberty: Time when the body is changing from the body of a child to the body of an adult. This process begins earlier in girls than in boys, usually between ages 8 and 13, and lasts 2 to 4 years.

radiation: Energy moving in the form of particles or waves. Familiar radiations are heat, light, radio, and microwaves.

rheumatoid arthritis (RA): An inflammatory disease that causes pain, swelling, stiffness, and loss of function in the joints. It occurs when the immune system, which normally defends the body from invading organisms, attacks the membrane lining the joints. Studies have found an increased risk of bone loss and fracture in individuals with RA.

rubella: Also called German measles. Rubella virus causes rash, mild fever, and arthritis. If a woman gets rubella while she is pregnant, she could have a miscarriage or her baby could be born with serious birth defects.

serum: The liquid part of blood that remains after clotting proteins and blood cells are removed.

smoking cessation: To quit smoking. Smoking cessation lowers the risk of multiple sclerosis and other serious health problems. Counseling, behavior therapy, medicines, and nicotine-containing products, such as nicotine patches, gum, lozenges, inhalers, and nasal sprays, may be used to help a person quit smoking.

sodium: A mineral and an essential nutrient needed by the human body in relatively small amounts (provided that substantial sweating does not occur).

solvent: A liquid capable of dissolving or dispersing another substance (for example, acetone or mineral spirits).

steroid: Any of a group of lipids (fats) that have a certain chemical structure. Steroids occur naturally in plants and animals or they may be made in the laboratory.

stimulants: A class of drugs that enhance the activity of monoamines (such as dopamine and norepinephrine) in the brain, increasing arousal, heart rate, blood pressure, and respiration, and decreasing appetite; includes some medications used to treat attention deficit hyperactivity disorder (e.g., methylphenidate and amphetamines), as well as cocaine and methamphetamine.

tobacco: A plant with leaves that have high levels of the addictive chemical nicotine. After harvesting, tobacco leaves are cured, aged, and processed in various ways. The resulting products may be smoked (in cigarettes, cigars, and pipes), applied to the gums (as dipping and chewing tobacco), or inhaled (as snuff).

toxic: Causing temporary or permanent effects detrimental to the functioning of a body organ or group of organs.

urinary tract infection: An infection anywhere in the urinary tract, or organs that collect and store urine and release it from your body (the kidneys, ureters, bladder, and urethra).

vagina: The muscular canal that extends from the cervix to the outside of the body. Its walls are lined with mucus membranes and tiny glands that make vaginal secretions.

virus: A small organism that can infect a person and cause illness or disease.

vitamin D: A nutrient that the body needs to absorb calcium.

withdrawal: Symptoms that occur after chronic use of a drug is reduced abruptly or stopped.

X-ray: A type of high-energy radiation. In low doses, X-rays are used to diagnose diseases by making pictures of the inside of the body.

yoga: A mind and body practice with origins in ancient Indian philosophy. The various styles of yoga typically combine physical postures, breathing techniques, and meditation or relaxation.

Chapter 71

Organizations with Additional Information about Multiple Sclerosis

Government Organizations That Provide Information about Multiple Sclerosis and Related Issues

Administration for Community Living (ACL)
330 C St. S.W.
Washington, DC 20201
Phone: 202-401-4634
Website: www.acl.gov

Agency for Healthcare Research and Quality (AHRQ)
Office of Communications and Knowledge Transfer (OCKT)
5600 Fishers Ln.
Seventh Fl.
Rockville, MD 20857
Phone: 301-427-1104
Website: www.ahrq.gov

Brain Resources and Information Network (BRAIN)
P.O. Box 5801
Bethesda, MD 20824
Toll-Free: 800-352-9424
Website: www.education.ninds.nih.gov
E-mail: braininfo@ninds.nih.gov

Resources in this chapter were compiled from several sources deemed reliable; all contact information was verified and updated in March 2019.

455

Centers for Medicare & Medicaid Services (CMS)
7500 Security Blvd.
Baltimore, MD 21244
Toll-Free: 877-267-2323
Phone: 410-786-3000
TTY: 410-786-0727
Toll-Free TTY: 866-226-1819
Website: www.cms.gov

Eunice Kennedy Shriver National Institute of Child Health and Human Development (NICHD)
NICHD Information Resource Center (IRC)
P.O. Box 3006
Rockville, MD 20847
Toll-Free: 800-370-2943
Toll-Free TTY: 888-320-6942
Toll-Free Fax: 866-760-5947
Website: www.nichd.nih.gov
E-mail: NICHDInformation
ResourceCenter@mail.nih.gov

Genetic and Rare Diseases Information Center (GARD)
P.O. Box 8126
Gaithersburg, MD 20898-8126
Toll-Free: 888-205-2311
Phone: 301-251-4925
Toll-Free TTY: 888-205-3223
Fax: 301-251-4911
Website: www.rarediseases.info.nih.gov

Healthfinder.gov
1101 Wootton Pkwy
Rockville, MD 20852
Website: www.healthfinder.gov
E-mail: healthfinder@hhs.gov

National Center for Complementary and Integrative Health (NCCIH)
NCCIH Clearinghouse
9000 Rockville Pike
Bethesda, MD 20892
Toll-Free: 888-644-6226
Toll-Free TTY: 866-464-3615
Website: www.nccih.nih.gov
E-mail: info@nccih.nih.gov

National Eye Institute (NEI)
Information Office
31 Center Dr. MSC 2510
Bethesda, MD 20892-2510
Phone: 301-496-5248
Website: www.nei.nih.gov
E-mail: 2020@nei.nih.gov

National Human Genome Research Institute (NHGRI)
Office of Communications and Public Liaison Branch (OCPL)
Bldg. 31, Rm. 4B09, 31 Center Dr., MSC 2152
9000 Rockville Pike
Bethesda, MD 20892-2152
Phone: 301-402-0911
Fax: 301-402-2218
Website: www.genome.gov
E-mail: nhgripressoffice@mail.nih.gov

**National Institute
of Arthritis and
Musculoskeletal and Skin
Diseases (NIAMS)**
NIAMS Information
Clearinghouse
1 AMS Cir.
Bethesda, MD 20892-3675
Toll-Free: 877-22-NIAMS
(877-226-4267)
Phone: 301-495-4484
TTY: 301-565-2966
Fax: 301-718-6366
Website: www.niams.nih.gov
E-mail: NIAMSinfo@mail.nih.
gov

**National Institute of
Diabetes, Digestive and
Kidney Diseases (NIDDK)**
Health Information Center
Toll-Free: 800-860-8747
Toll-Free TTY: 866-569-1162
Website: www.niddk.nih.gov
E-mail: healthinfo@niddk.nih.
gov

**National Institute of
Environmental Health
Sciences (NIEHS)**
P.O. Box 12233, MD K3-16
Research Triangle Park, NC 27709
Phone: 919-541-3345
Fax: 919-541-4395
Website: www.niehs.nih.gov

**National Institute of Mental
Health (NIMH)**
Office of Science Policy,
Planning, and Communications
(OSPPC)
6001 Executive Blvd.
Rm. 6200, MSC 9663
Bethesda, MD 20892-9663
Toll-Free: 866-615-NIMH
(866-615-6464)
TTY: 301-443-8431
Toll-Free TTY: 866-415-8051
Fax: 301-443-4279
Website: www.nimh.nih.gov
E-mail: nimhinfo@nih.gov

**National Institute of
Neurological Disorders and
Stroke (NINDS)**
NIH Neurological Institute
P.O. Box 5801
Bethesda, MD 20824
Toll-Free: 800-352-9424
Website: www.ninds.nih.gov

**National Institutes of Health
(NIH)**
9000 Rockville Pike
Bethesda, MD 20892
Phone: 301-496-4000
TTY: 301-402-9612
Website: www.nih.gov

Office on Women's Health (OWH)
U.S. Department of Health and Human Services (HHS)
200 Independence Ave. S.W.
Rm. 712E
Washington, DC 20201
Toll-Free: 800-994-9662
Phone: 202-690-7650
Fax: 202-205-2631
Website: www.womenshealth.gov

U.S. Department of Health and Human Services (HHS)
200 Independence Ave. S.W.
Washington, DC 20201
Toll-Free: 877-696-6775
Website: www.hhs.gov

U.S. Department of Justice (DOJ)
950 Pennsylvania Ave. N.W.
Washington, DC 20530-0001
Phone: 202-353-1555;
202-514-2000
Toll-Free TTY/TDD:
800-877-8339
Website: www.justice.gov

U.S. Department of Veterans Affairs (VA)
Toll-Free: 844-698-2311
Toll-Free TTY: 844-698-2711
Website: www.va.gov

U.S. Equal Employment Opportunity Commission (EEOC)
131 M St. N.E.
Fourth Fl., Ste. 4NWO2F
Washington, DC 20507-0100
Toll-Free: 800-669-4000
Phone: 202-663-4900
TTY: 202-663-4494
Toll-Free TTY: 800-669-6820
Fax: 202-419-0739
Website: www.eeoc.gov
E-mail: info@eeoc.gov

U.S. Food and Drug Administration (FDA)
10903 New Hampshire Ave.
Silver Spring, MD 20993-0002
Toll-Free: 888-INFO-FDA
(888-463-6332)
Website: www.fda.gov

U.S. National Library of Medicine (NLM)
8600 Rockville Pike
Bethesda, MD 20894
Toll-Free: 888-FIND-NLM
(888-346-3656)
Phone: 301-594-5983
Website: www.nlm.nih.gov

U.S. Social Security Administration (SSA)
Office of Public Inquiries
1100 W. High Rise 6401 Security Blvd.
Baltimore, MD 21235
Toll-Free: 800-772-1213
Toll-Free TTY: 800-325-0778
Website: www.ssa.gov

Private Organizations That Provide Information about Multiple Sclerosis and Related Issues

Accelerated Cure Project (ACP)
460 Totten Pond Rd.
Ste. 140
Waltham, MA 02451
Phone: 781-487-0008
Website: www.acceleratedcure.org
E-mail: info@acceleratedcure.org

Accessible Space, Inc. (ASI)
2550 University Ave. W.
Ste. 330N
St. Paul, MN 55114
Toll-Free: 800-466-7722
Phone: 651-645-7271
Toll-Free TTY: 800-627-3529
Fax: 651-645-0541
Website: www.accessiblespace.org
E-mail: info@accessiblespace.org

American Association of Retired Persons (AARP)
601 E. St. N.W.
Washington, DC 20049
Toll-Free: 888-OUR-AARP
(888-687-2277)
Phone: 202-434-3525
Toll-Free TTY: 877-434-7598
Website: www.aarp.org

American Autoimmune Related Diseases Association (AARDA)
22100 Gratiot Ave.
Eastpointe, MI 48021
Toll-Free: 800-598-4668
Phone: 586-776-3900
Fax: 586-776-3903
Website: www.aarda.org
E-mail: aarda@aarda.org

American Hospital Association (AHA)
155 N. Wacker Dr.
Chicago, IL 60606-3421
Toll-Free: 800-424-4301
Phone: 312-422-3000
Website: www.aha.org/front

The American Institute of Stress (AIS)
220 Adams Dr.
Ste. 280 – #224
Weatherford, TX 76086
Phone: 682-239-6823
Website: www.stress.org
E-mail: info@stress.org

Anxiety Disorders Association of America (ADAA)
8701 Georgia Ave.
Ste. 412
Silver Spring, MD 20910
Phone: 240-485-1001
Fax: 240-485-1035
Website: www.adaa.org
E-mail: information@adaa.org

Argentum
1650 King St.
Ste. 602
Alexandria, VA 22314
Phone: 703-894-1805
Fax: 703-894-1831
Website: www.argentum.org

Center for Universal Design (CUD)
College of Design North Carolina State University
CB 8613
Raleigh, NC 27695-8613
Toll-Free: 800-647-6777
Website: www.projects.ncsu.edu
E-mail: cud@ncsu.edu

The Clearing House
National Mental Health Consumers' Self-Help Clearinghouse
Toll-Free: 800-553-4539
Phone: 215-204-5593
Website: www.mhselfhelp.org
E-mail: selfhelpclearinghouse@gmail.com

Consortium of Multiple Sclerosis Centers (CMSC)
3 University Plaza Dr.
Ste. 116
Hackensack, NJ 07601
Phone: 201-487-1050
Fax: 862-772-7275
Website: www.mscare.org
E-mail: info@mscare.org

Family Caregiver Alliance (FCA)
National Center on Caregiving (NCC)
101 Montgomery St.
Ste. 2150
San Francisco, CA 94104
Toll-Free: 800-445-8106
Phone: 415-434-3388
Website: www.caregiver.org
E-mail: info@caregiver.org

The Foundation for Peripheral Neuropathy (FPN)
485 Half Day Rd.
Ste. 350
Buffalo Grove, IL 60089
Toll-Free: 877-883-9942
Fax: 847-883-9960
Website: www.foundationforpn.org
E-mail: info@TFFPN.org

The Human Brain and Spinal Fluid Resource Center (HBSFRC)
11301 Wilshire Blvd. (127A), Bldg. 115
Rm. 130
Los Angeles, CA 90073
Phone: 310-268-3536
Fax: 310-268-4768
Website: www.brainbank.ucla.edu
E-mail: brainbnk@ucla.edu

International Essential Tremor Foundation (IETF)
11111 W. 95th St.
Ste. 260
Overland Park, KS 66214
Toll-Free: 888-387-3667
Phone: 913-341-3880
Fax: 913-341-1296
Website: www.essentialtremor.org
E-mail: info@essentialtremor.org

Mental Health America (MHA)
500 Montgomery St.
Ste. 820
Alexandria, VA 22314
Toll-Free: 800-969-6642
Phone: 703-684-7722
Fax: 703-684-5968
Website: www.mentalhealthamerica.net

Multiple Sclerosis Association of America (MSAA)
375 Kings Hwy N.
Cherry Hill, NJ 08034
Toll-Free: 800-532-7667
Fax: 856-661-9797
Website: www.mymsaa.org
E-mail: msaa@mymsaa.com

Multiple Sclerosis Foundation
6350 N. Andrews Ave.
Ft. Lauderdale, FL 33309-2132
Toll-Free: 888-MSFOCUS
(888-673-6287)
Phone: 954-776-6805
Fax: 954-351-0630
Website: www.msfocus.org
E-mail: support@msfocus.org

National Association for Continence (NAFC)
P.O. Box 1019
Charleston, SC 29402
Toll-Free: 800-BLADDER
(800-252-3337)
Website: www.nafc.org

National Association for Home Care (NAHC)
228 Seventh St. S.E.
Washington, DC 20003
Phone: 202-547-7424
Fax: 202-547-3540
Website: www.nahc.org

National Ataxia Foundation (NAF)
600 Hwy 169 S.
Ste. 1725
Minneapolis, MN 55426
Phone: 763-553-0020
Fax: 763-553-0167
Website: www.ataxia.org
E-mail: naf@ataxia.org

National Center for Assisted Living (NCAL)
American Health Care Association (AHCA)
1201 L St. N.W.
Washington, DC 20005
Phone: 202-842-4444
Fax: 202-842-3860
Website: www.ahcancal.org/ncal/Pages/index.aspx

National Center on Health, Physical Activity and Disability (NCHPAD)
4000 Ridgeway Dr.
Birmingham, AL 35209
Toll-Free: 800-900-8086
Fax: 205-313-7475
Website: www.nchpad.org
E-mail: email@nchpad.org

National Hospice and Palliative Care Organization (NHPCO)
1731 King St.
Alexandria, VA 22314
Phone: 703-837-1500
Fax: 703-837-1233
Website: www.nhpco.org

National Multiple Sclerosis Society (NMSS)
733 Third Ave. Third Fl.
New York, NY 10017
Toll-Free: 800-FIGHTMS
(800-344-4867)
Phone: 212-463-7787
Fax: 212-986-7981
Website: www.nationalmssociety.org

National Organization for Rare Disorders (NORD)
55 Kenosia Ave.
Danbury, CT 06810
Toll-Free: 800-999-NORD
(800-999-6673)
Phone: 203-744-0100
Fax: 203-263-9938
Website: www.rarediseases.org

National Tay-Sachs and Allied Diseases Association (NTSAD)
2001 Beacon St.
Ste. 204
Boston, MA 02135
Toll-Free: 800-90-NTSAD
(800-906-8723)
Phone: 617-277-4463
Website: www.ntsad.org
E-mail: info@ntsad.org

Tremor Action Network (TAN)
P.O. Box 5013
Pleasanton, CA 94566-0513
Phone: 510-681-6565
Fax: 925-369-0485
Website: www.tremoraction.org

United Leukodystrophy Foundation (ULF)
224 N. Second St.
Ste. 2
DeKalb, IL 60115
Toll-Free: 800-SAV-LIVE
(800-728-5483)
Fax: 815-748-0844
Website: www.ulf.org
E-mail: office@ulf.org

Urology Care Foundation
American Urological Association
Foundation (AUA)
1000 Corporate Blvd.
Linthicum, MD 21090
Toll-Free: 800-828-7866
Phone: 410-689-3700
Fax: 410-689-3800; 410-689-3998
Website: www.urologyhealth.org
E-mail: info@
UrologyCareFoundation.org

Visiting Nurse Associations
of America (VNAA)
1800 Diagonal Rd.
Ste. 600
Alexandria, VA 22314
Phone: 571-527-1520
Website: www.vnaa.org

Well Spouse Association
(WSA)
63 W. Main St.
Ste. H
Freehold, NJ 07728
Toll-Free: 800-838-0879
Phone: 732-577-8899
Website: www.wellspouse.org
E-mail: info@wellspouse.org

Index

Index

Page numbers followed by 'n' indicate a footnote. Page numbers in *italics* indicate a table or illustration.

alcohol
  defined 445
  environmental factors 26
  hyperactive bladder 96
  restless leg syndrome 268
  self-management 343
  sexuality 293
  tremor 66
alcoholism
  cerebellar tremor 69
  defined 446
  electroencephalography 123
alemtuzumab
  chicken pox vaccine 247
  multiple sclerosis (MS) 147
alleles, *HLA-DRB1* gene 21
alprazolam, tranquilizers 71
ALS *see* amyotrophic lateral sclerosis
Alzheimer disease
  cognitive changes 165
  functional magnetic resonance
    imaging (fMRI) 127
  guardianship 397
  healthcare options 369
  tremors 74
amantadine
  fatigue 79
  multiple sclerosis (MS)
    treatment 163
ambulatory impairment, assistive
  technology 312
amenorrhea, defined 446
American Association of Retired
  Persons *see* AARP
American Autoimmune Related
  Diseases Association (AARDA),
  contact 459
American Hospital Association (AHA),
  contact 459
The American Institute of Stress
  (AIS), contact 459
Americans with Disabilities Act
  (ADA)
  described 373
  employment 343
amino acid
  defined 446
  gene variations 23
amitriptyline, pseudobulbar affect 164

amniocentesis, defined 119
amphetamine, defined 446
Ampyra *see* dalfampridine
amyotrophic lateral sclerosis,
  neurologists 136
anemia, defined 446
anesthetic, defined 446
angiography, neurological
  disorders 121
ankle-foot orthoses, mobility assistive
  technology 314
antianxiety, multiple sclerosis (MS) 107
antibiotic, defined 446
antibodies
  autoimmune and inflammatory
    processes 33
  defined 446
  laboratory screening tests 119
  plasmapheresis 227
  shingles vaccine 248
anticonvulsant
  focused ultrasound 72
  pain 163
antidepressant medications,
  sexuality 294
anti-inflammatory
  nutritional approach 411
  omega-3 fatty acid 220
antigen
  defined 446
  genes 19
antioxidant
  electromyography 125
  multiple sclerosis (MS) 411
  omega-3 fatty acid
    supplementation 220
antiseizure medications, tremor 71
anxiety, defined 446
Anxiety Disorders Association of
  America (ADAA), contact 459
aphasia
  multiple sclerosis (MS) 81
  Schilder disease 42
apoptosis, *TNFRSF1A* gene 22
Architectural Barriers Act (ABA)
  described 380
Argentum, contact 460
artificial hydration, advance
  directives 384

blurred vision
  driving 297
  plasmapheresis 229
  uveitis 92
BMI *see* body mass index
body mass index, defined 447
bone, defined 447
Botox (botulinum toxin), hyperactive
  bladder 97
brain
  cerebrospinal fluid analysis 122
  exacerbation 39
  magnetic resonance imaging
    (MRI) 90
  surgery 72
  see also central nervous system
BRAIN *see* Brain Resources and
  Information Network
Brain Resources and Information
  Network (BRAIN), contact 455
brain scans
  diagnostic tests 121
  myelin 17
brain tumor, defined 121
breast cancer
  defined 447
  Ocrevus (ocrelizumab) 154
breastfeeding, contraception 253
breath support
  speaking 283
  verbal communication 209
Bureau of Alcohol, Tobacco, Firearms
  and Explosives (ATF)
  publication
    employment support for
      disabled 353n

C

calcium
  CYP27B1 gene 20
  defined 447
  neurological examination 120
CAM *see* complementary and
  alternative medicine
Campath *see* alemtuzumab
cancer
  clinical trials 354
  defined 447

cannabinoids, complementary and
  alternative medicine 216
cannabis
  defined 447
  oral cannabinoids 217
carbamazepine, neuromyelitis
  optica 49
carbidopa, tremor 72
cardiopulmonary resuscitation (CPR),
  emergency treatments 384
caregivers, Gilenya 158
caregiving tips, overview 335–8
"Caregiving Tips—Multiple Sclerosis
  (MS)" (VA) 335n
cartilage, vocal fold paralysis 87
CAT scan *see* computed axial
  tomography scan
catheter
  chorionic villus sampling (CVS) 119
  intrathecal baclofen (ITB)
    therapy 174
  mechanical repair 138
  plasmapheresis 228
celiac disease, autoimmune diseases 8
cell body, depicted *14*
Center for Universal Design (CUD),
  contact 460
Centers for Disease Control and
  Prevention (CDC)
  publication
    contraception for women 251n
Centers for Medicare & Medicaid
  Services (CMS)
  contact 456
  publications
    advance directives and long-
      term care 383n
    Medicare coverage 321n
cerebellum
  plaques 18
  tremor 69
cerebral cortex, myoclonus 181
cerebrospinal fluid (CSF)
  magnetic resonance imaging
    (MRI) 116
  neuromyelitis optica 49
  ultrasound imaging 129
cerebrospinal fluid analysis,
  described 122

470

11/19

LINDENHURST MEMORIAL LIBRARY
One Lee Avenue
Lindenhurst, New York 11757